Bioactive Molecules from Extreme Environments

Bioactive Molecules from Extreme Environments

Editor

Daniela Giordano

MDPI • Basel • Beijing • Wuhan • Barcelona • Belgrade • Manchester • Tokyo • Cluj • Tianjin

Editor
Daniela Giordano
National Research Council
(CNR)
Italy

Editorial Office
MDPI
St. Alban-Anlage 66
4052 Basel, Switzerland

This is a reprint of articles from the Special Issue published online in the open access journal *Marine Drugs* (ISSN 1660-3397) (available at: https://www.mdpi.com/journal/marinedrugs/special_issues/Extreme_Environments).

For citation purposes, cite each article independently as indicated on the article page online and as indicated below:

LastName, A.A.; LastName, B.B.; LastName, C.C. Article Title. *Journal Name* **Year**, *Volume Number*, Page Range.

ISBN 978-3-0365-0564-0 (Hbk)
ISBN 978-3-0365-0565-7 (PDF)

Cover image courtesy of Daniela Giordano.

Contents

About the Editor . . . . **vii**

Daniela Giordano
Bioactive Molecules from Extreme Environments
Reprinted from: *Mar. Drugs* **2020**, *18*, 640, doi:10.3390/md18120640 . . . . **1**

Stefano Bruno, Daniela Coppola, Guido di Prisco, Daniela Giordano and Cinzia Verde
Enzymes from Marine Polar Regions and Their Biotechnological Applications
Reprinted from: *Mar. Drugs* **2019**, *17*, 544, doi:10.3390/md17100544 . . . . **9**

Stefano Varrella, Michael Tangherlini and Cinzia Corinaldesi
Deep Hypersaline Anoxic Basins as Untapped Reservoir of Polyextremophilic Prokaryotes of Biotechnological Interest
Reprinted from: *Mar. Drugs* **2020**, *18*, 91, doi:/10.3390/md18020091 . . . . **45**

Kezhen Liu, Haitao Ding, Yong Yu and Bo Chen
A Cold-Adapted Chitinase-Producing Bacterium from Antarctica and Its Potential in Biocontrol of Plant Pathogenic Fungi
Reprinted from: *Mar. Drugs* **2019**, *17*, 695, doi:10.3390/md17120695 . . . . **77**

Min Jin, Yingbao Gai, Xun Guo, Yanping Hou and Runying Zeng
Properties and Applications of Extremozymes from Deep-Sea Extremophilic Microorganisms: A Mini Review
Reprinted from: *Mar. Drugs* **2019**, *17*, 656, doi:10.3390/md17120656 . . . . **93**

Patricia Aguila-Torres, Jonathan Maldonado, Alexis Gaete, Jaime Figueroa, Alex González, Richard Miranda, Roxana González-Stegmaier, Carolina Martin and Mauricio González
Biochemical and Genomic Characterization of the Cypermethrin-Degrading and Biosurfactant-Producing Bacterial Strains Isolated from Marine Sediments of the Chilean Northern Patagonia
Reprinted from: *Mar. Drugs* **2020**, *18*, 252, doi:10.3390/md18050252 . . . . **109**

Muhammad Zain ul Arifeen, Yu-Nan Ma, Ya-Rong Xue and Chang-Hong Liu
Deep-Sea Fungi Could Be the New Arsenal for Bioactive Molecules
Reprinted from: *Mar. Drugs* **2020**, *18*, 9, doi:10.3390/md18010009 . . . . **123**

Paulina Corral, Mohammad A. Amoozegar and Antonio Ventosa
Halophiles and Their Biomolecules: Recent Advances and Future Applications in Biomedicine
Reprinted from: *Mar. Drugs* **2020**, *18*, 33, doi:10.3390/md18010033 . . . . **139**

Jun Young Choi, Kunjoong Lee and Pyung Cheon Lee
Characterization of Carotenoid Biosynthesis in Newly Isolated *Deinococcus* sp. AJ005 and Investigation of the Effects of Environmental Conditions on Cell Growth and Carotenoid Biosynthesis
Reprinted from: *Mar. Drugs* **2019**, *17*, 705, doi:10.3390/md17120705 . . . . **173**

Maria Sindhura John, Joseph Amruthraj Nagoth, Kesava Priyan Ramasamy, Alessio Mancini, Gabriele Giuli, Antonino Natalello, Patrizia Ballarini, Cristina Miceli and Sandra Pucciarelli
Synthesis of Bioactive Silver Nanoparticles by a *Pseudomonas* Strain Associated with the Antarctic Psychrophilic Protozoon *Euplotes focardii*
Reprinted from: *Mar. Drugs* **2020**, *18*, 38, doi:10.3390/md18010038 . . . . **183**

Fengjie Li, Christian Peifer, Dorte Janussen and Deniz Tasdemir
New Discorhabdin Alkaloids from the Antarctic Deep-Sea Sponge *Latrunculia biformis*
Reprinted from: *Mar. Drugs* **2019**, *17*, 439, doi:10.3390/md17080439 . . . . **197**

Yuting Huang, Chao Bian, Zhaoqun Liu, Lingling Wang, Changhu Xue, Hongliang Huang, Yunhai Yi, Xinxin You, Wei Song, Xiangzhao Mao, Linsheng Song and Qiong Shi
The First Genome Survey of the Antarctic Krill (*Euphausia superba*) Provides a Valuable Genetic Resource for Polar Biomedical Research
Reprinted from: *Mar. Drugs* **2020**, *18*, 185, doi:10.3390/md18040185 . . . . **217**

About the Editor

Daniela Giordano, Ph.D., is a CNR (National Research Council) Scientist in Biochemistry. She obtained a permanent position at CNR in 2011, working first at the Institute of Protein Biochemistry (IBP-CNR) and, since 2014, at the Institute of Biosciences and BioResources (IBBR-CNR) in Naples. She graduated in Pharmaceutical Chemistry at the University of Naples Federico II in 2002 and obtained a Ph.D. at the University of Sacro Cuore in Rome in 2007, spending a period of six months at Northeastern University in Boston. After receiving her Ph.D., she began her research experience with fellowships at the Institute of Protein Biochemistry (IBP-CNR) in Naples, focusing her research on the molecular basis of cold adaptation of oxygen-binding proteins in polar bacteria and fish. She spent many periods as a visiting scientist at the National Institute of Health and Medical Research (INSERM), Paris, the University of Antwerp, and the University of Buenos Aires, studying the recombinant expression of globins of Antarctic bacteria and fish and their kinetic and thermodynamic properties. In 2010, she participated in an Arctic cruise, the TUNU-IV expedition (TUNU is East Greenland in Inuit language), for the collection of Arctic samples. Her research interest is focused on Antarctic and Arctic marine organisms because they are amongst the most vulnerable species to climate change and are a valuable source of natural products that can function as start structures of new molecules for drug discovery. Indeed, she is now leading a new research line on the identification of bioactive compounds as promising industrial products (pharmacy, nutraceutics, cosmeceuticals) from marine polar organisms. The results of her research are summarized in over 60 publications on highly qualified international journals and book chapters.

marine drugs

MDPI

Commentary

Bioactive Molecules from Extreme Environments

Daniela Giordano [1,2]

[1] Institute of Biosciences and BioResources (IBBR), CNR, Via Pietro Castellino 111, 80131 Napoli, Italy; daniela.giordano@ibbr.cnr.it

[2] Department of Marine Biotechnology, Stazione Zoologica Anton Dohrn (SZN), Villa Comunale, 80121 Napoli, Italy

Received: 10 November 2020; Accepted: 17 November 2020; Published: 14 December 2020

Abstract: Marine organisms inhabiting extreme habitats are a promising reservoir of bioactive compounds for drug discovery. Extreme environments, i.e., polar and hot regions, deep sea, hydrothermal vents, marine areas of high pressure or high salinity, experience conditions close to the limit of life. In these marine ecosystems, "hot spots" of biodiversity, organisms have adopted a huge variety of strategies to cope with such harsh conditions, such as the production of bioactive molecules potentially valuable for biotechnological applications and for pharmaceutical, nutraceutical and cosmeceutical sectors. Many enzymes isolated from extreme environments may be of great interest in the detergent, textile, paper and food industries. Marine natural products produced by organisms evolved under hostile conditions exhibit a wide structural diversity and biological activities. In fact, they exert antimicrobial, anticancer, antioxidant and anti-inflammatory activities. The aim of this Special Issue "Bioactive Molecules from Extreme Environments" was to provide the most recent findings on bioactive molecules as well as enzymes isolated from extreme environments, to be used in biotechnological discovery pipelines and pharmaceutical applications, in an effort to encourage further research in these extreme habitats.

Keywords: Arctic/Antarctic; deep-sea; deep hypersaline anoxic basin; cold-adapted bacteria; halophilic microorganisms; marine natural product; enzyme; carotenoid; silver nanoparticle; marine bioprospecting

1. Foreword

Marine organisms produce a huge variety of natural products that confer important advantages, either as antibiotics or by allowing communication with other organisms and with the environment. These molecules have long been exploited in medical fields as antioxidants, antimicrobial and anticancer agents, and in biotechnological applications, attracting an increasing commercial interest from the biotech sector [1]. In 2016, 1277 new marine compounds were reported exerting interesting biological activities, and many of these are of bacterial origin [2]. The global market for marine-derived drugs is expected to be USD 2745.80 million by 2025 [3]. However, to date, few molecules isolated from marine organisms have been approved [4] and many marine ecosystems remain unexplored.

Due to the limited accessibility and remoteness, extreme marine environments are still largely underexploited in comparison with terrestrial ecosystems. Recent advances in the sampling and accessibility of extreme areas, together with the development of omics technologies, have opened new avenues for drug discovery. These remote habitats are promising reservoirs of biotechnological and biomedical applicability, and represent a good opportunity for compound discovery and bioprospecting. Marine organisms inhabiting extreme environments have adopted unique survival strategies for growing and reproducing under hostile conditions, biosynthesizing an array of biomolecules potentially valuable for many applications in the biotechnological sector, in the pharmaceutical and cosmeceutical industries and in the bioremediation.

Extreme environments are exposed to one or more environmental parameters, i.e., temperature, salinity, osmolarity, UV radiation, pressure or pH, showing values close to the limit of life. Polar and hot regions, deep sea, hydrothermal vents, marine areas of high pressure or high salinity, and acidic and alkaline regions are examples of extreme environments. In the Arctic and Antarctic regions, the sea ice can reach up to ~13% of the Earth's total surface. The Arctic Ocean is mainly characterized by light seasonality and cold temperatures with winter extremes, whereas Antarctica is considered as the driest, windiest and coldest place on Earth, completely isolated, geographically and thermally, from the other continents. Polar marine life has adapted to thrive in the ocean's most inhospitable conditions, where extremes of pressure and temperature and the absence of light have selected species with a unique range of bioactive compounds, either enzymes [5] or secondary metabolites [6].

The deep sea, below a depth of 1000 m, is recognized as an extreme environment. It is characterized by the absence of sunlight and the presence of low temperatures and high hydrostatic pressures. This environment becomes even more extreme in particular conditions, with extremely high temperatures of >400 °C in deep-sea hydrothermal vents, and with extremely high salinities and high pressures in deep hypersaline anoxic basins (DHABs). These habitats have been discovered on the sea floor in different oceanic regions, such as the Red Sea, the eastern Mediterranean Sea and the Gulf of Mexico. New DHABs, the Thetis, Kyros and Haephestus basins in the Mediterranean Sea, have been recently discovered. DHABs are microbial "hotspot", with dense microbial populations of unique bacterial lineages more metabolically active than those of the adjacent layers [7]. Deep-sea extremophiles, able to proliferate under these challenging parameters (pressure and temperature, pH, salinity and redox potential), have adopted a variety of strategies to cope with these extreme environments, such as the production of extremozymes, with thermal or cold adaptability, salt tolerance and/or pressure tolerance, and secondary metabolites with biomedical applications.

The majority of marine bioactive compounds comes from microorganisms as a prolific resource for novel chemistry and the sustainable production of bioactive compounds, bypassing the problem of the recollection of samples from the field, which is required for macroorganisms. Recently, the increasing number of whole microbial genomes and the development of genome mining approaches have accelerated the discovery of novel bioactive molecules, overcoming the requirement for the isolation or cultivation of microorganisms [8].

2. The Special Issue

The Special Issue "Bioactive Molecules from Extreme Environments" was aimed at collecting papers regarding bioactive molecules and enzymes isolated from organisms inhabiting extreme environments being used in biotechnological discovery pipelines and pharmaceutical applications. Special attention was paid to the species biodiversity of extreme habitats as a promising reservoir of untapped compounds with biotechnological potential.

In total, eleven articles were accepted and included in the Special Issue. Most of the articles in this Special Issue were focused on marine microorganisms, bacteria and fungi, with their chemical diversity and active metabolites able to cope with harsh habitats.

Five articles in this Special Issue were focused on enzymes from microorganisms in extreme environments. Many enzymes have been evaluated for industrial applications, for the production of pharmaceuticals, foods, beverages, paper, as well as in textile and leather processing and waste-water treatment. However, only a few of these are able to meet the industrial demands that include tolerance of harsh conditions of temperature, pH, salinity and pressure, maintaining high conversion rate and reproducibility. The market for enzymes is expected to reach USD 7.0 billion by 2023, from USD 5.5 billion in 2018 [9]. Enzymes currently on the market derive from mesophilic organisms. However, the enzymes isolated from extreme environments are endowed with unique catalytic properties, and might be of great interest in different sectors of biotechnology.

In Bruno et al. 2019 [5], the authors described microbial enzymes with a potential biotechnological interest isolated in either Arctic or Antarctic environments. Polar marine environments are a promising research area for the discovery of enzymes with a potential industrial application. Cold-adapted enzymes are characterized by unique catalytic properties in comparison to their mesophilic homologues, i.e., higher catalytic efficiency, improved flexibility and lower thermal stability. These features make them particularly interesting for a potential commercial use in the food industry, agricultural production, synthetic biology, and biomedicine. Oxidoreductases, transferases, hydrolases, lyases, isomerases and ligases, and their proposed biotechnological applications, were reviewed in this paper. Hydrolases are the most abundant class of cold-adapted enzymes with a potential industrial application in the detergent, textile, paper, and food industries. For example, lactases or β-galactosidases, due to their capacity to reduce lactose intolerance, have attracted the interest of many research group and industries, and some of these isolated from the Antarctic marine *P. haloplanktis* LMG P-19143 were patented [10] and produced in large quantities by NutrilabNV (Bekkevoort, Belgium). Other enzymes have found application in molecular biology; a cold-adapted uracil-DNA glycosylase isolated from a psychrophilic Antarctic marine bacterium was released by New England Biolabs [11], a cold-active nuclease, isolated from an Antarctic marine psychrophile, *Shewanella* sp. strain Ac10, was developed by Takara-Clontech [12], and a recombinant alkaline phosphatase isolated from the Antarctic bacterial strain TAB5 was developed by New England Biolabs [13].

In Liu et al. 2019 [14], samples of seal and penguin feces, soil and marine sediment, collected from Fildes Peninsula in Antarctica were used as sources for the bioprospecting of chitinase-producing microorganisms. After optimizing the medium components and culture conditions, a cold-adapted strain belonging to *Pseudomonas* was identified as the best producer of chitinase, exhibiting more than 50% of its catalytic activity even at 0 °C. The crude chitinase showed the significant inhibition of fungi *Verticillium dahlia* CICC 2534 and *Fusarium oxysporum* f. sp. *cucumerinum* CICC 2532, which can cause cotton wilt and cucumber blight, respectively, suggesting that the cold strain may be a competitive candidate for biological control in agriculture, especially at low temperatures.

Jin et al. 2019 [15] discussed the potential industrial applications of extremozymes, as thermophilic, psychrophilic, halophilic and piezophilic enzymes. Deep-sea thermophiles, able to grow at high temperatures of 41–120 °C, produce thermostable proteolytic enzymes, attractive for use in the detergent, food and feed industries. For example, an α-amylase from the thermophile *Thermococcus* sp., isolated from a deep-sea hydrothermal vent, is on the market, and is named Fuelzyme®, released by Verenium Corporation (San Diego, CA, USA) [16]. Deep-sea psychrophiles, exhibiting an active metabolism even at −25 °C, are a promising source of industrial cold-active enzymes with applicability in the textile, detergent, beverage, food and biofuel industries. Deep-sea halophilic enzymes have particularly great potential in the production of biodiesel, polyunsaturated fatty acids and food, or in the treatment of waste water containing high salt concentrations and starch residues. Deep-sea piezophilic enzymes, living up to 70–110 MPa, have shown high efficiency in applications for food production, where high pressures are used for the processing and sterilization of food materials.

Aguila-Torres and co-authors 2020 [17] reported a taxonomic identification and biochemical characterization of cypermethrin-degrading and biosurfactant-producing bacterial strains from samples collected in cypermethrin-contaminated marine sediment in Chilean northern Patagonia. This environment is considered extreme because of a wide range of temperatures, ranging from 4 to 20 °C, salinity, and a low nutrient availability. In addition, there has been an extensive use of cypermethrin as an antiparasitic pesticide in the salmon farming industry in northern Patagonia. Cypermethrin, used in agriculture and aquaculture, is considered a possible human carcinogen, able also to affect marine ecosystems. In northern Patagonia, a high concentration of cypermethrin has been reported in marine sediment. Among isolated strains, four strains exhibited the highest growth rate on cypermethrin, and high levels of biosurfactant production. An analysis of the genome sequence of these strains demonstrated the presence of genes encoding esterase, pyrethroid hydrolase and laccase, associated with the different biodegradation pathways of cypermethrin.

Bioremediation has become an important tool for removing pollutants from contaminated environments, taking advantage of the presence of microorganisms and their ability to clean contaminated environments. Hydrocarbon-degrading bacteria are able to metabolize contaminants, developing specific pathways for sustaining their energetic and carbon requirements in the presence of them.

Varrella and colleagues 2020 [7] in their review described the environmental characteristics of DHABs, highlighting the unique bacterial lineages found in these extreme habitats. DHAB-derived microorganisms represent promising candidates for the bioremediation of oil hydrocarbons thanks to the presence of enzymes involved in pathways associated with hydrocarbon degradation. Proteobacteria represented by sulfate-reducing Deltaproteobacteria, as well as sulfur-oxidizing Gamma- and Epsilonproteobacteria, Actinobacteria, Deferribacteres and Euryarchaeota, were found across DHABs worldwide. In addition, viruses, found to be well-preserved in DHAB sediments, were able to control prokaryotic dynamics in these ecosystems. The variety of prokaryotes inhabiting DHABs represents an important source of polyextreme enzymes, such as esterase, lipase, α-amilase, pullulanase and xylanase, with applications in pharmaceutical, food, and beverage industrial processes, and many bioactive compounds with antiviral, antimicrobial and antitumor activities.

The marine chemical diversity varies from simple peptides and linear fatty acids to complex compounds such as terpenes, alkaloids and polyketides, etc., incorporating elements used in the marine environment as chemical defenses against predators. Natural products with different structures, able to perform a wide range of biological activities, make marine biomolecules valuable alternatives to many pathogenic bacteria and fungi, especially in the era of antimicrobial resistance. The most commonly reported activity is toward pathogenic agents, including viruses. Discovering novel and efficient antimicrobial molecules is becoming essential for natural-product chemistry, because of antibiotic-resistant microorganisms or even multidrug-resistance, and the development of new emerging infections. One example is represented by a potent antiviral agent isolated from the ascidian *Aplidium albicans*, which is under clinical trials in patients affected by Corona Virus SARS-CoV-2 [18]. Many papers in this issue are related to antimicrobial activity as well as anticancer activity. Cancer is the leading cause of death globally, and finding new molecules with anticancer activities remains a major challenge in the pursuit for a cure.

Zain ul Arifeen et al. 2019 [19] wrote a review in which they described the structure, biological activity, and distribution of secondary metabolites produced by deep-sea fungi in the last five years. Fungi living in deep-sea environments produce unique secondary metabolites for defense and communication. Despite being the producer of many important bioactive molecules, deep-sea fungi have not been explored thoroughly due to methodological and technical limitations. However, their abundance and presence in all possible extreme ecosystems make them an ideal source of new bioactive molecules with many applications. Polyketide- and nitrogen-containing compounds, polypeptides, ester and phenolic derivatives, piperazine derivatives and terpenoid compounds were the bioactive molecules isolated from deep-sea fungi and showing antibiotic, antimicrobial, antiviral activities as well as cytotoxicity against cancer cells. Most of these compounds were isolated from two fungal genera, i.e., *Penicillium* and *Aspergillus*. Among these natural products, terpenoid derivatives were the most abundant compounds with the strongest antibiotic and cytotoxic activities with respect to other classes of molecules. In particular, breviones, isolated from the deepest sediment-derived fungus *Penicillium* sp. (5115 m depth), showing the strongest cytotoxic activity against cancer cells, have the potential to be good candidates for anticancer drugs.

Corral and co-authors 2019 [20] described the antimicrobial and anticancer molecules produced by microorganisms, illustrating their action mechanisms *in vitro*. Halophilic microorganisms, such as archaea, bacteria and fungi, widely distributed around the world, inhabit hypersaline ecosystems characterized by a salinity higher than seawater, i.e., 3.5% NaCl. They are a source of bioactive molecules with applications in biomedicine. The continuous increase in antibiotic resistance establishes an urgent need for the exploiting of natural and sustainable resources to find novel antimicrobial molecules. Bacteria of the genus *Nocardiopsis* and *Streptomyces*, belonging to the phylum Actinobacteria, were found to be the main producers of antimicrobial compounds, whereas among fungi the genus

Aspergillus was the most prolific. Likewise, *Nocardiopsis*, *Streptomyces*, *Bacillus*, *Halomonas* and *Aspergillus* were the most frequent producers of antitumoral molecules. Some of these compounds are promising candidates for preclinical trials.

Choi et al. 2019 [21] reported the characterization of deinoxanthin from a novel reddish *Deinococcus* sp. AJ005 isolated from seawater near King George Island in Antarctica, whose genome was recently completely sequenced. *Deinococcus* strains, Gram-positive bacteria, live in different habitats such as air, soils, and seas, and also at high altitudes and in Antarctic environments. They cope with these extreme habitats thanks to a variety of metabolic pathways, including the biosynthesis of antioxidants such as deinoxanthin. This carotenoid is particularly interesting for its use as an antioxidant, a cosmetic ingredient, and a food or feed additive, it being an efficient scavenger of reactive oxygen species and an anticancer agent. On the basis of genome annotation analysis, the authors proposed the deinoxanthin biosynthetic pathway, investigating the effects of culture conditions on the deinoxanthin biosynthesis in this strain.

John et al. 2020 [22] used a new *Pseudomonas* strain associated with the Antarctic marine ciliate *Euplotes focardii* to obtain silver nanoparticles (AgNPs) after incubation with 1 mM of $AgNO_3$ within 24 h. Nanoparticles (NPs) have become particularly interesting in biomedical sciences, drug-gene delivery, space industries, cosmetics and chemical industries. AgNPs show general antibacterial and bactericidal features, thus becoming promising tools in biomedical applications. Since the physiochemical methods used for AgNP synthesis are not convenient given their high energy consumption and the use of toxic reagents, there has been a growing need to develop a simple and low-cost approach to AgNP synthesis without toxic chemicals. An alternative to the chemical synthesis method is to use microbes to obtain nanoparticles. This easy and efficient biological method to synthesize AgNPs may be used against drug-resistant pathogenic bacteria, contributing to solving the problem of antibiotic resistance. The authors characterized the size and morphology of AgNPs and demonstrated that *Pseudomonas* AgNPs showed a higher antibacterial activity against *Escherichia coli*, *Staphylococcus aureus* and *Candida albicans* with respect to the chemically synthesized NPs. The results of this paper are related to the patent number 102019000014121 deposited in 06/08/2019.

Only two articles in this Special Issue are focused on macroorganisms, specifically the deep-sea Antarctic sponge *Latrunculia biformis*, collected from the Antarctic Weddell Sea shelf at a depth of 291 m, and the Antarctic krill *Euphausia superba* that represents the most abundant biomass in cold environments at the base of the Antarctic food chain.

In Li et al. 2019 [23], the authors isolated diverse discorhabdin alkaloids from the Antarctic deep-sea sponge *L. biformis*. Three known discorhabdins, (−)-discorhabdin L, (+)-discorhabdin A and (+)-discorhabdin Q, and three new discorhabdin analogs (−)-2-bromo-discorhabdin D, (−)-1-acetyl-discorhabdin L and (+)-1-octacosatrienoyl-discorhabdin L, were identified and characterized by bioactivity and molecular networking-based metabolomics and the chemical structures elucidated by extensive spectroscopy analyses. (−)-discorhabdin L, (−)-1-acetyl-discorhabdin L and (+)-1-octacosatrienoyl-discorhabdin L showed promising anticancer activities, demonstrated by the molecular modeling of the potential binding of discorhabdins to the anticancer targets involved in their anticancer activity. (−)-1-acetyl-discorhabdin L and (+)-1-octacosatrienoyl-discorhabdin L are the first discorhabdin analogs with an ester function at C-1 with (+)-1-octacosatrienoyl-discorhabdin L, which is the first discorhabdin bearing a long-chain fatty acid at this position.

The experimental article by Huang et al. 2020 [24] reported the first genome survey of the Antarctic krill *E. superba*, a very important marine organism in the Antarctic food chain. The high-throughput comparative identification of putative antimicrobial peptides (AMPs) and antihypertensive peptides (AHTPs) from whole-body transcriptomes of the Antarctic krill and its mesophilic counterpart, the whiteleg shrimp *Penaeus vannamei*, revealed that AMPs/AMP precursors and AHTPs were generally conserved, with interesting variations between the two crustacean species due to cold adaptation. This paper is a preliminary exploration of bioactive peptides in a polar key species of the trophic chain for the development of novel marine drugs.

3. Perspectives and Conclusions

The papers included in this Special Issue provide an overview of the growing interest in species biodiversity, highlighting the importance of marine extreme environments as sources of a unique marine chemical diversity of molecules. It is worth noting that six articles in this Issue are focused on molecules and enzymes isolated from Antarctica. This means that there is an increasing interest in this habitat because it is perceived as an important source of drug discovery. In fact, the unique environment and ecological pressures of marine polar regions might be the major drivers of a selection of unique biological communities able to biosynthesize new compounds with diverse biological activities. It is expected that, in the near future, more marine molecules from polar regions as well as from other extreme habitats will find their way into biomedical and biotechnological applications.

In conclusion, the Guest Editor thanks all the authors that contributed with their interesting articles to this Special Issue, all the reviewers for evaluating the submitted manuscripts, and the Editorial board of Marine Drugs, the Editor-in-Chief of the Journal Orazio Taglialatela-Scafati for their support, especially in this difficult period of the 2020 pandemic SARS CoV-2.

Funding: This research received no external funding.

Acknowledgments: I dedicate this book to the memory of Guido di Prisco, passed away in Sep-tember 2019. He was my mentor, contributing to inspire my interest on the life in Antarctic and Arctic environments.

Conflicts of Interest: The author declares no conflict of interest.

References

1. Martins, A.; Vieira, H.; Gaspar, H.A.; Santos, S. Marketed Marine Natural Products in the Pharmaceutical and Cosmeceutical Industries: Tips for Success. *Mar. Drugs* **2014**, *12*, 1066–1101. [CrossRef] [PubMed]
2. Blunt, J.W.; Carroll, A.R.; Copp, B.R.; Davis, R.A.; Keyzers, R.A.; Prinsep, M.R. Marine natural products. *Nat. Prod. Rep.* **2018**, *35*, 8–53. [CrossRef] [PubMed]
3. Market Research Engine. Marine Derived Drugs Market Research Report. Available online: https://www.marketresearchengine.com/marine-derived-drugs-market (accessed on 28 October 2020).
4. Tomorrow's Healthcare Team. Clinical Pipeline Marine Pharmacology. Available online: https://www.midwestern.edu/departments/marinepharmacology/clinical-pipeline.xml (accessed on 3 November 2020).
5. Bruno, S.; Coppola, D.; Di Prisco, G.; Giordano, D.; Verde, C. Enzymes from Marine Polar Regions and Their Biotechnological Applications. *Mar. Drugs* **2019**, *17*, 544. [CrossRef] [PubMed]
6. Núñez-Pons, L.; Shilling, A.; Verde, C.; Baker, B.J.; Giordano, D. Marine Terpenoids from Polar Latitudes and Their Potential Applications in Biotechnology. *Mar. Drugs* **2020**, *18*, 401. [CrossRef] [PubMed]
7. Varrella, S.; Tangherlini, M.; Corinaldesi, C. Deep Hypersaline Anoxic Basins as Untapped Reservoir of Polyextremophilic Prokaryotes of Biotechnological Interest. *Mar. Drugs* **2020**, *18*, 91. [CrossRef] [PubMed]
8. Ziemert, N.; Alanjaryab, M.; Weber, T. The evolution of genome mining in microbes—A review. *Nat. Prod. Rep.* **2016**, *33*, 988–1005. [CrossRef] [PubMed]
9. BCC. *Global Markets for Enzymes in Industrial Applications*; BCC Publishing: Wellesley, MA, USA, 2018.
10. Gerday, C.; Hoyoux, A.; Marie Francois, J.M.; Dubois, P.; Baise, E.; Jennes, I.; Genicot, S. Cold-Active Beta Galactosidase, the Process for its Preparation and the Use Thereof. U.S. Patent WO2001004276A1, 9 July 1999.
11. New England Biolabs Inc. Antarctic Thermolabile UDG. Available online: https://international.neb.com/products/m0372-antarctic-thermolabile-udg#Product%20Information (accessed on 3 November 2020).
12. Available online: https://www.takarabio.com/products/cloning/modifying-enzymes/nucleases/cryonase-cold-active-nuclease?catalog=2670A (accessed on 10 December 2020).
13. New England Biolabs Inc. Antarctic Phosphatase. Available online: https://www.neb.com/products/m0289-antarctic-phosphatase#Product%20Information (accessed on 3 November 2020).
14. Liu, K.; Ding, H.; Yu, Y.; Chen, B. A Cold-Adapted Chitinase-Producing Bacterium from Antarctica and Its Potential in Biocontrol of Plant Pathogenic Fungi. *Mar. Drugs* **2019**, *17*, 695. [CrossRef] [PubMed]
15. Jin, M.; Gai, Y.; Guo, X.; Hou, Y.; Zeng, R. Properties and Applications of Extremozymes from Deep-Sea Extremophilic Microorganisms: A Mini Review. *Mar. Drugs* **2019**, *17*, 656. [CrossRef] [PubMed]

16. Callen, W.; Richardson, T.; Frey, G.; Miller, C.; Kazaoka, M.; Mathur, E.; Short, J. Amylases and Methods for Use in Starch Processing. U.S. Patent No. 8,338,131, 25 December 2012.
17. Aguila-Torres, P.; Maldonado, J.; Gaete, A.; Figueroa, J.; González, A.R.; Miranda, R.; González-Stegmaier, R.; Martin, C.; González, M. Biochemical and Genomic Characterization of the Cypermethrin-Degrading and Biosurfactant-Producing Bacterial Strains Isolated from Marine Sediments of the Chilean Northern Patagonia. *Mar. Drugs* **2020**, *18*, 252. [CrossRef] [PubMed]
18. U.S. National Library of Medicine. Proof of Concept Study to Evaluate the Safety Profile of Plitidepsin in Patients With COVID-19 (APLICOV-PC). Available online: https://clinicaltrials.gov/ct2/show/study/NCT04382066 (accessed on 7 November 2020).
19. Arifeen, M.Z.U.; Ma, Y.-N.; Xue, Y.-R.; Liu, C. Deep-Sea Fungi Could Be the New Arsenal for Bioactive Molecules. *Mar. Drugs* **2019**, *18*, 9. [CrossRef] [PubMed]
20. Corral, P.; Amoozegar, M.A.; Ventosa, A. Halophiles and Their Biomolecules: Recent Advances and Future Applications in Biomedicine. *Mar. Drugs* **2019**, *18*, 33. [CrossRef] [PubMed]
21. Choi, J.Y.; Lee, K.; Lee, P.; Lee, S. Characterization of Carotenoid Biosynthesis in Newly Isolated *Deinococcus* sp. AJ005 and Investigation of the Effects of Environmental Conditions on Cell Growth and Carotenoid Biosynthesis. *Mar. Drugs* **2019**, *17*, 705. [CrossRef] [PubMed]
22. John, M.S.; Amruthraj, N.J.; Ramasamy, K.P.; Mancini, A.; Giuli, G.; Natalello, A.; Ballarini, P.; Miceli, C.; Pucciarelli, S. Synthesis of Bioactive Silver Nanoparticles by a Pseudomonas Strain Associated with the Antarctic Psychrophilic Protozoon Euplotes focardii. *Mar. Drugs* **2020**, *18*, 38. [CrossRef] [PubMed]
23. Li, F.; Peifer, C.; Janussen, D.; Tasdemir, D. New Discorhabdin Alkaloids from the Antarctic Deep-Sea Sponge Latrunculia biformis. *Mar. Drugs* **2019**, *17*, 439. [CrossRef] [PubMed]
24. Huang, Y.; Bian, C.; Liu, Z.; Wang, L.; Xue, C.; Huang, H.; Yi, Y.; You, X.; Song, W.; Mao, X.; et al. The First Genome Survey of the Antarctic Krill (*Euphausia superba*) Provides a Valuable Genetic Resource for Polar Biomedical Research. *Mar. Drugs* **2020**, *18*, 185. [CrossRef] [PubMed]

marine drugs

Review

Enzymes from Marine Polar Regions and Their Biotechnological Applications

Stefano Bruno [1], Daniela Coppola [2,3], Guido di Prisco [2], Daniela Giordano [2,3] and Cinzia Verde [2,3,*]

1 Department of Food and Drug, University of Parma, Parco Area delle Scienze 23A, 43124 Parma, Italy; stefano.bruno@unipr.it
2 Institute of Biosciences and BioResources (IBBR), CNR, Via Pietro Castellino 111, 80131 Napoli, Italy; daniela.coppola@ibbr.cnr.it (D.C.); guido.diprisco@ibbr.cnr.it (G.d.P.); daniela.giordano@ibbr.cnr.it (D.G.)
3 Department of Marine Biotechnology, Stazione Zoologica Anton Dohrn, Villa Comunale, 80121 Napoli, Italy
* Correspondence: c.verde@ibp.cnr.it or cinzia.verde@ibbr.cnr.it

Received: 2 August 2019; Accepted: 18 September 2019; Published: 23 September 2019

Abstract: The microorganisms that evolved at low temperatures express cold-adapted enzymes endowed with unique catalytic properties in comparison to their mesophilic homologues, i.e., higher catalytic efficiency, improved flexibility, and lower thermal stability. Cold environments are therefore an attractive research area for the discovery of enzymes to be used for investigational and industrial applications in which such properties are desirable. In this work, we will review the literature on cold-adapted enzymes specifically focusing on those discovered in the bioprospecting of polar marine environments, so far largely neglected because of their limited accessibility. We will discuss their existing or proposed biotechnological applications within the framework of the more general applications of cold-adapted enzymes.

Keywords: Arctic/Antarctic environment; biocatalysis; cold-adaptation; marine biotechnology

1. Introduction

The economic progress in the "Era of Biotech" demands new biocatalysts for a wide range of applications, from therapy to industrial manufacturing. Particularly, biocatalysis is an attractive alternative to chemical synthesis, as biocatalysts are biodegradable and non-toxic, they originate from renewable sources, they have high selectivity and they provide products in high yields [1]. Up to 40% of the industrially relevant chemical reactions that require organic solvents harmful to the environment could be substituted by enzymatic catalysis by 2030 [2]. Many industrial processes already benefit from the use of enzymes (e.g., proteases, amylases, cellulases, carboxymethylcellulases, xylanases) in the production of pharmaceuticals, foods, beverages, confectionery, paper, as well as in textile and leather processing and waste-water treatment. Most of these enzymes are microbial in origin because they are relatively more thermostable than their counterparts from plants and animals [3]. Their market is expected to reach $7.0 billion by 2023 from $5.5 billion in 2018, with an annual growth rate of 4.9% for the period 2018–2023 [4]. In this market, industrial detergents will reach $10.8 billion by 2022, with an annual growth rate of 4.2% for the period 2017–2022 [4], whereas the global market for enzymes in the food and beverages industries is expected to grow from $1.8 billion in 2017 to nearly $2.2 billion by 2022, with an annual growth rate of 4.6% from 2017 to 2022 [4].

The increasing demand for new or better biocatalysts with different substrate selectivity, chiral selectivity, stability and activity at various pH and temperatures is likely to be met through the investigation of microorganisms, the largest reservoir of biological activities in Nature. Marine microorganisms are particularly promising in this respect and it is predicted [5] that the global market for marine biotechnology, estimated at $4.1 billion in 2015, may reach $4.8 billion by 2020 and $6.4 billion by 2025, with the identification of new marine-derived enzymes [6]. The bioprospecting of marine environments, i.e., the systematic search for new bioactive compounds or biomolecules, has been traditionally focused on temperate/tropical latitudes [7], and polar marine environments have been mostly neglected, mainly due to their limited accessibility. These habitats include not only seawater but also sediments and sea ice, where internal fluids remain liquid in winter. Although both polar regions contain freezing seas, their microorganisms have different evolutionary histories due to their different geography and land-sea distribution [8]. The northern polar region is characterized by extensive, shallow shelves of landmasses that surround a partially land-locked ocean [9], whereas the Antarctic region consists in a dynamic open ocean that surrounds the continent [10,11]. The opening of the Drake Passage between Tierra del Fuego and the Antarctic Peninsula 23.5–32.5 million years ago was the key event for the development of the Antarctic Circumpolar Current (ACC), partially responsible for cooling of the Antarctic waters. The Antarctic Polar Front, the northern boundary of the ACC, promoted the isolation of the Antarctic marine fauna [10,11]. In both polar regions, the constantly low temperatures have driven the evolution of cold-adapted microorganisms, which are classified as psychrophilic and psychrotolerant according to the physiological features of their growth [12]. In this review, the general term "cold-adapted" will be used to indicate "psychrophile" organisms indigenous to cold environments [13].

In view of recent breakthroughs in sampling methodologies, sequencing, and bioinformatics, polar marine environments have recently come into the scientific spotlight—also because of growing concerns about their role in global climate change dynamics. An increasing number of works demonstrated their biological diversity [14–19], which includes bacteria, archaea, yeasts, fungi and algae [20,21]. Among polar microorganisms, those defined as 'cold-adapted' are those that thrive in permanently cold environments, even at subzero temperatures in super-cooled liquid water, and that evolved the physiological and biochemical capability to survive and reproduce under these extreme conditions [22]. With a better knowledge of marine microorganisms of polar regions, previously inaccessible bio-products, both in terms of new bioactive metabolites and proteins/enzymes with potential commercial applications, have been described [23,24]. Their biotechnological use can take many forms, from agricultural production to industrial processes, food chemistry [25], synthetic biology, and biomedical uses [26,27]. It is expected that, in the near future, more cold-adapted bacteria and their enzymes will find their way to biotechnological applications.

In this review, we will describe recent findings in enzymes isolated in either Arctic or Antarctic regions, some of which are of potential biotechnological interest. Unlike previous reviews, we particularly focused on enzymes isolated from marine polar environments. Cold-adapted enzymes from non-marine environments (i.e., from soil or lakes) or from non-polar sources (i.e., deep sea) will be reported to suggest potential future applications for enzymes isolated from marine polar microorganisms or to highlight structure-function relationships common to all cold-adapted enzymes, regardless of their origin.

2. Methods for Enzyme Discovery and Engineering

The identification of enzymes from cultured or uncultured marine microorganisms have been carried out through several '-omics' techniques. Additionally, natural enzymes have been optimized through enzyme engineering to improve their biotechnological properties (Figure 1).

Omics techniques. The overall knowledge on polar microorganisms has recently increased through the application of "omic" approaches (environmental shotgun sequencing, metatranscriptomics, proteomics) that have revealed the peculiar properties of their communities [28].

High-throughput metagenomic screening approaches, using both sequence-based and function-driven screenings, are contributing to the identification of a large number of enzymes, with most industrial enzymes having being identified by traditional functional screening of (meta)genomic libraries [29–31]. Recently, rapid technological developments in bioinformatics have revolutionized the exploration of the microbial diversity for the discovery of enzymes with commercial impact [32].

The sequence-based analysis of their (meta)genomic DNA by high-throughput sequencing methods followed by in silico analysis was used to predict enzyme function [33] allowing an increase in the rate of discovery. Sequence-based metagenomic approaches represents a powerful tool by avoiding the intensive, expensive, and time-consuming lab work associated to classic screening by reducing the number of targets to be functionally tested. Nevertheless, the latter approach is only limited to the discovery of genes with high similarities to already deposited sequences, making the discovery of new enzymatic functions difficult [34].

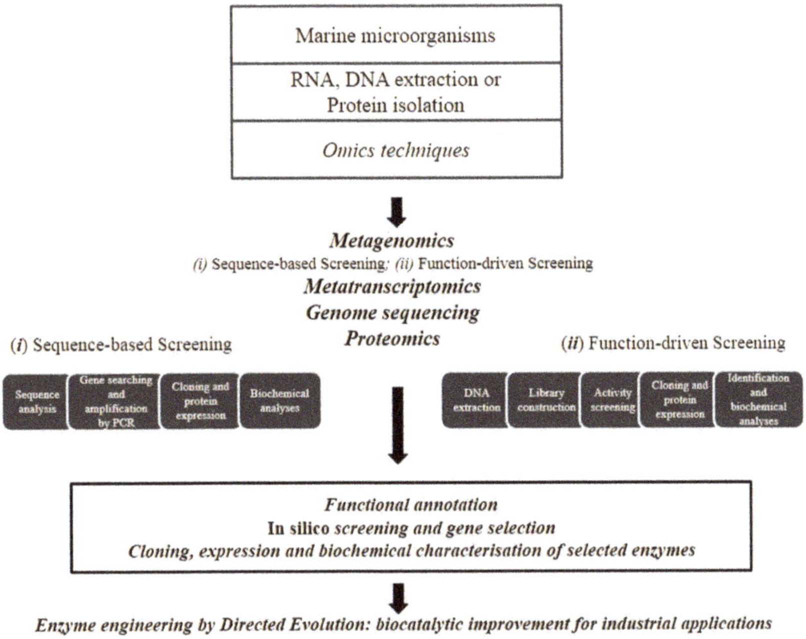

Figure 1. Workflow for the discovery of novel industrial enzymes by *omics* technologies.

Some recent EU FP7-funded projects (e.g., MACUMBA and PHARMASEA) made valuable efforts in exploiting the potential of microorganisms (mostly bacteria and microalgae) for pharmaceutical, cosmeceutical, and nutraceutical applications [35]. In order to explore marine biodiversity in several environments, including extreme habitats, a pan-European consortium was instituted in 2015 [36] for the creation of one of the largest collections of marine enzymes, with a focus on those of interest for the industrial market [32]. At present, this collection contains about 1000 enzymes, of which around 94% are available in ready-to-use expression systems and 32% have been completely characterized [2,32,37]. However, the publication of gene/genome sequences is faster than the identification of new protein functions, the most important challenge in modern biology due to the lack of experimental evidence to support functional annotation of a large fraction of genes and proteins [38,39]. Indeed, there is a gap between the numbers of biological activities predicted in silico and the number of new enzymes described experimentally, with the proportion of the latter ones approaching 0% [38,39], despite successful approaches of enzyme screen programmes through metagenomic approaches [40].

In addition to genomic screenings, recent technological developments in the complementary fields of transcriptomics have developed tools suitable for further discoveries. Indeed, advances within the field of RNA sequencing [41] have allowed analysis of whole (meta)transcriptomes and made them available for the generation of high-quality protein sequence databases, facilitating enzyme identification. The functional annotation of selected genomes and transcriptomes is relevant to infer associated biological functions and application of proteomics studies in the discovery of bioactive proteins.

As for proteomics approaches, the most commonly used method for enzyme discovery is bottom-up shotgun proteomics [42], in which proteins are enzymatically digested and the obtained peptides are analysed either by liquid chromatography coupled to electrospray ionization (ESI–LC–MS/MS) or by matrix-assisted laser desorption/ionization followed by time of flight mass spectrometry (MALDI–TOF–MS). A further direct method for enzyme discovery is activity-based proteomics, which takes advantage of enzyme class-specific substrates for the identification of groups of enzymes [43,44].

Enzyme Engineering

The ultimate value of biotechnology is the production and delivery of molecules or processes of interest for many applications; the emerging requirement for biotechnological products is to be energy saving, thus reducing environmental impacts [45]. Therefore, enzymes from cold-adapted organisms are important because their properties meet the ongoing efforts and needs to decrease energy consumption [46].

The ability of enzymes to catalyze a diverse set of reactions with exquisite specificity makes these proteins essential for reactions useful to humankind. Due their structural and functional complexity, the use of natural enzymes in biotechnology has been limited over the past decades. In fact, natural enzymes generally require modification for industrial use [47], given the improvements in catalytic efficiency, stereo-selectivity, and stability that can be reached through combinatorial engineering strategies [48]. Recent advances in science and technology have led to activity improvements for native and non-native substrates, synthesis of new chemistries and functional characterization of promising novel enzymes.

In the past, enzyme-based industrial processes were designed around the limitations of natural enzymes discovered in nature; today, enzymes can be engineered to fit the process specifications through enzyme engineering [1]. Enzyme engineering can be pursued by either rational site-directed mutagenesis based on currently available sequence and 3D structures deposited in the RCSB Protein Data Bank, or by directed evolution. Directed evolution is a key technology at the base of the development of new industrial biocatalysts [49–52] by random amino acid residues changes in the enzyme, largely carried out using PCR-based methods, followed by selection or screening of resulting libraries for variants with improved enzymatic properties. Changes in enzyme properties usually require simultaneous multiple amino-acid substitutions, creating exponentially more variants for testing. However, modern high-throughput screening methods, such as fluorescence-activated cell sorting [53–55] allow the screening of tens of millions of variants in a short time. Moreover, the best approach to create multiple mutations is to limit the choices by statistical or bioinformatic methods, such as the statistical correlation approach based on the ProSAR (protein structure-activity relationship) algorithm [56], to identify if a particular substitution is beneficial or not.

Furthermore, the development of synthetic biology methodology, through which large DNA sequences can be synthesized de novo, is increasing the ability for designing and engineering enzymes with new functions. Moreover, the possibility to synthesize whole-gene synthesis can also be used to build high-quality DNA libraries [1].

3. Cold-Adapted Enzymes and Their Biotechnological Applications

The bioprospecting of microorganisms living in extreme environmental conditions has already led to the discovery of several enzymes endowed with catalytic properties potentially useful for biotechnological applications [57], including some isolated from marine polar regions [23]. Moreover, the systematic investigation of the relationship between the structure and function of these enzymes—in comparison with their mesophilic homologs—has allowed recognising specific structural features associated with cold adaptation, which can be applied to the design of non-natural enzymes endowed with high activity at low/room temperatures. New catalytic activities are expected to arise from the Enzyme Function Initiative (EFI), which was recently established to address the challenge of assigning reliable functions to enzymes discovered in bacterial genome projects [58]. The main aim of the initiative is the computation-based prediction of substrate specificity for functional assignment of unknown enzymes.

3.1. Applications of Cold-Adapted Enzymes

The ultimate value of biotechnology is the production and delivery of molecules or processes of interest for many applications; the emerging requirement for biotechnological products is to be energy saving, thus reducing environmental impacts. Therefore, enzymes from cold-adapted organisms are important because their properties meet the ongoing efforts and needs to decrease energy consumption.

The ability of enzymes to catalyze a diverse set of reactions with exquisite specificity makes these proteins essential for biochemical studies, as well as promising catalysts for reactions useful to humankind. Due to their structural and functional complexity, the use of natural enzymes in biotechnology has been limited over the past decades. In fact, natural enzymes generally require modification for industrial use, given the improvements in catalytic efficiency, stereo-selectivity, and stability that can be reached through combinatorial engineering strategies. Recent advances in science and technology have led to activity improvements for native and non-native substrates, synthesis of new chemistries and functional characterization of promising novel enzymes.

Protein engineering technologies make it possible to develop enzymes that are highly active on non-natural targets, in the presence of organic solvents, and even enzymes for chemical transformations not found in nature. Application of these advanced engineering technologies to the creation of biocatalysts typically starts with an integrated approach with iterative cycles of DNA mutation and selection to create—by directed evolution—enzymes with novel functions for biotechnological approaches [59]. Due to our enhanced understanding of how these enzymes work in extreme environments, we can look forward to increasingly use computational tools, such as Artificial Intelligence, and to design enzymes with new structures and functions [60].

Cold-adapted enzymes have been suggested as biotechnological tools for several reasons:

(1) They are cost-effective, e.g., lower amounts are required, due to higher catalytic efficiency at low temperature;
(2) They can catalyze reactions at temperatures where competitive, undesirable chemical reactions are slowed down. This property is particularly relevant in the food industry, where deterioration and loss of thermolabile nutrients can occur at room temperature;
(3) They catalyze the desired reactions at temperatures where bacterial contamination is reduced. There is a number of advantages in working at lower temperature (around 10–15 °C) than those currently used for large-scale industrial production;
(4) Most cold-adapted enzymes can be inactivated by moderate heat due to their thermolability, avoiding chemical-based inactivation. A striking application of this property has been described for the design of live vaccines. Mesophilic pathogens were engineered for production of thermolabile homologs of essential enzymes, making them temperature-sensitive (TS). The engineered strains are inactivated at mammalian body temperatures, thus losing pathogenicity, but retaining their entire antigenic repertoire. Duplantis and colleagues [61] were able to entirely shift the lifestyle of *Francisella* (*F. novicida*), responsible for tularaemia disease in mice, by substituting its genes encoding essential enzymes with those identified in an Arctic bacterium. The authors applied the same approach to *Salmonella enterica* and the Gram-positive *Mycobacterium* [62]. The TS *S. enterica* strains were shown to be safe in research or diagnostic laboratories but were still capable of stimulating a protective immune response [63]. The TS strain of *M. tuberculosis* could be a safe research or diagnostic strain that is incapable of causing serious disease in humans while being identical to wild-type *M. tuberculosis* except for the TS phenotype [62].

The isolation of cold-adapted enzymes from natural sources is mostly unfeasible and their recombinant expression through standard protocols is hindered by the relatively high growth temperature of the commonly used expression hosts, including *E. coli*. However, several recombinant expression systems have been devized for the production of cold-adapted enzymes [64], mostly aimed at the stabilization and solubilization of heat-sensitive proteins. Development of low-temperature expression system has been attempted in the psychrophilic *Arthrobacter* sp. isolated from a Greenland glacier [65]. An alternative strategy is to use the engineered Arctic Express Cells which co-express cold-adapted homologues of the *E. coli* GroELS chaperonines, Cpn60 and Cpn10, from *O. antarctica* [66]. This system allows protein processing at very low temperatures (4–12 °C), potentially increasing the yield of active, soluble recombinant protein.

3.2. Structural Features of Cold-Adapted Enzymes

A basic requirement of evolutionary cold adaptation is that the enzyme should afford metabolic rates comparable to those of mesophilic organisms at its working temperature. Indeed, the temperature-dependence of the catalyzed reaction constants is described by the Arrhenius Equation (1)

$$k = Ae^{-E/(RT)} \quad (1)$$

where k is the reaction rate, E is the activation energy of the reaction, R is the gas constant, T is temperature and A is a collision frequency factor. It shows that a decrease of 10 °C brings about a decrease of 2–3 fold in the reaction rate. Therefore, a mesophilic enzyme with an optimal working temperature around 37 °C is expected to work 16–80 times slower when brought to 0 °C [67]. Increases in enzyme expression in psychrophilic microorganisms to compensate for the slower reactivity have been observed only in a small number of cases. Rather, the most common evolutionary adaptation consists in the evolution of enzyme homologs endowed with increased catalytic efficiency, the k_{cat}/K_M ratio, either by an increase of k_{cat}—particularly for enzymes working at saturating concentrations of substrate—or by a decrease in K_M—particularly for enzymes working at sub-saturating concentrations of substrate. k_{cat} is almost invariably increased in cold-adapted enzymes, up to 10-fold. The trade-off between k_{cat} and K_M in cold-adapted enzymes has been comprehensively reviewed [68].

From a structural point of view, it is widely accepted that these kinetic parameters are associated with the increased flexibility of these enzymes [69,70]. This dynamics adaptation allows for the conformational rearrangements required for catalysis at low temperatures, making it possible for cold-adapted enzymes to maintain the same conformational space accessible to their mesophilic and thermophilic homologs at higher temperatures. Indeed, for the latter enzymes, the kinetic energy associated with low temperatures would be insufficient to overcome the kinetic barriers required for the conformational rearrangements associated with catalysis. The turnover number, or k_{cat}, is a good index of enzyme flexibility, as it reflects the rate of transition between all conformational states involved in the catalytic cycle.

Multiple structural features are usually associated with increased flexibility, involving both the active site and the peripheral regions. Commonly observed structural features are: Decreased core hydrophobicity, fewer prolyl residues in loops, increased hydrophobicity of the surface, more glycyl residues, lower arginyl/lysyl ratio, weaker interactions between subunits and domains, longer loops, decreased secondary-structure content, more prolyl residues in α-helices, fewer and weaker metal-binding sites, fewer disulfide bridges, fewer electrostatic interactions, reduced oligomerization and increase in conformational entropy of the unfolded state [71,72]. Many of these structural adaptations are summarized in Table 1. The crystal structures of 11 proteins isolated from the Antarctic marine oil-degrading bacterium *Oleispira antarctica* (α/β hydrolase, phosphodiesterase, transaldolase, isochorismatase, amidohydrolase, fumarylacetoacetate isomerase/hydrolase, 2-keto-3-deoxy-6-phosphogluconate aldolase, phoshonoacetaldehyde hydrolase, inorganic pyrophosphatase, and protein with unknown function) revealed that the most dominant structural feature is an increase in surface hydrophobicity and negative charge, with higher Glu+Asp/Arg+Lys ratio compared to their mesophilic counterparts [73].

Table 1. Structural adaptations in cold-adapted enzymes and their effects on protein structure.

Molecular Adaptation	Effect	Reference
Decreased number of hydrogen bonds and salt bridges	Increased flexibility	[69,72]
Reduced proline and arginine content	Increased molecular entropy	[23,74]
Increased surface charged residues	Increased conformational flexibility	[23]
Reduced frequency of surface, inter-domain and inter-subunit ionic linkages and ion-network	Increased conformational flexibility and reduced enthalphic contribution to stability	[75]
Reduced core hydrophobicity/increased surface hydrophobicity	Reduced hydrophobic effect/ entropic destabilization	[70]
Increased accessibility of active site	Increased flexibility for substrate and cofactor binding	[76]
Loop extensions	Reduced stability	[77]

Adapted from [22].

In other instances, however, a small number of specific residues was recognized as solely responsible for the cold adaptation of enzymes. In the β-galactosidase from the polyextremophilic Antarctic archaeon *Halorubrum lacusprofundi*, the mutation of only six amino-acid residues in comparison to its mesophilic homologs resulted in altered temperature activity profiles, suggesting that a small number of mutations can indeed account for cold adaptation [71]. In other proteins, a limited number of regions were associated to cold adaptation: the characterization of chimeric derivatives of monomeric isocitrate dehydrogenases of *Colwellia maris* and *Pseudomonas psychrophila*—cold adapted and mesophilic, respectively—led to the identification of two regions responsible for their different thermal properties [78]. The relative contribution of local and global protein flexibility in determining cold adaptation was assessed by performing molecular dynamics simulations on cytosolic malate dehydrogenases orthologous from marine mollusks adapted to different temperatures [79]. A convergent evolution trend was observed, with a significant negative correlation between the adaptation temperature of the organism and overall protein flexibility, with regions involved in ligand binding and catalysis showing the largest fluctuation differences [79].

Generally, the higher flexibility at low temperatures brings about low stability at higher temperatures. However, thermolability, although common [70], is not universal in cold-adapted enzymes. Three superoxide dismutases from the Antarctic psychrophilic ciliate *Euplotes focardii* were recently showed to exhibit a melting temperature of around 50–70 °C, suggesting a combination of cold adaptation and relative tolerance to high temperatures [80]. GroEL and thioredoxin from the Antarctic bacterium *Pseudoalteromonas haloplanktis* TAC125 were shown to be only marginally less stable than their *Escherichia coli* homologs [81].

It should also be highlighted that cold adaptation does not only consist in altered kinetic parameters of individual enzymes. For instance, sequencing and functional analysis of the genome the Antarctic marine oil-degrading bacterium *O. antarctica* revealed an array of alkane monooxygenases, osmoprotectants, siderophores and micronutrient-scavenging pathways [73] associated to cold adaptation.

3.3. Examples of Biotechnological Applications of Polar Enzymes

According to the type of catalyzed reaction, enzymes are classified into six main classes, i.e., oxidoreductases, transferases, hydrolases, lyases, isomerases and ligases, as reported in Table 2. The proposed biotechnological applications of cold-adapted enzymes belonging to several of these classes have been extensively reviewed [23,25,82–85].

Table 2. Polar-active enzymes isolated from Antarctic and Arctic marine polar environments.

Marine Polar-Active Enzymes	Reaction	Organism Source	Origin of Sample	Applications/Potential Uses	References
HYDROLASES: EC 3 (Type of reaction: Hydrolytic cleavage AB + $H_2O \rightarrow$ AOH + BH)					
β-galactosidase	Hydrolysis of lactose into its constituent monosaccharides	*Pseudoalteromonas* sp. 22b	Alimentary tract of Antarctic krill *Thyssanoessa macrura*	Candidates for lactose removal from dairy products at low temperatures	[86,87]
β-galactosidase		*Pseudoalteromonas haloplanktis* TAE 79	Antarctic seawater		[88]
β-galactosidase		*Pseudoalteromonas haloplanktis* LMG P-19143	Antarctic seawater		[89]
β-galactosidase		*Guehomyces pullulans*	Antarctic sea sediment		[90]
β-galactosidase		*Enterobacter ludwigii*	Sediment samples of Kongsfgord, Arctic		[91]
β-galactosidase		*Alkalilactibacillus ikkense*	Ikka columns in South-West Greenland		[92]
α-Amylase	Cleavage of α-1,4-glycosidic linkages in starch molecules to generate smaller polymers of glucose units	*Pseudoalteromonas* sp. M175	Antarctic sea-ice	Detergent additive for its stain removal efficiency	[93]
α-Amylase§		*Glaciozyma antarctica* PI12	Antarctic sea-ice	Additives in processed food, in detergents for cold washing, in waste-water treatment, in bioremediation in cold climates and in molecular biology applications	[94]
α-Amylase		Bacterial strains	Sediment samples from Midtre Lovènbreen Arctic glacier		[95]
α-Amylase		*Alteromonas* sp. TAC 240B	Antarctic seawater		[96]
α-Amylase		*Pseudoalteromonas haloplanktis* *	Antarctic seawater		[97,98]
Xylanase	Hydrolysis of the main chain of xylan to oligosaccharides, which in turn are degraded to xylose	*Cladosporium* sp.	Antarctic marine sponges	Additives in textile and food industries, and bioremediation	[99]
Xylanase		*Flavobacterium frigidarium* sp.	Antarctic shallow-water marine sediment		[100]

Table 2. *Cont.*

Marine Polar-Active Enzymes	Reaction	Organism Source	Origin of Sample	Applications/Potential Uses	References
HYDROLASES: EC 3 (Type of reaction: Hydrolytic cleavage AB + $H_2O \rightarrow$ AOH + BH)					
Serine protease (Subtilisin)	Cleavage of peptide bonds	*Bacillus* TA39	Antarctic seawater	Additives in low-temperature food processing, food and textile industries, leather processing, detergent industry	[101,102]
Serine protease (Subtilisin)		*Bacillus* TA41	Antarctic seawater		[101,103]
Serine protease		*Colwellia* sp. NJ341	Antarctic sea-ice		[104]
Serine alkaline protease		*Shewanella* sp. Ac10u	Antarctic seawater		[105]
Acid protease		*Rhodotorula mucilaginosa* L7	Antarctic marine alga		[106]
Subtilisin-like serine protease		*Pseudoalteromonas* sp., *Marinobacter* sp., *Psychrobacter* sp., *Polaribacter* sp.	Antarctic seawater and thorax, abdomen and head of krill (*Euphausia superba* Dana)		[107]
Protease		*Pseudoalteromonas* sp. NJ276	Antarctic sea-ice		[108]
Subtilisin-like Serine proteinase		*Leucosporidium antarcticum* 171	Antarctic sub-glacial waters		[109]
Aminopeptidase		*Pseudoalteromonas haloplanktis* TAC125	Antarctic seawater		[110]
Aminopeptidase		*Colwellia psychrerythraea* 34H	Greenland continental shelf sediment samples		[111,112]
Serine peptidase		*Lysobacter* sp. A03	Penguin feathers in Antarctica		[113]
Serine peptidase		*Serratia* sp.	Coastal seawater in Northern Norway		[114]
Metalloprotease		*Pseudoalteromonas* sp. SM495	Arctic sea-ice (Canadian Basin)		[115]
Metalloprotease		*Sphingomonas paucimobilis*	Stomach of Antarctic krill, *Euphausia superba* Dana		[116]
Metalloprotease		*Psychrobacter proteolyticus* sp.	Stomach of Antarctic krill *Euphausia superba* Dana		[117]
Endopeptidase		Microbial source	Arctic marine microbial source	Candidate for molecular biology application: digestion of chromatin (ArcticZymes)	[118]

Table 2. *Cont.*

Marine Polar-Active Enzymes	Reaction	Organism Source	Origin of Sample	Applications/Potential Uses	References
HYDROLASES: EC 3 (Type of reaction: Hydrolytic cleavage AB + $H_2O \rightarrow$ AOH + BH)					
Lipase	Hydrolysis of long-chain triacylglycerol substances with the formation of an alcohol and a carboxylic acid	*Bacillus pumilus* ArcL5	Arctic seawater (Chukchi Sea)	Detergent additives used at low temperatures and biocatalysts for the biotransformation of heat-labile compounds	[119]
Lipase		*Pseudoalteromonas haloplanktis* TAC125	Antarctic seawater		[120]
Lipase		*Colwellia psychrerythraea* 34H	Arctic seawater		[121]
Lipase		*Polaromonas vacuolata*	Antarctic seawater		[122]
Lipase		*Psychrobacter* sp.	Antarctic seawater		[123,124]
Lipase		*Shewanella frigidimarina*	Antarctic seawater		[125]
Lipase		Bacterial strains	Arctic sediment samples from the snout of Midtre Lovènbreen glacier up to the convergence point with the sea		[95]
Lipase		*Psychrobacter* sp. TA144 **	Antarctic seawater		[126]
Lipase		*Psychrobacter* sp. 7195	Antarctic deep-sea sediment (Prydz Bay)		[127]
Lipase		*Moritella* sp. 2-5-10-1	Antarctic deep-sea water		[128]
Lipase		*Pseudoalteromonas* sp., *Psychrobacter* sp., *Vibrio* sp.	Antarctic seawater samples (Ross Sea)		[129]
Phytase	Hydrolysis of phytate to phosphorylated myo-inositol derivatives	*Rhodotorula mucilaginosa* JMUY14	Antarctic deep-sea sediment	Candidate for feed applications, especially in aquaculture	[130]
Esterase	Hydrolysis of simple esters, usually only triglycerides composed of fatty acids shorter than C 8	*Pseudoalteromonas arctica*	Arctic sea-ice from Spitzbergen, Norway	Additives in laundry detergents and biocatalysts for the biotransformation of labile compounds at low temperatures	[131]
Esterase		*Thalassospira* sp.	Arctic sea fan (*Paramuricea placomus*), Vestfjorden area (Northern Norway)		[132]
Esterase		*Oleispira antarctica*	Antarctic coastal waters		[73,133]
Esterase		*Pseudoalteromas haloplanktis* TAC125	Antarctic seawater		[134,135]
Esterase		*Pseudoalteromas* sp. 643A	Alimentary tract of Antarctic krill *Euphasia superba* Dana		[136]
Esterase		Marine Arctic metagenomics libraries	Arctic seawater and sediment from Barents Sea and Svalbard	Candidate for organic synthesis reactions and cheese ripening processes	[137,138]

Table 2. *Cont.*

Marine Polar-Active Enzymes	Reaction	Organism Source	Origin of Sample	Applications/Potential Uses	References
HYDROLASES: EC 3 (Type of reaction: Hydrolytic cleavage AB + $H_2O \rightarrow$ AOH + BH)					
Epoxide hydrolase	Hydrolysis of an epoxide to its corresponding vicinal diol with the addition of a water molecule to the oxirane ring	*Sphingophyxis alaskensis*	Arctic seawater	Candidate for the production of enantiopure epoxides in the pharmaceutical industry	[139]
S-formylglutathione hydrolase	Hydrolysis of S-formylglutathione to formic acid and glutathione	*Pseudoalteromonas haloplanktis* TAC125	Antarctic seawater	Candidates for chemical synthesis and industrial pharmaceutics	[140]
S-formylglutathione hydrolase		*Shewanella frigidimarina*	Antarctic marine environment		[141]
Polygalacturonase (pectin depolymerase)	Cleavage of glycosidic bonds between galacturonic acid residues	*Pseudoalteromonas haloplanktis*	Antarctic seawater	Additive in food industries, such as clarification of juice, in the process of vinification, yield and color enhancement and in the mashing of fruits	[142]
Pullulanase	Hydrolysis of α-1,6-glycosidic bonds in pullulan to produce maltotriose	*Shewanella arctica*	Seawater samples in Spitsbergen, Norway	Additive in food and biofuel industries	[143]
Invertase	Hydrolysis of the terminal non-reducing β-fructofuranoside residue in sucrose, raffinose and related β-D-fructofuranosides	*Leucosporidium antarcticum*	Antarctic seawater	Not defined (ND)	[144]
α-glucosidase	Hydrolysis of the non-reducing terminal α-glucopyranoside residues from various α-glucosides and related compounds	*Leucosporidium antarcticum*	Antarctic seawater	Additive in detergent and food industries	[144]
Cellulase	Hydrolysis of the β-1,4-D-glycosidic linkages in cellulose	*Pseudoalteromonas haloplanktis*	Antarctic seawater	Additive in detergent industry	[145]
Chitobiase	Hydrolysis of chitobiose to N-acetylglucosamine	*Arthrobacter* sp. TAD20	Antarctic sea sediments	ND	[146]

Table 2. *Cont.*

Marine Polar-Active Enzymes	Reaction	Organism Source	Origin of Sample	Applications/Potential Uses	References
HYDROLASES: EC 3 (Type of reaction: Hydrolytic cleavage AB + $H_2O \rightarrow$ AOH + BH)					
Alkaline phosphatase	Hydrolysis and transphosphorylation of a wide variety of phosphate monoesters	TAB5 strain	Antarctica^	Candidate for molecular biology application: dephosphorylation of DNA (New England Biolabs)	[147–149]
Alkaline phosphatase		*Shewanella* sp.	Intestine of Antarctic shellfish	Candidate for molecular biology application	[150]
Pyrophosphatase	Catalysis of the conversion of one ion of pyrophosphate to two phosphate ions	*Oleispira antarctica*	Antarctic deep sea	ND	[73]
Glycerophosphodiesterase	Catalysis of the hydrolysis of a glycerophosphodiester	*Oleispira antarctica*	Antarctic deep sea	ND	[73]
Endonuclease (Cryonase)	Cleavage of the phosphodiester bond the middle of a polynucleotide chain	*Shewanella* sp. Ac10	Antarctic seawater	Candidate for molecular biology application: digestion of all types of DNA and RNA at cold temperatures (Takara-Clontech)	[151]
Exonuclease	Cleavage of the phosphodiester bond at either the 3′ or the 5′ end	Arctic marine bacterium	Arctic marine microbial source	Candidate for molecular biology application: 3′-5′ exonuclease specific for single stranded DNA (ArcticZymes)	[152]
Ribonuclease	Hydrolysis of the phosphodiester bonds among the nucleic acid residues of RNA	*Psychrobacter* sp. ANT206	Antarctic sea-ice	Candidate for molecular biology applications	[153]
Uracil-DNA glycosylase	Hydrolysis of the N-glycosidic bond from deoxyuridine to release uracil	Antarctic marine bacterium	Antarctic marine microbial source	Candidate for molecular biology application: release of free uracil from uracil-containing single-stranded or double-stranded DNA (New England Biolabs)	[154]

Table 2. *Cont.*

Marine Polar-Active Enzymes	Reaction	Organism Source	Origin of Sample	Applications/Potential Uses	References
OXIDOREDUCTASES: EC 1 (Type of reaction: Transfer of hydrogen or oxygen or electrons between molecules AH + B → A + BH; A + O → AO; A⁻+B→A+B⁻)					
Phenylalanine hydroxylase	Catalysis of the hydroxylation of L-Phe to form tyrosine	*Colwellia psychrerythraea* 34H	Arctic marine sediments	ND	[76]
Alcohol dehydrogenase	Catalysis of the interconversion of alcohols to their corresponding carbonyl compounds	*Moraxella* sp. TAE123	Antarctic seawater	Candidate for asymmetric synthesis	[155]
Alanine dehydrogenase	Catalysis of reversible deamination of L-alanine to pyruvate	*Shewanella* sp. Ac10u, *Carnobacterium* sp. St2	Antarctic seawater	Candidate for enantioselective production of optically active amino acids	[156]
Leucine dehydrogenase	Catalysis of reversible L-leucine and other branched chain L-amino acids deamination reaction to the corresponding α-keto acid	*Pseudoalteromonas* sp. ANT178	Antarctic sea-ice	Candidate for medical and pharmaceutical industry applications	[157]
Malate dehydrogenase	Catalysis of reversible oxidation of malate to oxalacetate	*Flavobacterium frigidimaris* KUC-1	Antarctic seawater	Candidate for detection and production of malate under cold conditions	[158]
Isocitrate dehydrogenase	Catalysis of decarboxylation of isocitrate to α-ketoglutarate and CO_2	*Desulfotalea psychrophila*	Arctic marine sediments	ND	[159]
L-threonine dehydrogenase	Catalysis of dehydrogenation at the β-carbon (C3) position of L-threonine	*Flavobacterium frigidimaris* KUC-1 ***	Antarctic seawater	ND	[160]
Superoxide dismutase	Catalysis of the dismutation of superoxide anion radicals into molecular oxygen and hydrogen peroxide	*Pseudoalteromonas haloplanktis*	Antarctic seawater	Candidates for applications in agriculture, cosmetics, food, healthcare products and medicines	[161]
Superoxide dismutase		*Marinomonas* sp. NJ522	Antarctic sea-ice		[162]
Superoxide dismutase		*Pseudoalteromonas* sp. ANT506	Antarctic sea-ice		[163]
Superoxide dismutase		*Psychromonas arctica*	Arctic sea-ice and sea-water samples		[164]
Superoxide dismutase		*Rhodotorula mucilaginosa* AN5	Antarctic sea-ice		[165]

Table 2. *Cont.*

Marine Polar-Active Enzymes	Reaction	Organism Source	Origin of Sample	Applications/Potential Uses	References
OXIDOREDUCTASES: EC 1 (Type of reaction: Transfer of hydrogen or oxygen or electrons between molecules $AH + B \rightarrow A + BH$; $A + O \rightarrow AO$; $A^- + B \rightarrow A + B^-$)					
Catalase	Catalysis of degradation of hydrogen peroxide into water and molecular oxygen	*Bacillus* sp. N2a	Antarctic seawater	Candidate for textile and cosmetic industries	[166,167]
Glutathione reductase	Catalysis of the reduction of oxidized glutathione to produce reduced glutathione	*Colwellia psychrerythraea*	Antarctic seawater	Candidate as an antioxidant enzyme in heterologous systems	[168]
Glutathione peroxidase	Catalysis of the reduction of hydrogen peroxide and other organic peroxides	*Pseudoalteromonas* sp. ANT506	Antarctic sea-ice	ND	[169]
Thioredoxin reductase	Catalysis of the reduction of thioredoxin	*Pseudoalteromonas haloplanktis* TAC125	Antarctic seawater	ND	[170]
Glutaredoxin	Catalysis of the reduction of protein disulfides in glutathione-dependent reactions	*Pseudoalteromonas* sp. AN178	Antarctic sea-ice	ND	[171]
Peroxiredoxin	Catalysis of the reduction of hydrogen peroxide, peroxynitrite and a wide range of organic hydroperoxides	*Psychrobacter* sp. ANT206	Antarctic sea-ice	Candidate for food and pharmaceutical industries	[172]
Dihydroorotate oxidase	Catalysis of the stereospecific oxidation of (S)-dihydroorotate to orotate	*Oleispira antarctica*	Antarctic deep sea	ND	[73]

Table 2. *Cont.*

Marine Polar-Active Enzymes	Reaction	Organism Source	Origin of Sample	Applications/Potential Uses	References
TRANSFERASES: EC 2 (Type of reaction: Transfer of groups of atoms AB + C → A + BC)					
Aspartate aminotransferase	Catalysis of transamination reaction of L-aspartate and α-ketoglutarate into the corresponding oxaloacetate and L-glutamate	*Pseudoalteromonas haloplanktis* TAC125 ****	Antarctic seawater	ND	[173]
Glutathione S-transferase	Catalysis of conjugation of reduced glutathione with various electrophilic compounds and ROS	*Pseudoalteromonas* sp. ANT506	Antarctic sea-ice	ND	[174]
Hydroxymethyl-transferase	Catalysis of reversible conversion of L-serine and tetrahydropteroylglutamate to glycine and 5,10-methylenetetrahydropteroylglutamate. Cleavage of many 3-hydroxyamino acids and decarboxylation of aminomalonate	*Psychromonas ingrahamii*	Arctic polar sea-ice	Candidate as a pharmaceutical, agrochemicals and food additive	[175]
LIGASES: EC 6 (Type of reaction: Covalent joining of two molecules coupled with the hydrolysis of an energy rich bond in ATP or similar triphosphates A + B+ ATP → AB + ADP + Pi)					
Glutathione synthetase	Catalysis of formation of glutathione from L-γ-glutamylcysteine and glycine	*Pseudoalteromonas haloplanktis*	Antarctic seawater	ND	[176]
DNA ligase	Catalysis of the formation of a phosphodiester bond between adjacent 5′-phosphoryl and 3′-hydroxyl groups in double stranded DNA	*P. haloplanktis* TAE 72	Antarctic seawater	Candidate for applications in molecular biology	[177]

Table 2. *Cont.*

Marine Polar-Active Enzymes	Reaction	Organism Source	Origin of Sample	Applications/Potential Uses	References
LYASES: EC 4 (Type of reaction: Cleavage of C-C, C-O, C-S, C-N or other bonds by other means than by hydrolysis or oxidation RCOCOOH → RCOH + CO_2)					
γ-carbonic anhydrase	Catalysis of CO_2 hydration to bicarbonate and protons	*Colwellia psychrerythraea*	Antarctic cold ice sediments	Candidates for biomedical applications	[178]
γ-carbonic anhydrase		*Pseudoalteromonas haloplanktis*	Antarctic seawater		[179,180]
Pectate lyase	Cleavage of the α-1,4 glycosidic bonds of polygalacturonic acid into simple sugars	*Pseudoalteromonas haloplanktis* ANT/505	Antarctic sea-ice	Candidate for detergent industry	[167,181]
Acid decarboxylase	Catalysis of decarboxylation of 3-octaprenyl-4-hydroxybenzoate to produce 2-polyprenylphenol	*Colwellia psychrerythraea* 34H	Arctic marine sediments	ND	[182,183]
ISOMERASES: EC 5 (Type of reaction: Transfer of group from one position to another within one molecule AB → BA)					
Sedoheptulose 7-phosphate isomerase	Catalysis of the conversion of sedoheptulose 7-phosphate to D-glycero-D-mannoheptose 7-phosphate	*Colwellia psychrerythraea 34H*	Arctic marine sediments	Candidate for biocatalysis under low water conditions	[184]
Triose phosphate isomerase§	Catalysis of the isomerization of dihydroxyacetone phosphate to D-glyceraldehyde 3-phosphate	*Pseudomonas* sp. π9	Antarctic sea-ice		[185]
Triose phosphate isomerase		*Moraxella* sp. TA137	Intestine of Antarctic fish		[186]

* previously known as *Alteromonas haloplanktis* [187], ** previously known as *Moraxella* TA144 [188], *** formerly known as *Cytophaga sp.* KUC-1 [189], **** formerly known as *Moraxella* TAC 125 [190]. ^it was isolated from Dumont d'Urville Antarctic Station but it was not possible to ascertain the marine origin. § only characterization of genes.

Currently, approximately 65% of more than 3000 enzymes with an industrial application are hydrolases, used in the detergent, textile, paper, and food industries [167,191]. Hydrolases, classified as Class 3 (EC 3) by the Nomenclature Committee of the International Union of Biochemistry and Molecular Biology (NC-IUBMB), catalyze the hydrolysis of chemical bonds. Herein, we focus on some recent examples of cold-adapted enzymes, particularly hydrolases, isolated from marine polar microorganisms. More examples of microbial enzymes isolated in Arctic or Antarctic marine polar regions are reported in Table 2. To our knowledge, this is the first table including only cold-active enzymes isolated from marine polar microorganisms. Indeed, several recent reviews do not distinguish between polar and non-polar enzymes or between marine and non-marine origin. The latter distinction is crucial to guide bioprospecting in search for novel activities.

3.3.1. Glycoside Hydrolases

Glycoside hydrolases (GH; EC 3.2.1.), or glycosidases, hydrolyse the glycosidic bond between two or more carbohydrates, or between a carbohydrate and a non-carbohydrate moiety (Scheme 1a), overall processing a wide variety of complex substrates [192]. They are extremely common in nature, with more than 100 GH families currently recognized and grouped in the Carbohydrate-Active Enzymes database (CAZy), which provides a continuously updated list of families [193]. Their function ranges from the degradation of complex carbohydrates for their metabolic use (cellulases, amylases), to the defense against pathogens (lysozyme, chitosanase), to the synthesis of the oligosaccharide groups of glycoproteins. Their biotechnological applications are manifold, especially in the food processing industry, where enzyme activity at low temperatures is desirable to slow down spoilage and loss of nutrients. For this reason, cold-adapted hydrolases are usually in need [194].

Lactases or β-galactosidases (EC 3.2.1.23) (Scheme 1b) offer a clear example in this respect: with more than 70% of the world population suffering from lactose intolerance, the enzymatic removal of lactose from milk and dairy products using β-galactosidases is now common. The enzyme catalysing the hydrolysis of lactose into its constituent monosaccharides, glucose, and galactose, has drawn the interest of many research groups and enterprizes due to nutritional (lactose intolerance) and technological (crystallization), challenges associated with lactose [195]. The isolation of several cold-adapted β-galactosidases has been reported. Among them, some are from Antarctic organisms, e.g., *H. lacusprofundi*, isolated from the hypersaline Deep Lake [71,196], *Arthrobacter* species from soil samples [197,198], and marine *Pseudoalteromonas* species [86–88,199]. Other enzymes were isolated from marine organisms from the Arctic region, including those from *Enterobacter ludwigii* [91] and *Alkalilactibacillus ikkense* [92]. A cold-active β-galactosidase from the Antarctic marine bacterium *P. haloplanktis* TAE 79 was applied to lactose hydrolysis at low temperatures during milk storage [88] and was proposed for the production of tagatose, a natural monosaccharide with low caloric value and glycemic index [200]. A cold-active lactase isolated from the Antarctic marine *P. haloplanktis* LMG P-19143 was patented [89] and is also produced in large quantities by Nutrilab NV (Bekkevoort, Belgium). Yeasts are important sources for β-galactosidase production. *Guehomyces pullulans* 17-1, isolated from the Antarctic sea sediment, synthesize both extracellular and cell-bound β-galactosidases [90]. A 1,3-α-3,6-anhydro-L-galactosidase—an enzyme involved in the final steps of the agarolytic pathway and used in the industrial processing of agar—was identified in the agarolytic marine bacterium *Gayadomonas joobiniege* G7 and was shown to be active between 7.0 and 15 C [201].

Amylases (Scheme 1c) are also interesting enzymes for industrial processes, in detergent formulations and in food industry for beer and wine fermentation and for the preparation of bread and fruit juice. They hydrolyse starch to maltose, maltotriose, glucose monomers and limit dextrins. They can be classified in exoamylases (β-amylase EC 3.2.1.2; glucoamylase, EC 3.2.1.3; α-glucosidase, EC 3.2.1.20) endoamylases (α-amylase, EC 3.2.1.1) and debranching (pullulanases, EC 3.2.1.41; isoamylases, EC 3.2.1.68; dextrinases, EC 3.2.1.142) according to the specificity of the hydrolysis reaction they catalyze [194]. In the detergent industry, cold-active amylases not isolated from polar regions are already available on the market [167], i.e., Stainzyme® (active at temperatures between 30 and 70 °C) and Stainzyme® Plus (active below 20 °C) released by Novozymes and Preferenz™ S100 (active at 16 °C) released by DuPont Industrial Biosciences. In the textile industry, Genencor-DuPont developed Optisize® COOL, using a cold-active amylase for the desizing of woven fabrics at low temperatures. Other cold-active, detergent-stable α-amylases, not isolated from polar regions, were identified from *Bacillus cereus* GA6 [202] and from the marine bacterium *Zunongwangia profunda* [203]. The latter was isolated from surface seawater in the costal area of Fujian, China, but shows a cold-adapted and salt-tolerant α-amylase activity. An α-amylase produced by the psychrophilic yeast *Glaciozyma antarctica* PI12 was recently characterized [94].

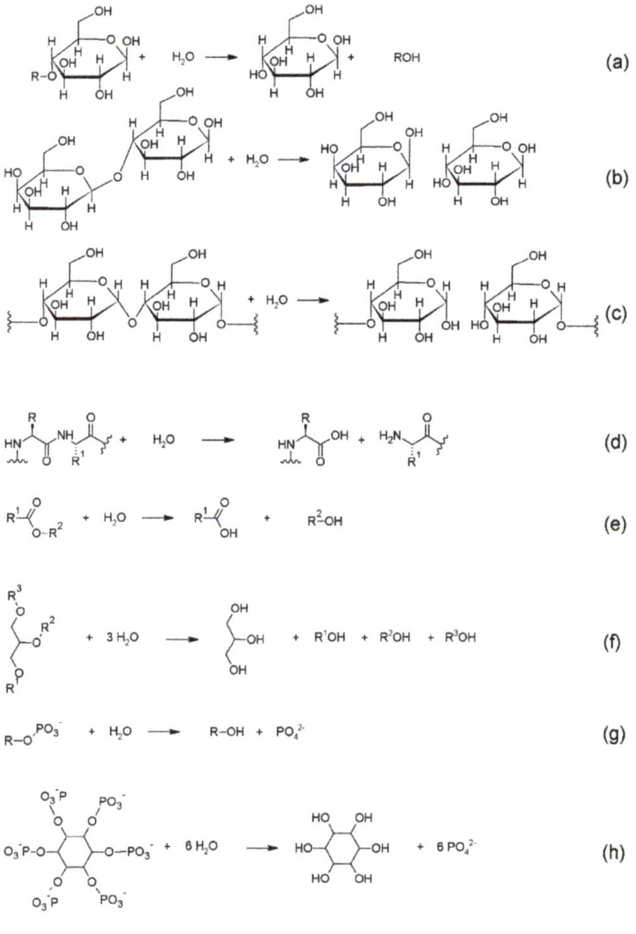

Scheme 1. Principal enzymatic activities of cold-adapted enzymes investigated for biotechnological applications. (**a**) Generic reaction catalyzed by glycoside hydrolases, with a glucose derivative as substrate. (**b**) Reaction catalyzed by lactases, with conversion of lactose to galactose and glucose. (**c**) Reaction catalyzed by amylases on glucose polymers, with glucose or maltooligosaccharides as final products. (**d**) Generic reaction catalyzed by proteases, which catalyze the hydrolysis of peptide bonds of proteins or peptides. (**e**) Generic reaction catalyzed by esterases, which hydrolyse ester bonds. (**f**) Reaction catalyzed by lipases, with the hydrolysis of fatty acids from acyl glycerol. In this case, the full hydrolysis of a triglyceride to glycerol is represented. (**g**) Generic reaction catalyzed by phosphatases with the hydrolysis of phosphate monoesters. (**h**) Reaction catalyzed by phytases. In this case, the full hydrolysis to phosphate ions and inositol is represented.

Cold-adapted enzymes from marine polar regions could successfully be employed in these applications, and some of them are already under investigation or in use. A cold-adapted α-amylases from the Antarctic sea-ice bacterium *Pseudoalteromonas* sp. M175 exhibited resistance towards all the tested commercial detergents and was shown to improve their stain removal efficiency [93]. Heat-labile α-amylases displaying high activity at low temperature isolated from bacteria of Antarctic seawater were structurally studied [96,97].

Pullulanases (EC 3.2.1.41), debranching enzymes that hydrolyse α-1,6-and α-1,4-linkages in pullulan, starch, amylopectin and various related oligosaccharides are interesting enzymes in starch processing. There are different pullulanase groups according to their substrate specificities and reaction products. Pul13A is a type-I pullulanase isolated from Arctic seawater strain *Shewanella arctica* in Spitsbergen, Norway. It is able to hydrolase α-1,6-glycosidic bonds in pullulan to produce maltotriose at low temperature, displaying low thermostability at elevated temperatures. It represents a potential candidate for industrial applications such as starch degradation for ethanol-based biofuel production [143].

Although poorly studied, cold-active xylanases (EC 3.2.1.8) are also interesting in the food industry for bread making, as they convert the insoluble hemicellulose of dough into soluble sugars, thus yielding soft and elastic bread. Three cold-adapted xylanases from psychrophilic bacteria were shown to improve dough properties and bread volume with respect to mesophilic orthologues [204]. The xylanase pXyl from *P. haloplanktis,* isolated from soil samples [205], was very efficient in improving the dough properties and bread volume due to its high activity at low temperature [205]. The psychrophilic enzyme is now sold by Puratos (Grand-Bigard, Belgium). Antarctic marine fungi from marine sponges, which are the dominant macroinvertebrates in many benthic communities, are considered new and promising sources of cold-active xylanases. *Cladosporium* sp. isolated from marine sponges collected in King George Island, Antarctica, showed high xylanase activity at low temperature and very low thermal stability [99]. Also *Flavobacterium frigidarium* sp. nov., an aerobic psychrophilic and halotolerant bacterium isolated from marine sediment of shallow waters surrounding Adelaide Island in Antarctica, exhibited xylanolytic activity [100].

Cellulases, used in detergents for color and brightness care, have been classified according to their activity into endo- (EC 3.2.1.4) and exo-cellulases with exo-β-1,4-glucan cellobiohydrolase (EC 3.2.1.91) and β-glucosidase (EC 3.2.1.21). *P. haloplanktis* is able to convert the cellulose into an immediate nutritive compound for plants by hydrolysis. *P. haloplanktis* secretes a multi-modular endocellulase composed N-terminal catalytic module, a linker region and the cellulose-binding module. Structural adaptations to cellulose hydrolysis at low temperatures have been identified in the catalytic module and unusually long linker region by using both X-ray diffraction and small angle X-ray scattering methods [145].

Leucosporidium antarcticum strain 171, widespread in the cold marine waters below the Antarctic ice, was isolated from a seawater sample collected at a depth of 100 m in Admiralty Bay, King George Island. The yeast was found to produce cold-adapted invertases (β-D-fructofuranoside fructohydrolases, EC 3.2.1.26) and glucosidases (α-D-glucoside glucohydrolases, EC 3.2.1.20). Their synthesis may facilitate assimilation of β-fructofuranosides and α-glucopyranosides in cold environments where nutrient availability is fluctuating [144].

Chitin, one of the most abundant organic compounds in nature, is a structural polysaccharide composed of N-acetylglucosamine (GlcNAc) residues. Chitobiases (EC 3.2.1.29) found in bacteria, fungi, and eukaryotes, hydrolyse chitobiose to GlcNAc, which is further converted to glucosamine by a deacetylase. A cell-bound chitobiase was isolated from the marine psychrophile *Arthrobacter* sp. TAD20 collected along the Antarctic ice. The cold-adapted chitobiase overexpressed in *E. coli* displayed four functionally independent domains: (i) The catalytic domain, (ii) the galactose-binding domain, and (iii) the immunoglobulin-like domain followed by (iv) the cell-wall anchorage signal. The enzyme exhibited features that are typical of cold-adapted enzymes, with unusually low-K_m and high-k_{cat} values, with improved flexibility around the active site for efficient activity at low temperatures [146].

3.3.2. Proteases

Proteases (EC 3.4) catalyze the hydrolysis of peptide bonds (Scheme 1d). This catalytic activity has evolved multiple times, yielding enzymes with different catalytic mechanisms [206]. These enzymes are classified as exo-peptidases (EC 3.4.11-19), when they cleave the terminal amino acid, and as endo-peptidases (EC 3.4.21-99), when the peptide bonds they hydrolysed is internal. Proteases have several industrial applications, particularly in the food industry and as components of laundry detergents [207,208]. Both thermophilic [209] and cold-adapted homologs [210] are of biotechnological interest, depending on the intended working temperature of the process. To obtain cold-active proteases, two approaches have been pursed: mutagenesis of mesophilic enzymes or identification and expression of naturally occurring psychrophilic proteases. The former approach was applied to subtilisins from *Bacillus* species, mutated to increase their activity at low temperature. Particularly, the subtilisin savinase from *Bacillus* was mutated to produce a thermostable variant with increased activity at low temperature [211]. The latter approach has also been investigated.

Commercially exploited cold-adapted proteases include a protease from *Bacillus amyloliquefaciens*—a non-polar soil bacterium—commercialized as Purafect Prime L^{TM}, which is active at 20 °C, and the protease Properase^{TM} from *B. alcalophilus*, which combines activity at high pH and low temperature and Excellase^{TM}. They are commercialized by Genencor (Genencor International Inc., Palo Alto, CA, USA). A cold-adapted extracellular aspartic protease was isolated from the yeast *Sporobolomyces roseus* isolated from an underground water sample drawn from the disused silver and lead mine "Luiza" (Zabrze, Poland) and was proposed as biocatalyst in the food industry, particularly in cheese and soy-sauce production, meat tenderization, and as bread additive [212]. It was also proposed in the production of antioxidant peptides from dairy and animal proteins, as hydrolysis of beef casein by this enzyme yielded peptides endowed with antioxidant activity [212].

Bioprospecting of cold-adapted bacteria from the polar regions could further increase the variety of cold-active proteases for industrial use. Several recent examples of such enzymes have been reported. Particularly, Antarctic fungi capable of producing proteases have been recently reviewed [85]. Two cold-adapted subtilisins from Antarctic marine *Bacillus* TA39 [102] and TA41 [103] showed high activity at low temperatures but also limited stability. A mutant with unaltered activity at low temperatures but higher stability was obtained through directed evolution [101]. A subtilisin-like cold-adapted serine peptidase was isolated from the Antarctic bacterium *Lysobacter* sp. A03, and is both active at low temperatures and resistant to higher temperatures [113].

A protease from the Antarctic bacterium *Janthinobacterium lividum* obtained from the Polar BioCenter (Korea Polar Research Institute) [213], recombinantly expressed and purified, was reported. Among the fungal proteases identified from polar marine samples, the extracellular subtilase lap2, from the Antarctic yeast *Leucosporidium antarcticum* 171, exhibited a low optimal temperature (25 °C) poor thermal stability, and high catalytic efficiency in the temperature range 0–25 °C [109].

The extracellular protease released by *Rhodotorula mucilaginosa* L7 strain was isolated from an Antarctic marine alga and was shown to be stable in the presence of high concentrations of NaCl [106]. A new cold-adapted protease with a potential biotechnological application, largely represented amongst Antarctic bacterial genus (*Pseudoalteromonas* sp., *Marinobacter* sp., *Psychrobacter* sp., *Polaribacter* sp.), exhibits a higher catalytic efficiency at lower temperatures compared to its mesophilic counterpart [107]. The extracellular cold-active protease from the marine psychrophilic bacterium *Pseudoalteromonas* sp. NJ276, for its catalytic activity and broad substrate specificities, has a potential application in low-temperature food processing, in particular in the preservation of milk at low temperature [108]. A secreted a cold-active serine protease identified in *Colwellia* sp. NJ341, isolated from Antarctic sea-ice, showing a 30% of activity at 0 °C and a better thermostability than other cold-active proteases, represents a good candidate for industrial applications, particularly in processes where there may be a risk of microbial contamination or a temperature instability of reactants or products [104].

An aminopeptidase produced by the marine psychrophile *Colwellia psychrerythraea* strain 34H was structurally investigated, displaying structural features (fewer proline residues, fewer ion pairs, and lower hydrophobic residue content) related to the cold adaptation and able to increase the flexibility for activity in the cold [111].

Besides their industrial applications, proteases have also long been used for therapeutic applications, particularly in the treatment of cardiovascular diseases, sepsis, digestive disorders, inflammation, cystic fibrosis, retinal disorders, and psoriasis [214]. The proteases so far approved by the US FDA derive from mesophilic organisms. However, the cold-adapted ones are endowed with a higher catalytic efficiency [215] and might, therefore, be of great interest. Indeed, they evolved to be efficient at low temperatures and, if thermostable enough, they would further increase their reaction rates at 37 °C, the intended temperatures for therapeutic applications. To overcome their thermal instability, mutational studies have been conducted [83].

As for general applications in molecular biology, proteinase, an endopeptidase from an Arctic marine microbial source, was developed by ArcticZymes [118] for the digestion of chromatin, thus releasing naked DNA. As it is thermolable, it can be inactivated at temperatures compatible with RNA integrity and DNA as double strands.

3.3.3. Lipases and Esterases

Esterases (EC 3.1.1) hydrolyse ester bonds (Scheme 1e). Lipases in particular (EC 3.1.1.3) are glycerol-ester hydrolases that catalyze the hydrolysis of triglycerides to fatty acids and glycerol (Scheme 1f). They are widely used in organic synthesis and as laundry detergents [216]. Although thermophilic homologs might appear more promising for industrial applications for their higher stability under harsh conditions, cold-adapted homologs are also actively investigated for their high activity at low temperatures [217]. Moreover, lipases are promising tools for the preparation of chiral molecules in the pharmaceutical industry, where low working temperatures are desirable to reduce the rate of non-catalytic side reactions. Particularly, the predictable enantiopreference of lipases allows the determination of the absolute configuration of secondary alcohols using the lipase-catalyzed kinetic resolution and the use of cold-active lipases in organic solvents is excellent for the preparation of single-isomer chiral drugs, and the enantioselective or regioselective preparation of alcohol and amine intermediates in the synthesis of pharmaceuticals [218].

There are already examples of lipases identified in organisms isolated from the polar regions which are currently on the market. Lipozyme® CALB is a non-specific lipase from *Candida antarctica* which was successfully used in the resolution of racemic alcohols, amines, and acids, and in the preparation of optically active compounds from meso substrates, as well as for the regio-selective catalysis in the selective acylation of different carbohydrates [219]. Lipases from *C. antarctica* catalyze hydrolysis on several substrates and are thermostable, a surprising property considering their origin. CALB is currently commercialized by Novozyme (Bagsværd, Denmark). The lipase from *C. antarctica* is also available in an immobilized form and commercialized as Novozym 435 (Novozyme, Bagsværd, Denmark).

More cold-adapted lipases were recently discovered in Arctic and Antarctic microorganisms. A lipase from the psychrotolerant yeast *Rhodotorula* sp. Y-23 isolated in the Nella Lake, East Antarctica, exhibited the highest V_{max} at 15 °C and high compatibility with commercial detergents, which brought about an increase in activity, making it a potential candidate in detergent formulation active at low temperatures [220]. The Gram-positive psychrotrophic Arctic bacterium *Arthrobacter gangotriensis*, obtained from an soil sample, was recently shown to exhibit lipolytic activity associated with a lipase that can work in a wide pH range and that exhibits good stability [221]. The bacterium *Bacillus pumilus* ArcL5 with lipolytic activity was isolated from the Chukchi Sea within the Arctic Ocean; the lipase BpL5, was recombinantly expressed in *E. coli* and was shown to retain 85% of its activity at 5 °C. Two mutants active against tricaprylin were also characterized [119].

Other lipases were identified in Antarctic soils [222]. The lipase LipG7 from the Antarctic filamentous fungus *Geomyces* sp. P7 was unusually thermostable and was proposed as an enantioselective biocatalyst [223].

Other cold-active lipases were identified in the Antarctic marine *P. haloplanktis* TAC125 [120], in the Arctic marine bacterium *C. psychrerythraea* 34H [121], *Psychrobacter* sp. of Antarctic marine origin [123,124,126] and Antarctic deep-sea water strain *Moritella* sp.2-5-10-1 [127,128].

Esterases (EC 3.1.1.1), hydrolases that catalyze the cleavage of simple esters such as triglycerides with short chains of fatty acids (less than eight carbon atoms) (Scheme 1e) [194], are interesting enzymes in organic synthesis and cheese ripening processes [137]. Cold-adapted esterases were identified in Arctic marine bacteria *Pseudoalteromonas arctica*, [131] and *Thalassospira* sp. [132] and the Antarctic marine bacteria *O. antarctica* [133] and *P. haloplanktis* TAC125 [134,135]. Moreover, a cold-adapted esterase was identified from *Pseudoalteromonas* sp. strain 643A, isolated from the alimentary tract of Antarctic krill *Euphasia superba* Dana. It displayed 20–50% of maximum activity at 0–20 °C, and the optimal temperature was close to 35 °C. The optimal pH for enzyme activity was around 8.0; however, it was stable between pH 9 and 11.5 [136].

3.3.4. Phosphatases

Alkaline phosphatases (EC 3.1.3.1), which catalyze the hydrolysis of phosphate monoesters (Scheme 1g), have an important application in molecular biology for the dephosphorylation of DNA linearized at the 5′ end to avoid its re-circularization during cloning processes. A recombinant alkaline phosphatase isolated from the Antarctic bacterial strain TAB5 [147,148] was developed by New England Biolabs [149]. The crystal structure of a cold-active alkaline phosphatase from a psychrophile, *Shewanella* sp. isolated from the intestine of an Antarctic shellfish, revealed local flexibility, responsible for the high catalytic efficiency at low temperatures [150].

Phytic acid is the phosphate ester of inositol. The phosphate groups in this form are not available for absorption by animals, with the partial exception of ruminants, where the hydrolysis is carried out by the rumen microbiota. Phytases (EC 3.1.3.) have been used for decades to enrich animal food of absorbable phosphate groups, both for non-ruminant livestock and fish [224] (Scheme 1h). Thermophilic phytases have been suggested for industrial use [225], but cold-adapted homologs were also proposed, especially in aquaculture, where low temperatures might be limiting for the activity of the mesophilic orthologues. In this view, the purification and characterization of novel cold-adapted phytases from the Antarctic marine *R. mucilaginosa* strain JMUY14 [130] and *Pseudomonas sp.* strain JPK1 isolated from soil were reported [226].

3.3.5. Other Hydrolases

A cold-adapted uracil-DNA glycosylase (EC 3.2.2.27 and EC 3.2.2.28) of Antarctic marine source was released by New England Biolabs as thermolabile uracil-DNA glycosylase [154]. This hydrolase, isolated from a psychrophilic marine bacterium, catalyzes the release of free uracil from uracil-containing single-stranded or double-stranded DNA; it is sensitive to heat and can be inactivated at temperatures above 50 °C.

Cryonase, a cold-active nuclease, isolated from an Antarctic marine psychrophile, *Shewanella* sp. strain Ac10 and patented by Awazu and colleagues [227] was developed by Takara-Clontech [151]. It is a recombinant endonuclease that can digest all types of DNA and RNA (single-stranded, double-stranded, linear or circularized) at low temperatures, frequently used during DNA digestion of samples in the presence of heat-labile proteins. A 3′–5′ exonuclease specific for single-stranded DNA and derived from an Arctic marine bacterium was released by ArcticZymes [152].

Antimicrobial enzymes endowed with bactericidal or bacteriostatic properties are an emerging strategy to combat pathogens, particularly by degrading their DNA, polysaccharides, and proteins, or by interfering with biofilm formation, or by catalysing reactions which result in the production of antimicrobial compounds [228]. For example, N-acyl homoserine lactones are signaling molecules involved in bacterial quorum sensing and their hydrolysis can reduce growth and biofilm formation of bacterial pathogens. A cold-adapted N-acylhomoserine lactonase (EC 3.1.1.81) was recently identified in Antarctic *Planococcus* sp. isolated from a soil sample collected on Lagoon Island (Antarctica) and was shown to attenuate the pathogenicity of *Pectobacterium carotovorum*, a plant pathogen that causes soft-rot disease [229]. As the enzyme was shown to be thermolabile at the human body temperature, it was suggested as a safe antimicrobial agent in the treatment of crops, as it would be inactivated upon ingestion.

3.3.6. Other Enzymes

Besides hydrolases, other enzymes have been isolated in marine microorganisms from the polar regions and, for some of them, a biotechnological application has been proposed.

Recently, few enzymes showing signatures of cold adaptation in their activity and structure have been isolated and fully characterized from the Arctic marine bacterium *C. psychrerythraea* strain 34H and also included a phenylalanine hydroxylase (PAH), an oxidoreductase, with high-catalytic efficiency at 10 °C, high thermostability and low affinity for substrate, probably due to enhanced flexibility of the active site [76]. PAH (EC 1.14.16.1) catalyzes the conversion of L-Phe to L-Tyr by para-hydroxylation of the aromatic side-chain and recently there has been an increased number of studies on the structure and function of PAH from bacteria and lower eukaryote organisms. Almost all characterized bacterial PAHs are monomeric and display a fold similar to the catalytic domain of mammalian PAHs.

Many oxidoreductases that catalyze redox reactions of industrial interest have been described in cold-adapted bacteria. The crystal structure of a Fe-superoxide dismutase, Fe-SOD (EC 1.15.1.1) isolated from the marine *P. haloplanktis*, revelead that cold-adapted enzyme displays high catalysis at low temperature increasing the flexibility of its active site without modifying the overall structure [161]. SODs have been used in the pharmaceutical and cosmetic industries, food, agricultural, and chemical industries [169]. Antioxidant defense is an important component of evolutionary adaptations in the cold to face increased levels of reactive oxygen species (ROS). The cold waters of the polar regions promote the formation of ROS and would be expected to lead to enhanced ROS damage of DNA and membrane lipid peroxidation in polar species [72]. *P. haloplanktis* TAC125 copes with increased O_2 solubility by deleting entire metabolic pathways that generate ROS as side products [230]. In contrast, the Arctic bacterium *C. psychrerythraea* has developed an enhanced antioxidant capacity, owing to the presence of three copies of catalase genes, as well as two superoxide-dismutase genes, one of which codes for a nickel-containing superoxide-dismutase, never reported before in proteobacteria [231].

A recombinant form of glutathione reductase (EC 1.8.1.7) from the Antarctic *C. psychrerythraea*, was recently characterized [168]. Since the cold-adapted enzyme displays activity also at moderate temperatures when overexpressed in *E. coli*, it may have some potential for industrial applications to protect cells and tissues from oxidative stress. Malato dehydrogenase (MDH) (EC 1.1.1.37) was purified from the Antarctic marine bacterium *Flavobacterium frigidimaris* KUC-1 and, among cold-adapted MDHs, was shown to be the most thermolabile and cold-active [158]. Thioredoxin and thioredoxin reductase (EC 1.8.1.9) from *P. haloplanktis* TAC125 were obtained as recombinant proteins. Both proteins exhibit activity at 10 °C [170]. The recombinat cold-adapted peroxiredoxin (EC 1.11.1.15) was biochemically characterized from the Antarctic marine psychrophilic bacterium *Psychrobacter* sp. ANT206, which had an optimum growth temperature of 10–12 °C. These enzymes may be relevant for many applications in food and medicine, mostly for their ability to protect super-coiled DNA from oxidative stress [172].

A cold-adapted leucine dehydrogenase (EC 1.4.1.9), a NAD^+-dependent oxidoreductase, with unique substrate specificity was cloned from the Antarctic marine psychrotrophic bacterium *Pseudoalteromonas* sp. ANT178 and was shown to retain 40% of its maximal activity at 0 °C. Being the key enzyme in the enzymatic conversion of L-leucine and other branched chain L-amino acids in the corresponding α-keto acid, it was suggested as biocatalyst in the pharmaceutical industry [157].

Aminotransferases (EC 2.6.1.), belonging to the class of transferases, have also been isolated from marine polar microorganisms, although no industrial application has been suggested so far. The aspartate aminotransferase, a ubiquitous transaminase enzyme that catalyzes the conversion of aspartate and α-ketoglutarate to oxaloacetate and glutamate, was isolated from the marine psychrophilic bacterium *P. haloplanktis* TAC125 and characterized from a structural and functional point of view [173].

It was shown to be thermolable, being inactivated at 50 °C. Its optimal working temperature is 10 °C lower than its *E. coli* homolog.

Photolyases (EC 4.1.99.3) were identified in the genera *Pseudomonas*, *Hymenobacter* and *Sphingomonas*, isolated in fresh waters in Antarctica (King George Island, Fildes Peninsula). Present in all living forms, except placental mammals and some marsupials, they are resistant to UV-radiations, being able to reverse DNA lesions (cyclobutane pyrimidine dimers and pyrimidine photoproducts [232] and, as UV radiations are known to be linked to skin cancer, they may have some potential in the cosmetic and pharmaceutical industries.

Cold-active γ-carbonic anhydrases (EC 4.2.1.1), able to catalyze the physiologic reaction of CO_2 hydration to bicarbonate and protons, were isolated from the psychrophilic marine bacteria *C. psychrerythraea* [178] and *P. haloplanktis* [179] cloned and characterized.

A cold-active DNA ligase from the psychrophile *P. haloplanktis* TAE72, isolated from Antarctic seawater at the Dumont d'Urville Antarctic Station, displays activity at temperatures as low as 4 °C [177]. DNA ligases (EC 6.5.1.) are enzymes involved in DNA replication, DNA recombination and DNA repair. They are commonly used in molecular biology to catalyze the formation of a phosphodiester bond between adjacent 5′-phosphoryl and 3′-hydroxyl groups in double stranded DNA. Currently, DNA ligases on the market, such as the recombinant versions of bacteriophage-derived DNA ligases, T4 and T7 ligases, and *E. coli* DNA ligases, are enzymes active at temperatures above 15 °C, where residual nucleases may interfere with the ligation process [167]. The possibility to use psychrophilic DNA ligases active at low temperature may guarantee high specific activity at low temperatures, thus avoiding unwanted reactions, carrying out the reaction in shorter times with respect to mesophilic ligases.

The crystal structure of the sedoheptulose 7-phosphate isomerase from the marine psychrophilic organism *C. psychrerythraea* 34H was determined. The Arctic bacterium produces extracellular polysaccharide substances to cope with cold and the isomerase is essential for producing D-glycero-D-mannoheptose 7-phosphate, a key mediator in the lipopolysaccharide biosynthetic pathway [184]. Other polar enzymes belonging to the class of isomerase are triose phosphate isomerases (EC 5.3.1.1), enzymes involved in the glycolytic pathway, identified in the Antarctic marine bacteria *Pseudomonas* sp. π9 [185], isolated from sea-ice and *Moraxella* sp. TA137 [186], isolated from the intestine of fish caught in Terre d'Adelie in Antarctica.

4. Perspectives and Conclusions

Marine microorganisms, whose immense genetic and biochemical diversity is only beginning to be appreciated, may become a rich source of novel enzyme activities in the near future. The marine bioprospecting of polar regions has begun only relatively recently but has already yielded success stories. Taking into account the evidence that the total number of species, and thus most likely biochemical diversity in the oceans, is higher than on land, there is a good reason to believe that a larger number of marine natural products from low-temperature environments may reach different sectors of biotechnology in the near future. For those reasons, a large number of research and development programmes in oceans are in progress worldwide. Although the genomic, functional and physiological knowledge of individual organisms is necessary to understand how enzymes and products work, more efficient strategies are needed to overcome the limits of the cultivation of microbes, especially those living in extreme environments such as the polar ones. The specific properties of polar marine microorganisms that make them unique and biotechnologically interesting are also responsible for their resistance to handling and cultivation. The most significant challenges are (i) the current lack of ability to produce extreme compounds (including enzymes) on large scale; (ii) the need to generate stronger synergies among marine scientists and industries at earlier levels to compensate the chronic underfunding of basic research and before large-scale production; (iii) the need to develop or improve technology transfer pathways for data and to secure access to fair and equitable benefit sharing of marine genetic resources. Metagenomics, genome engineering and systems biology will be fundamental to efficiently produce larger quantities of known and novel bioresources.

In the race to find new products for biotechnology, although there are good reasons to be optimistic, diverse strategies need to be adequately supported and funded in the academic context. The future perspectives require active collaboration between academia and industry at the beginning to support the research thus reducing the time lapse from the discovery to the industrial applications.

Author Contributions: All authors gave an important contribution in the consideration of the available bibliographic information for the review and in the preparation of the final version of the manuscript. S.B. and C.V. developed the original idea and organized all the materials.

Funding: This study was financially supported by the Italian National Programme for Antarctic Research (PNRA) (2016/AZ1.06-Project PNRA16_00043 and 2016/AZ1.20-Project PNRA16_00128). It was carried out in the framework of the SCAR Programme "Antarctic Thresholds–Ecosystem Resilience and Adaptation" (AnT-ERA).

Acknowledgments: We thank the Reviewers for the time and effort they have spent in reviewing the manuscript.

Conflicts of Interest: The authors declare no conflict of interest

References

1. Bornscheuer, U.T.; Huisman, G.W.; Kazlauskas, R.J.; Lutz, S.; Moore, J.C.; Robins, K. Engineering the third wave of biocatalysis. *Nature* **2012**, *485*, 185–194. [CrossRef] [PubMed]
2. Martinez-Martinez, M.; Coscolin, C.; Santiago, G.; Chow, J.; Stogios, P.J.; Bargiela, R.; Gertler, C.; Navarro-Fernandez, J.; Bollinger, A.; Thies, S.; et al. Determinants and Prediction of Esterase Substrate Promiscuity Patterns. *ACS Chem. Biol.* **2018**, *13*, 225–234. [CrossRef] [PubMed]
3. Raveendran, S.; Parameswaran, B.; Ummalyma, S.B.; Abraham, A.; Mathew, A.K.; Madhavan, A.; Rebello, S.; Pandey, A. Applications of Microbial Enzymes in Food Industry. *Food Technol. Biotechnol.* **2018**, *56*, 16–30. [CrossRef] [PubMed]
4. BCC. *Global Markets for Enzymes in Industrial Applications*; BCC Publishing: Wellesley, MA, USA, 2018.
5. SmithersGroup. *The Future of Marine Biotechnology for Industrial Applications to 2025*; SmithersGroup: Akron, OH, USA, 2015.
6. Di Donato, P.; Buono, A.; Poli, A.; Finore, I.; Abbamondi, G.R.; Nicolaus, B.; Lama, L. Exploring Marine Environments for the Identification of Extremophiles and Their Enzymes for Sustainable and Green Bioprocesses. *Sustainability* **2019**, *11*, 149. [CrossRef]
7. Gerwick, W.H.; Moore, B.S. Lessons from the past and charting the future of marine natural products drug discovery and chemical biology. *Chem. Biol.* **2012**, *19*, 85–98. [CrossRef] [PubMed]
8. Verde, C.; Giordano, D.; Bellas, C.M.; di Prisco, G.; Anesio, A.M. Chapter Four—Polar Marine Microorganisms and Climate Change. *Adv. Microb. Physiol.* **2016**, *69*, 187–215.
9. Jakobsson, M. Hypsometry and volume of the Arctic Ocean and its constituent seas. *Geochem. Geophys. Geosyst.* **2002**, *3*, 1–18. [CrossRef]
10. Scher, H.D.; Whittaker, J.M.; Williams, S.E.; Latimer, J.C.; Kordesch, W.E.; Delaney, M.L. Onset of Antarctic Circumpolar Current 30 million years ago as Tasmanian Gateway aligned with westerlies. *Nature* **2015**, *523*, 580–583. [CrossRef]
11. Maldonado, A.; Bohoyo, F.; Galindo-Zaldívar, J.; Hernández-Molina, F.J.; Lobo, F.J.; Lodolo, E.; Martos, Y.M.; Pérez, L.F.; Schreider, A.A.; Somoza, L. A model of oceanic development by ridge jumping: Opening of the Scotia Sea. *Glob. Planet. Chang.* **2014**, *123*, 152–173. [CrossRef]
12. Russell, N.J. Molecular adaptations in psychrophilic bacteria: Potential for biotechnological applications. *Adv. Biochem. Eng. Biotechnol.* **1998**, *61*, 1–21.
13. Cavicchioli, R. On the concept of a psychrophile. *ISME J.* **2015**, *10*, 793. [CrossRef] [PubMed]
14. Lebar, M.D.; Heimbegner, J.L.; Baker, B.J. Cold-water marine natural products. *Nat. Prod. Rep.* **2007**, *24*, 774–797. [CrossRef]
15. Wilson, Z.E.; Brimble, M.A. Molecules derived from the extremes of life. *Nat. Prod. Rep.* **2009**, *26*, 44–71. [CrossRef] [PubMed]
16. Liu, J.T.; Lu, X.L.; Liu, X.Y.; Gao, Y.; Hu, B.; Jiao, B.H.; Zheng, H. Bioactive natural products from the antarctic and arctic organisms. *Mini Rev. Med. Chem.* **2013**, *13*, 617–626. [CrossRef] [PubMed]
17. Skropeta, D.; Wei, L. Recent advances in deep-sea natural products. *Nat. Prod. Rep.* **2014**, *31*, 999–1025. [CrossRef] [PubMed]

18. Tian, Y.; Li, Y.L.; Zhao, F.C. Secondary Metabolites from Polar Organisms. *Mar. Drugs* **2017**, *15*, 28. [CrossRef]
19. Nunez-Montero, K.; Barrientos, L. Advances in Antarctic Research for Antimicrobial Discovery: A Comprehensive Narrative Review of Bacteria from Antarctic Environments as Potential Sources of Novel Antibiotic Compounds Against Human Pathogens and Microorganisms of Industrial Importance. *Antibiotics* **2018**, *7*, 90. [CrossRef]
20. Murray, A.E.; Grzymski, J.J. Diversity and genomics of Antarctic marine micro-organisms. *Philos. Trans. R. Soc. Lond. B Biol. Sci.* **2007**, *362*, 2259–2271. [CrossRef]
21. Margesin, R.; Miteva, V. Diversity and ecology of psychrophilic microorganisms. *Res. Microbiol.* **2011**, *162*, 346–361. [CrossRef]
22. Casanueva, A.; Tuffin, M.; Cary, C.; Cowan, D.A. Molecular adaptations to psychrophily: The impact of 'omic' technologies. *Trends Microbiol.* **2010**, *18*, 374–381. [CrossRef]
23. Cavicchioli, R.; Siddiqui, K.S.; Andrews, D.; Sowers, K.R. Low-temperature extremophiles and their applications. *Curr. Opin. Biotechnol.* **2002**, *13*, 253–261. [CrossRef]
24. de Pascale, D.; De Santi, C.; Fu, J.; Landfald, B. The microbial diversity of Polar environments is a fertile ground for bioprospecting. *Mar. Genom.* **2012**, *8*, 15–22. [CrossRef] [PubMed]
25. Joseph, B.; Kumar, V.; Ramteke, P.W. Chapter 47—Psychrophilic Enzymes: Potential Biocatalysts for Food Processing. *Enzym. Food Biotechnol.* **2019**, 817–825. [CrossRef]
26. Dhamankar, H.; Prather, K.L. Microbial chemical factories: Recent advances in pathway engineering for synthesis of value added chemicals. *Curr. Opin. Struct. Biol.* **2011**, *21*, 488–494. [CrossRef] [PubMed]
27. Weber, W.; Fussenegger, M. Emerging biomedical applications of synthetic biology. *Nat. Rev. Genet.* **2011**, *13*, 21–35. [CrossRef]
28. Cavicchioli, R. Microbial ecology of Antarctic aquatic systems. *Nat. Rev. Microbiol.* **2015**, *13*, 691–706. [CrossRef] [PubMed]
29. Uchiyama, T.; Miyazaki, K. Functional metagenomics for enzyme discovery: Challenges to efficient screening. *Curr. Opin. Biotechnol.* **2009**, *20*, 616–622. [CrossRef]
30. Ferrer, M.; Beloqui, A.; Timmis, K.N.; Golyshin, P.N. Metagenomics for mining new genetic resources of microbial communities. *J. Mol. Microbiol. Biotechnol.* **2009**, *16*, 109–123. [CrossRef]
31. Pena-Garcia, C.; Martinez-Martinez, M.; Reyes-Duarte, D.; Ferrer, M. High Throughput Screening of Esterases, Lipases and Phospholipases in Mutant and Metagenomic Libraries: A Review. *Comb. Chem. High Throughput Screen.* **2016**, *19*, 605–615. [CrossRef]
32. Ferrer, M.; Mendez-Garcia, C.; Bargiela, R.; Chow, J.; Alonso, S.; Garcia-Moyano, A.; Bjerga, G.E.K.; Steen, I.H.; Schwabe, T.; Blom, C.; et al. Decoding the ocean's microbiological secrets for marine enzyme biodiscovery. *FEMS Microbiol. Lett.* **2019**, *366*. [CrossRef]
33. Zallot, R.; Oberg, N.O.; Gerlt, J.A. 'Democratized' genomic enzymology web tools for functional assignment. *Curr. Opin. Chem. Biol.* **2018**, *47*, 77–85. [CrossRef] [PubMed]
34. Behrens, G.A.; Hummel, A.; Padhi, S.K.; Schätzle, S.; Bornscheuer, U.T. Discovery and Protein Engineering of Biocatalysts for Organic Synthesis. *Adv. Synth. Catal.* **2011**, *353*, 1615–4150. [CrossRef]
35. Lauritano, C.; Ianora, A. Overview of Recent EU-Funded Projects. In *Grand Challenges in Marine Biotechnology*; Springer: Berlin, Germany, 2018; pp. 425–449.
36. Available online: http://www.inmare-h2020.eu/ (accessed on 15 July 2019).
37. Popovic, A.; Hai, T.; Tchigvintsev, A.; Hajighasemi, M.; Nocek, B.; Khusnutdinova, A.N.; Brown, G.; Glinos, J.; Flick, R.; Skarina, T.; et al. Activity screening of environmental metagenomic libraries reveals novel carboxylesterase families. *Sci. Rep.* **2017**, *7*, 44103. [CrossRef] [PubMed]
38. Bastard, K.; Smith, A.A.; Vergne-Vaxelaire, C.; Perret, A.; Zaparucha, A.; De Melo-Minardi, R.; Mariage, A.; Boutard, M.; Debard, A.; Lechaplais, C.; et al. Revealing the hidden functional diversity of an enzyme family. *Nat. Chem. Biol.* **2014**, *10*, 42–49. [CrossRef] [PubMed]
39. Chistoserdova, L. Is metagenomics resolving identification of functions in microbial communities? *Microb. Biotechnol.* **2014**, *7*, 1–4. [CrossRef] [PubMed]
40. Ferrer, M.; Martinez-Martinez, M.; Bargiela, R.; Streit, W.R.; Golyshina, O.V.; Golyshin, P.N. Estimating the success of enzyme bioprospecting through metagenomics: Current status and future trends. *Microb. Biotechnol.* **2016**, *9*, 22–34. [CrossRef] [PubMed]
41. McGettigan, P.A. Transcriptomics in the RNA-seq era. *Curr. Opin. Chem. Biol.* **2013**, *17*, 4–11. [CrossRef] [PubMed]

42. Sturmberger, L.; Wallace, P.W.; Glieder, A.; Birner-Gruenberger, R. Synergism of proteomics and mRNA sequencing for enzyme discovery. *J. Biotechnol.* **2016**, *235*, 132–138. [CrossRef] [PubMed]
43. Cravatt, B.F.; Wright, A.T.; Kozarich, J.W. Activity-based protein profiling: From enzyme chemistry to proteomic chemistry. *Annu. Rev. Biochem.* **2008**, *77*, 383–414. [CrossRef]
44. Schittmayer, M.; Birner-Gruenberger, R. Lipolytic proteomics. *Mass Spectrom. Rev.* **2012**, *31*, 570–582. [CrossRef]
45. Perfumo, A.; Banat, I.M.; Marchant, R. Going Green and Cold: Biosurfactants from Low-Temperature Environments to Biotechnology Applications. *Trends Biotechnol.* **2018**, *36*, 277–289. [CrossRef] [PubMed]
46. Chen, G.Q.; Jiang, X.R. Next generation industrial biotechnology based on extremophilic bacteria. *Curr. Opin. Biotechnol.* **2018**, *50*, 94–100. [CrossRef] [PubMed]
47. Longwell, C.K.; Labanieh, L.; Cochran, J.R. High-throughput screening technologies for enzyme engineering. *Curr. Opin. Biotechnol.* **2017**, *48*, 196–202. [CrossRef] [PubMed]
48. Lalonde, J. Highly engineered biocatalysts for efficient small molecule pharmaceutical synthesis. *Curr. Opin. Biotechnol.* **2016**, *42*, 152–158. [CrossRef] [PubMed]
49. Porter, J.L.; Rusli, R.A.; Ollis, D.L. Directed Evolution of Enzymes for Industrial Biocatalysis. *ChemBioChem* **2016**, *17*, 197–203. [CrossRef] [PubMed]
50. Tyzack, J.D.; Furnham, N.; Sillitoe, I.; Orengo, C.M.; Thornton, J.M. Understanding enzyme function evolution from a computational perspective. *Curr. Opin. Struct. Biol.* **2017**, *47*, 131–139. [CrossRef] [PubMed]
51. Acevedo-Rocha, C.G.; Gamble, C.G.; Lonsdale, R.; Li, A.; Nett, N.; Hoebenreich, S.; Lingnau, J.B.; Wirtz, C.; Fares, C.; Hinrichs, H.; et al. P450-Catalyzed Regio- and Diastereoselective Steroid Hydroxylation: Efficient Directed Evolution Enabled by Mutability Landscaping. *ACS Catal.* **2018**, *8*, 3395–3410. [CrossRef]
52. Agostini, F.; Völler, J.-S.; Koksch, B.; Acevedo-Rocha, C.G.; Kubyshkin, V.; Budisa, N. Biocatalysis with Unnatural Amino Acids: Enzymology Meets Xenobiology. *Angew. Chem. Int. Ed.* **2017**, *56*, 9680–9703. [CrossRef]
53. Bernath, K.; Hai, M.; Mastrobattista, E.; Griffiths, A.D.; Magdassi, S.; Tawfik, D.S. In vitro compartmentalization by double emulsions: Sorting and gene enrichment by fluorescence activated cell sorting. *Anal. Biochem.* **2004**, *325*, 151–157. [CrossRef]
54. Becker, S.; Hobenreich, H.; Vogel, A.; Knorr, J.; Wilhelm, S.; Rosenau, F.; Jaeger, K.E.; Reetz, M.T.; Kolmar, H. Single-cell high-throughput screening to identify enantioselective hydrolytic enzymes. *Angew. Chem. Int. Ed. Engl.* **2008**, *47*, 5085–5088. [CrossRef]
55. Fernandez-Alvaro, E.; Snajdrova, R.; Jochens, H.; Davids, T.; Bottcher, D.; Bornscheuer, U.T. A combination of in vivo selection and cell sorting for the identification of enantioselective biocatalysts. *Angew. Chem. Int. Ed. Engl.* **2011**, *50*, 8584–8587. [CrossRef]
56. Fox, R.J.; Davis, S.C.; Mundorff, E.C.; Newman, L.M.; Gavrilovic, V.; Ma, S.K.; Chung, L.M.; Ching, C.; Tam, S.; Muley, S.; et al. Improving catalytic function by ProSAR-driven enzyme evolution. *Nat. Biotechnol.* **2007**, *25*, 338–344. [CrossRef] [PubMed]
57. Coker, J.A. Extremophiles and biotechnology: Current uses and prospects. *F1000Res* **2016**, *5*. [CrossRef] [PubMed]
58. Gerlt, J.A.; Allen, K.N.; Almo, S.C.; Armstrong, R.N.; Babbitt, P.C.; Cronan, J.E.; Dunaway-Mariano, D.; Imker, H.J.; Jacobson, M.P.; Minor, W.; et al. The Enzyme Function Initiative. *Biochemistry* **2011**, *50*, 9950–9962. [CrossRef] [PubMed]
59. Devine, P.N.; Howard, R.M.; Kumar, R.; Thompson, M.P.; Truppo, M.D.; Turner, N.J. Extending the application of biocatalysis to meet the challenges of drug development. *Nat. Rev. Chem.* **2018**, *2*, 409–421. [CrossRef]
60. Liszka, M.J.; Clark, M.E.; Schneider, E.; Clark, D.S. Nature versus nurture: Developing enzymes that function under extreme conditions. *Annu. Rev. Chem. Biomol. Eng.* **2012**, *3*, 77–102. [CrossRef] [PubMed]
61. Duplantis, B.N.; Osusky, M.; Schmerk, C.L.; Ross, D.R.; Bosio, C.M.; Nano, F.E. Essential genes from Arctic bacteria used to construct stable, temperature-sensitive bacterial vaccines. *Proc. Natl. Acad. Sci. USA* **2010**, *107*, 13456–13460. [CrossRef]
62. Pinto, C.T.; Nano, F.E. Stable, temperature-sensitive recombinant strain of Mycobacterium smegmatis generated through the substitution of a psychrophilic ligA gene. *FEMS Microbiol. Lett.* **2015**, *362*, fnv152. [CrossRef] [PubMed]
63. Duplantis, B.N.; Puckett, S.M.; Rosey, E.L.; Ameiss, K.A.; Hartman, A.D.; Pearce, S.C.; Nano, F.E. Temperature-Sensitive *Salmonella enterica* Serovar Enteritidis PT13a Expressing Essential Proteins of Psychrophilic Bacteria. *Appl. Environ. Microbiol.* **2015**, *81*, 6757–6766. [CrossRef]

64. Santiago, M.; Ramirez-Sarmiento, C.A.; Zamora, R.A.; Parra, L.P. Discovery, Molecular Mechanisms, and Industrial Applications of Cold-Active Enzymes. *Front. Microbiol.* **2016**, *7*, 1408. [CrossRef]
65. Miteva, V.; Lantz, S.; Brenchley, J. Characterization of a cryptic plasmid from a Greenland ice core *Arthrobacter* isolate and construction of a shuttle vector that replicates in psychrophilic high G+C Gram-positive recipients. *Extremophiles* **2008**, *12*, 441–449. [CrossRef] [PubMed]
66. Ferrer, M.; Chernikova, T.N.; Yakimov, M.M.; Golyshin, P.N.; Timmis, K.N. Chaperonins govern growth of *Escherichia coli* at low temperatures. *Nat. Biotechnol.* **2003**, *21*, 1266–1267. [CrossRef] [PubMed]
67. Georlette, D.; Blaise, V.; Collins, T.; D'Amico, S.; Gratia, E.; Hoyoux, A.; Marx, J.C.; Sonan, G.; Feller, G.; Gerday, C. Some like it cold: Biocatalysis at low temperatures. *FEMS Microbiol. Rev.* **2004**, *28*, 25–42. [CrossRef] [PubMed]
68. Feller, G. Psychrophilic enzymes: From folding to function and biotechnology. *Scientifica* **2013**, *2013*, 512840. [CrossRef] [PubMed]
69. Feller, G.; Gerday, C. Psychrophilic enzymes: Hot topics in cold adaptation. *Nat. Rev. Microbiol.* **2003**, *1*, 200–208. [CrossRef]
70. Siddiqui, K.S.; Cavicchioli, R. Cold-adapted enzymes. *Annu. Rev. Biochem.* **2006**, *75*, 403–433. [CrossRef] [PubMed]
71. Laye, V.J.; Karan, R.; Kim, J.M.; Pecher, W.T.; DasSarma, P.; DasSarma, S. Key amino acid residues conferring enhanced enzyme activity at cold temperatures in an Antarctic polyextremophilic beta-galactosidase. *Proc. Natl. Acad. Sci. USA* **2017**, *114*, 12530–12535. [CrossRef] [PubMed]
72. Giordano, D.; Coppola, D.; Russo, R.; Tinajero-Trejo, M.; di Prisco, G.; Lauro, F.; Ascenzi, P.; Verde, C. The globins of cold-adapted *Pseudoalteromonas haloplanktis* TAC125: From the structure to the physiological functions. *Adv. Microb. Physiol.* **2013**, *63*, 329–389. [CrossRef]
73. Kube, M.; Chernikova, T.N.; Al-Ramahi, Y.; Beloqui, A.; Lopez-Cortez, N.; Guazzaroni, M.E.; Heipieper, H.J.; Klages, S.; Kotsyurbenko, O.R.; Langer, I.; et al. Genome sequence and functional genomic analysis of the oil-degrading bacterium Oleispira antarctica. *Nat. Commun.* **2013**, *4*, 2156. [CrossRef]
74. D'Amico, S.; Claverie, P.; Collins, T.; Georlette, D.; Gratia, E.; Hoyoux, A.; Meuwis, M.A.; Feller, G.; Gerday, C. Molecular basis of cold adaptation. *Philos. Trans. R. Soc. Lond. B Biol. Sci.* **2002**, *357*, 917–925. [CrossRef]
75. D'Amico, S.; Collins, T.; Marx, J.C.; Feller, G.; Gerday, C. Psychrophilic microorganisms: Challenges for life. *EMBO Rep.* **2006**, *7*, 385–389. [CrossRef] [PubMed]
76. Leiros, H.K.; Pey, A.L.; Innselset, M.; Moe, E.; Leiros, I.; Steen, I.H.; Martinez, A. Structure of phenylalanine hydroxylase from *Colwellia psychrerythraea* 34H, a monomeric cold active enzyme with local flexibility around the active site and high overall stability. *J. Biol. Chem.* **2007**, *282*, 21973–21986. [CrossRef] [PubMed]
77. Sonan, G.K.; Receveur-Brechot, V.; Duez, C.; Aghajari, N.; Czjzek, M.; Haser, R.; Gerday, C. The linker region plays a key role in the adaptation to cold of the cellulase from an Antarctic bacterium. *Biochem. J.* **2007**, *407*, 293–302. [CrossRef] [PubMed]
78. Mouri, Y.; Takada, Y. Contribution of Three Different Regions of Isocitrate Dehydrogenases from Psychrophilic and Psychrotolerant Bacteria to Their Thermal Properties. *Curr. Microbiol.* **2018**, *75*, 1523–1529. [CrossRef] [PubMed]
79. Dong, Y.W.; Liao, M.L.; Meng, X.L.; Somero, G.N. Structural flexibility and protein adaptation to temperature: Molecular dynamics analysis of malate dehydrogenases of marine molluscs. *Proc. Natl. Acad. Sci. USA* **2018**, *115*, 1274–1279. [CrossRef] [PubMed]
80. Pischedda, A.; Ramasamy, K.P.; Mangiagalli, M.; Chiappori, F.; Milanesi, L.; Miceli, C.; Pucciarelli, S.; Lotti, M. Antarctic marine ciliates under stress: Superoxide dismutases from the psychrophilic Euplotes focardii are cold-active yet heat tolerant enzymes. *Sci. Rep.* **2018**, *8*, 14721. [CrossRef] [PubMed]
81. Tosco, A.; Birolo, L.; Madonna, S.; Lolli, G.; Sannia, G.; Marino, G. GroEL from the psychrophilic bacterium *Pseudoalteromonas haloplanktis* TAC 125: Molecular characterization and gene cloning. *Extremophiles* **2003**, *7*, 17–28. [CrossRef] [PubMed]
82. Joshi, S.; Satyanarayana, T. Biotechnology of cold-active proteases. *Biology* **2013**, *2*, 755–783. [CrossRef] [PubMed]
83. Marx, J.C.; Collins, T.; D'Amico, S.; Feller, G.; Gerday, C. Cold-adapted enzymes from marine Antarctic microorganisms. *Mar. Biotechnol.* **2007**, *9*, 293–304. [CrossRef]
84. Cavicchioli, R.; Charlton, T.; Ertan, H.; Mohd Omar, S.; Siddiqui, K.S.; Williams, T.J. Biotechnological uses of enzymes from psychrophiles. *Microb. Biotechnol.* **2011**, *4*, 449–460. [CrossRef]

85. Duarte, A.W.F.; Dos Santos, J.A.; Vianna, M.V.; Vieira, J.M.F.; Mallagutti, V.H.; Inforsato, F.J.; Wentzel, L.C.P.; Lario, L.D.; Rodrigues, A.; Pagnocca, F.C.; et al. Cold-adapted enzymes produced by fungi from terrestrial and marine Antarctic environments. *Crit. Rev. Biotechnol.* **2018**, *38*, 600–619. [CrossRef] [PubMed]
86. Cieslinski, H.; Kur, J.; Bialkowska, A.; Baran, I.; Makowski, K.; Turkiewicz, M. Cloning, expression, and purification of a recombinant cold-adapted beta-galactosidase from antarctic bacterium *Pseudoalteromonas* sp. 22b. *Protein Expr. Purif.* **2005**, *39*, 27–34. [CrossRef] [PubMed]
87. Turkiewicz, M.; Kur, J.; Bialkowska, A.; Cieslinski, H.; Kalinowska, H.; Bielecki, S. Antarctic marine bacterium *Pseudoalteromonas* sp. 22b as a source of cold-adapted beta-galactosidase. *Biomol. Eng.* **2003**, *20*, 317–324. [CrossRef]
88. Hoyoux, A.; Jennes, I.; Dubois, P.; Genicot, S.; Dubail, F.; Francois, J.M.; Baise, E.; Feller, G.; Gerday, C. Cold-adapted beta-galactosidase from the Antarctic psychrophile *Pseudoalteromonas haloplanktis*. *Appl. Environ. Microbiol.* **2001**, *67*, 1529–1535. [CrossRef] [PubMed]
89. Gerday, C.; Hoyoux, A.; Marie Francois, J.M.; Dubois, P.; Baise, E.; Jennes, I.; Genicot, S. Cold-Active Beta Galactosidase, the Process for its Preparation and the Use Thereof. U.S. Patent WO2001004276A1, 9 July 1999.
90. Song, C.; Chi, Z.; Li, J.; Wang, X. beta-Galactosidase production by the psychrotolerant yeast *Guehomyces pullulans* 17-1 isolated from sea sediment in Antarctica and lactose hydrolysis. *Bioprocess. Biosyst. Eng.* **2010**, *33*, 1025–1031. [CrossRef] [PubMed]
91. Alikkunju, A.P.; Sainjan, N.; Silvester, R.; Joseph, A.; Rahiman, M.; Antony, A.C.; Kumaran, R.C.; Hatha, M. Screening and Characterization of Cold-Active beta-Galactosidase Producing Psychrotrophic *Enterobacter ludwigii* from the Sediments of Arctic Fjord. *Appl. Biochem. Biotechnol.* **2016**, *180*, 477–490. [CrossRef]
92. Schmidt, M.; Stougaard, P. Identification, cloning and expression of a cold-active beta-galactosidase from a novel Arctic bacterium, *Alkalilactibacillus ikkense*. *Environ. Technol.* **2010**, *31*, 1107–1114. [CrossRef] [PubMed]
93. Wang, X.; Kan, G.; Ren, X.; Yu, G.; Shi, C.; Xie, Q.; Wen, H.; Betenbaugh, M. Molecular Cloning and Characterization of a Novel alpha-Amylase from Antarctic Sea Ice Bacterium *Pseudoalteromonas* sp. M175 and Its Primary Application in Detergent. *BioMed Res. Int.* **2018**, *2018*, 3258383. [CrossRef] [PubMed]
94. Ramli, A.N.; Azhar, M.A.; Shamsir, M.S.; Rabu, A.; Murad, A.M.; Mahadi, N.M.; Illias, R.M. Sequence and structural investigation of a novel psychrophilic alpha-amylase from *Glaciozyma antarctica* PI12 for cold-adaptation analysis. *J. Mol. Model.* **2013**, *19*, 3369–3383. [CrossRef] [PubMed]
95. Vardhan Reddy, P.V.; Shiva Nageswara Rao, S.S.; Pratibha, M.S.; Sailaja, B.; Kavya, B.; Manorama, R.R.; Singh, S.M.; Radha Srinivas, T.N.; Shivaji, S. Bacterial diversity and bioprospecting for cold-active enzymes from culturable bacteria associated with sediment from a melt water stream of Midtre Lov´enbreen glacier, an Arctic glacier. *Res. Microbiol.* **2009**, *160*, 538–546. [CrossRef] [PubMed]
96. Chessa, J.P.; Feller, G.; Gerday, C. Purification and characterization of the heat-labile alpha-amylase secreted by the psychrophilic bacterium TAC 240B. *Can. J. Microbiol.* **1999**, *45*, 452–457. [CrossRef] [PubMed]
97. Feller, G.; D'Amico, D.; Gerday, C. Thermodynamic stability of a cold-active alpha-amylase from the Antarctic bacterium Alteromonas haloplanctis. *Biochemistry* **1999**, *38*, 4613–4619. [CrossRef] [PubMed]
98. Kuddus, M.; Roohi, J.M.A.; Ramteke, P.W. An Overview of Cold-active Microbial α-amylase: Adaptation Strategies and Biotechnological Potentials. *Biotechnol. Biotechnol. Equip.* **2011**, *10*, 246–258.
99. Del-Cid, A.; Ubilla, P.; Ravanal, M.C.; Medina, E.; Vaca, I.; Levican, G.; Eyzaguirre, J.; Chavez, R. Cold-active xylanase produced by fungi associated with Antarctic marine sponges. *Appl. Biochem. Biotechnol.* **2014**, *172*, 524–532. [CrossRef] [PubMed]
100. Humphry, D.R.; George, A.; Black, G.W.; Cummings, S.P. *Flavobacterium frigidarium* sp. nov., an aerobic, psychrophilic, xylanolytic and laminarinolytic bacterium from Antarctica. *Int. J. Syst. Evol. Microbiol.* **2001**, *51*, 1235–1243. [CrossRef] [PubMed]
101. Miyazaki, K.; Wintrode, P.L.; Grayling, R.A.; Rubingh, D.N.; Arnold, F.H. Directed evolution study of temperature adaptation in a psychrophilic enzyme. *J. Mol. Biol.* **2000**, *297*, 1015–1026. [CrossRef] [PubMed]
102. Narinx, E.; Davail, S.; Feller, G.; Gerday, C. Nucleotide and derived amino acid sequence of the subtilisin from the antarctic psychrotroph *Bacillus* TA39. *Biochim. Biophys. Acta* **1992**, *1131*, 111–113. [CrossRef]
103. Davail, S.; Feller, G.; Narinx, E.; Gerday, C. Cold adaptation of proteins. Purification, characterization, and sequence of the heat-labile subtilisin from the antarctic psychrophile *Bacillus* TA41. *J. Biol. Chem.* **1994**, *269*, 17448–17453.

104. Wang, Q.F.; Miao, J.L.; Hou, Y.H.; Ding, Y.; Wang, G.D.; Li, G.Y. Purification and characterization of an extracellular cold-active serine protease from the psychrophilic bacterium *Colwellia* sp. NJ341. *Biotechnol. Lett.* **2005**, *27*, 1195–1198. [CrossRef]
105. Kulakova, L.; Galkin, A.; Kurihara, T.; Yoshimura, T.; Esaki, N. Cold-active serine alkaline protease from the psychrotrophic bacterium *Shewanella* strain ac10: Gene cloning and enzyme purification and characterization. *Appl. Environ. Microbiol.* **1999**, *65*, 611–617.
106. Lario, L.D.; Chaud, L.; Almeida, M.D.G.; Converti, A.; Duraes Sette, L.; Pessoa, A., Jr. Production, purification, and characterization of an extracellular acid protease from the marine Antarctic yeast *Rhodotorula mucilaginosa* L7. *Fungal Biol.* **2015**, *119*, 1129–1136. [CrossRef] [PubMed]
107. Acevedo, J.P.; Rodriguez, V.; Saavedra, M.; Munoz, M.; Salazar, O.; Asenjo, J.A.; Andrews, B.A. Cloning, expression and decoding of the cold adaptation of a new widely represented thermolabile subtilisin-like protease. *J. Appl. Microbiol.* **2013**, *114*, 352–363. [CrossRef] [PubMed]
108. Wang, Q.-F.; Hou, Y.-H.; Xu, Z.; Miao, J.-L.; Li, G.-Y. Purification and properties of an extracellular cold-active protease from the psychrophilic bacterium *Pseudoalteromonas* sp. NJ276. *Biochem. Eng. J.* **2008**, *38*, 362–368. [CrossRef]
109. Turkiewicz, M.; Pazgier, M.; Kalinowska, H.; Bielecki, S. A cold-adapted extracellular serine proteinase of the yeast Leucosporidium antarcticum. *Extremophiles* **2003**, *7*, 435–442. [CrossRef] [PubMed]
110. de Pascale, D.; Giuliani, M.; De Santi, C.; Bergamasco, N.; Amoresano, A.; Carpentieri, A.; Parrilli, E.; Tutino, M.L. PhAP protease from *Pseudoalteromonas haloplanktis* TAC125: Gene cloning, recombinant production in E. coli and enzyme characterization. *Polar Sci.* **2010**, *4*, 285–294. [CrossRef]
111. Huston, A.L.; Methe, B.; Deming, J.W. Purification, characterization, and sequencing of an extracellular cold-active aminopeptidase produced by marine psychrophile *Colwellia psychrerythraea* strain 34H. *Appl. Environ. Microbiol.* **2004**, *70*, 3321–3328. [CrossRef] [PubMed]
112. Huston, A.L.; Haeggstrom, J.Z.; Feller, G. Cold adaptation of enzymes: Structural, kinetic and microcalorimetric characterizations of an aminopeptidase from the Arctic psychrophile *Colwellia psychrerythraea* and of human leukotriene A(4) hydrolase. *Biochim. Biophys. Acta* **2008**, *1784*, 1865–1872. [CrossRef]
113. Pereira, J.Q.; Ambrosini, A.; Passaglia, L.M.P.; Brandelli, A. A new cold-adapted serine peptidase from Antarctic *Lysobacter* sp. A03: Insights about enzyme activity at low temperatures. *Int. J. Biol. Macromol.* **2017**, *103*, 854–862. [CrossRef]
114. Larsen, A.N.; Moe, E.; Helland, R.; Gjellesvik, D.R.; Willassen, N.P. Characterization of a recombinantly expressed proteinase K-like enzyme from a psychrotrophic *Serratia* sp. *FEBS J.* **2006**, *273*, 47–60. [CrossRef]
115. Xie, B.B.; Bian, F.; Chen, X.L.; He, H.L.; Guo, J.; Gao, X.; Zeng, Y.X.; Chen, B.; Zhou, B.C.; Zhang, Y.Z. Cold adaptation of zinc metalloproteases in the thermolysin family from deep sea and arctic sea ice bacteria revealed by catalytic and structural properties and molecular dynamics: New insights into relationship between conformational flexibility and hydrogen bonding. *J. Biol. Chem.* **2009**, *284*, 9257–9269. [CrossRef]
116. Turkiewicz, M.; Gromek, E.; Kalinowska, H.; Zielińska, M. Biosynthesis and properties of an extracellular metalloprotease from the Antarctic marine bacterium Sphingomonas paucimobilis. *J. Biotechnol.* **1999**, *70*, 53–60. [CrossRef]
117. Denner, E.B.; Mark, B.; Busse, H.J.; Turkiewicz, M.; Lubitz, W. *Psychrobacter proteolyticus* sp. nov., a psychrotrophic, halotolerant bacterium isolated from the Antarctic krill Euphausia superba Dana, excreting a cold-adapted metalloprotease. *Syst. Appl. Microbiol.* **2001**, *24*, 44–53. [CrossRef] [PubMed]
118. Available online: https://arcticzymes.com/technology/proteinase/ (accessed on 15 July 2019).
119. Wi, A.R.; Jeon, S.J.; Kim, S.; Park, H.J.; Kim, D.; Han, S.J.; Yim, J.H.; Kim, H.W. Characterization and a point mutational approach of a psychrophilic lipase from an arctic bacterium, *Bacillus pumilus*. *Biotechnol. Lett.* **2014**, *36*, 1295–1302. [CrossRef] [PubMed]
120. de Pascale, D.; Cusano, A.M.; Autore, F.; Parrilli, E.; di Prisco, G.; Marino, G.; Tutino, M.L. The cold-active Lip1 lipase from the Antarctic bacterium *Pseudoalteromonas haloplanktis* TAC125 is a member of a new bacterial lipolytic enzyme family. *Extremophiles* **2008**, *12*, 311–323. [CrossRef] [PubMed]
121. Do, H.; Lee, J.H.; Kwon, M.H.; Song, H.E.; An, J.Y.; Eom, S.H.; Lee, S.G.; Kim, H.J. Purification, characterization and preliminary X-ray diffraction analysis of a cold-active lipase (CpsLip) from the psychrophilic bacterium *Colwellia psychrerythraea* 34H. *Acta Crystallogr. Sect. F Struct. Biol. Cryst. Commun.* **2013**, *69*, 920–924. [CrossRef] [PubMed]

122. Irgens, R.L.; Gosink, J.J.; Staley, J.T. *Polaromonas vacuolata* gen. nov., sp. nov., a psychrophilic, marine, gas vacuolate bacterium from Antarctica. *Int. J. Syst. Bacteriol.* **1996**, *46*, 822–826. [CrossRef]
123. Parra, L.P.; Reyes, F.; Acevedo, J.P.; Salazar, O.; Andrews, B.A.; Asenjo, J.A. Cloning and fusion expression of a cold-active lipase from marine Antarctic origin. *Enzym. Microb. Technol.* **2008**, *42*, 371–377. [CrossRef]
124. Xuezheng, L.; Shuoshuo, C.; Guoying, X.; Shuai, W.; Ning, D.; Jihong, S. Cloning and heterologous expression of two cold-active lipases from the Antarctic bacterium *Psychrobacter* sp. G. *Polar Res.* **2010**, *29*, 421–429. [CrossRef]
125. Parra, L.P.; Espina, G.; Devia, J.; Salazar, O.; Andrews, B.; Asenjo, J.A. Identification of lipase encoding genes from Antarctic seawater bacteria using degenerate primers: Expression of a cold-active lipase with high specific activity. *Enzym. Microb. Technol.* **2015**, *68*, 56–61. [CrossRef]
126. Feller, G.; Thiry, M.; Arpigny, J.L.; Gerday, C. Cloning and expression in *Escherichia coli* of three lipase-encoding genes from the psychrotrophic antarctic strain *Moraxella* TA144. *Gene* **1991**, *102*, 111–115. [CrossRef]
127. Zhang, J.; Lin, S.; Zeng, R. Cloning, expression, and characterization of a cold-adapted lipase gene from an antarctic deep-sea psychrotrophic bacterium, *Psychrobacter* sp 7195. *J. Microbiol. Biotechnol.* **2007**, *17*, 604–610. [PubMed]
128. Yang, X.; Lin, X.; Fan, T.; Bian, J.; Huang, X. Cloning and expression of lipP, a gene encoding a cold-adapted lipase from *Moritella* sp.2-5-10-1. *Curr. Microbiol.* **2008**, *56*, 194–198. [CrossRef]
129. Lo Giudice, A.; Michaud, L.; de Pascale, D.; De Domenico, M.; di Prisco, G.; Fani, R.; Bruni, V. Lipolytic activity of Antarctic cold-adapted marine bacteria (Terra Nova Bay, Ross Sea). *J. Appl. Microbiol.* **2006**, *101*, 1039–1048. [CrossRef] [PubMed]
130. Yu, P.; Wang, X.T.; Liu, J.W. Purification and characterization of a novel cold-adapted phytase from *Rhodotorula mucilaginosa* strain JMUY14 isolated from Antarctic. *J. Basic Microbiol.* **2015**, *55*, 1029–1039. [CrossRef] [PubMed]
131. Al Khudary, R.; Venkatachalam, R.; Katzer, M.; Elleuche, S.; Antranikian, G. A cold-adapted esterase of a novel marine isolate, *Pseudoalteromonas arctica*: Gene cloning, enzyme purification and characterization. *Extremophiles* **2010**, *14*, 273–285. [CrossRef] [PubMed]
132. De Santi, C.; Leiros, H.K.; Di Scala, A.; de Pascale, D.; Altermark, B.; Willassen, N.P. Biochemical characterization and structural analysis of a new cold-active and salt-tolerant esterase from the marine bacterium *Thalassospira* sp. *Extremophiles* **2016**, *20*, 323–336. [CrossRef]
133. Lemak, S.; Tchigvintsev, A.; Petit, P.; Flick, R.; Singer, A.U.; Brown, G.; Evdokimova, E.; Egorova, O.; Gonzalez, C.F.; Chernikova, T.N.; et al. Structure and activity of the cold-active and anion-activated carboxyl esterase OLEI01171 from the oil-degrading marine bacterium Oleispira antarctica. *Biochem. J.* **2012**, *445*, 193–203. [CrossRef]
134. D'Auria, S.; Aurilia, V.; Marabotti, A.; Gonnelli, M.; Strambini, G. Structure and dynamics of cold-adapted enzymes as investigated by phosphorescence spectroscopy and molecular dynamics studies. 2. The case of an esterase from *Pseudoalteromonas haloplanktis*. *J. Phys. Chem. B* **2009**, *113*, 13171–13178. [CrossRef]
135. Aurilia, V.; Parracino, A.; Saviano, M.; Rossi, M.; D'Auria, S. The psychrophilic bacterium *Pseudoalteromonas halosplanktis* TAC125 possesses a gene coding for a cold-adapted feruloyl esterase activity that shares homology with esterase enzymes from gamma-proteobacteria and yeast. *Gene* **2007**, *397*, 51–57. [CrossRef]
136. Cieslinski, H.; Bialkowska, A.M.; Dlugolecka, A.; Daroch, M.; Tkaczuk, K.L.; Kalinowska, H.; Kur, J.; Turkiewicz, M. A cold-adapted esterase from psychrotrophic *Pseudoalteromas* sp. strain 643A. *Arch. Microbiol.* **2007**, *188*, 27–36. [CrossRef]
137. De Santi, C.; Altermark, B.; Pierechod, M.M.; Ambrosino, L.; de Pascale, D.; Willassen, N.P. Characterization of a cold-active and salt tolerant esterase identified by functional screening of Arctic metagenomic libraries. *BMC Biochem.* **2016**, *17*, 1. [CrossRef] [PubMed]
138. Jeon, J.H.; Kim, J.T.; Kang, S.G.; Lee, J.H.; Kim, S.J. Characterization and its potential application of two esterases derived from the arctic sediment metagenome. *Mar. Biotechnol.* **2009**, *11*, 307–316. [CrossRef]
139. Kang, J.H.; Woo, J.H.; Kang, S.G.; Hwang, Y.O.; Kim, S.J. A cold-adapted epoxide hydrolase from a strict marine bacterium, Sphingophyxis alaskensis. *J. Microbiol. Biotechnol.* **2008**, *18*, 1445–1452. [PubMed]
140. Alterio, V.; Aurilia, V.; Romanelli, A.; Parracino, A.; Saviano, M.; D'Auria, S.; De Simone, G. Crystal structure of an S-formylglutathione hydrolase from *Pseudoalteromonas haloplanktis* TAC125. *Biopolymers* **2010**, *93*, 669–677. [CrossRef] [PubMed]

141. Lee, C.W.; Yoo, W.; Park, S.-H.; Le, L.T.H.L.; Jeong, C.-S.; Ryu, B.H.; Shin, S.C.; Kim, H.-W.; Park, H.; Kim, K.K.; et al. Structural and functional characterization of a novel cold-active S-formylglutathione hydrolase (SfSFGH) homolog from *Shewanella frigidimarina*, a psychrophilic bacterium. *Microb. Cell Fact.* **2019**, *18*, 140. [CrossRef] [PubMed]
142. Ramya, L.N.; Pulicherla, K.K. Molecular insights into cold active polygalacturonase enzyme for its potential application in food processing. *J. Food Sci. Technol.* **2015**, *52*, 5484–5496. [CrossRef] [PubMed]
143. Elleuche, S.; Qoura, F.M.; Lorenz, U.; Rehn, T.; Brück, T.; Antranikian, G. Cloning, expression and characterization of the recombinant cold-active type-I pullulanase from *Shewanella arctica*. *J. Mol. Catal. B Enzym.* **2015**, *116*, 70–77. [CrossRef]
144. Turkiewicz, M.; Pazgier, M.; Donachie, S.; Kalinowska, H. Invertase and a-glucosidase production by the endemic Antarctic marine yeast Leucosporidium antarcticum. *Pol. Polar Res.* **2005**, *26*, 125–136.
145. Violot, S.; Aghajari, N.; Czjzek, M.; Feller, G.; Sonan, G.K.; Gouet, P.; Gerday, C.; Haser, R.; Receveur-Brechot, V. Structure of a full length psychrophilic cellulase from *Pseudoalteromonas haloplanktis* revealed by X-ray diffraction and small angle X-ray scattering. *J. Mol. Biol.* **2005**, *348*, 1211–1224. [CrossRef]
146. Lonhienne, T.; Zoidakis, J.; Vorgias, C.E.; Feller, G.; Gerday, C.; Bouriotis, V. Modular structure, local flexibility and cold-activity of a novel chitobiase from a psychrophilic Antarctic bacterium. *J. Mol. Biol.* **2001**, *310*, 291–297. [CrossRef]
147. Rina, M.; Pozidis, C.; Mavromatis, K.; Tzanodaskalaki, M.; Kokkinidis, M.; Bouriotis, V. Alkaline phosphatase from the Antarctic strain TAB5. Properties and psychrophilic adaptations. *Eur. J. Biochem.* **2000**, *267*, 1230–1238. [CrossRef] [PubMed]
148. Koutsioulis, D.; Wang, E.; Tzanodaskalaki, M.; Nikiforaki, D.; Deli, A.; Feller, G.; Heikinheimo, P.; Bouriotis, V. Directed evolution on the cold adapted properties of TAB5 alkaline phosphatase. *Protein Eng. Des. Sel.* **2008**, *21*, 319–327. [CrossRef] [PubMed]
149. Available online: https://www.neb.com/products/m0289-antarctic-phosphatase#Product%20Information (accessed on 15 July 2019).
150. Tsuruta, H.; Mikami, B.; Higashi, T.; Aizono, Y. Crystal structure of cold-active alkaline phosphatase from the psychrophile *Shewanella* sp. *Biosci. Biotechnol. Biochem.* **2010**, *74*, 69–74. [CrossRef] [PubMed]
151. Available online: https://www.takarabio.com/products/cloning/modifying-enzymes/nucleases/cryonase-cold-active-nuclease (accessed on 15 July 2019).
152. Available online: https://arcticzymes.com/technology/hl-exol/ (accessed on 15 July 2019).
153. Wang, Y.; Hou, Y.; Nie, P.; Wang, Y.; Ren, X.; Wei, Q.; Wang, Q. A Novel Cold-Adapted and Salt-Tolerant RNase R from Antarctic Sea-Ice Bacterium *Psychrobacter* sp. ANT206. *Molecules* **2019**, *24*, 2229. [CrossRef] [PubMed]
154. Available online: https://international.neb.com/products/m0372-antarctic-thermolabile-udg#Product%20Information (accessed on 15 July 2019).
155. Tsigos, I.; Velonia, K.; Smonou, I.; Bouriotis, V. Purification and characterization of an alcohol dehydrogenase from the Antarctic psychrophile *Moraxella* sp. TAE123. *Eur. J. Biochem.* **1998**, *254*, 356–362. [CrossRef]
156. Galkin, A.; Kulakova, L.; Ashida, H.; Sawa, Y.; Esaki, N. Cold-adapted alanine dehydrogenases from two antarctic bacterial strains: Gene cloning, protein characterization, and comparison with mesophilic and thermophilic counterparts. *Appl. Environ. Microbiol.* **1999**, *65*, 4014–4020.
157. Wang, Y.; Hou, Y.; Wang, Y.; Zheng, L.; Xu, X.; Pan, K.; Li, R.; Wang, Q. A Novel Cold-Adapted Leucine Dehydrogenase from Antarctic Sea-Ice Bacterium *Pseudoalteromonas* sp. ANT178. *Mar. Drugs* **2018**, *16*, 359. [CrossRef] [PubMed]
158. Oikawa, T.; Yamamoto, N.; Shimoke, K.; Uesato, S.; Ikeuchi, T.; Fujioka, T. Purification, characterization, and overexpression of psychrophilic and thermolabile malate dehydrogenase of a novel antarctic psychrotolerant, Flavobacterium frigidimaris KUC-1. *Biosci. Biotechnol. Biochem.* **2005**, *69*, 2146–2154. [CrossRef]
159. Fedoy, A.E.; Yang, N.; Martinez, A.; Leiros, H.K.; Steen, I.H. Structural and functional properties of isocitrate dehydrogenase from the psychrophilic bacterium Desulfotalea psychrophila reveal a cold-active enzyme with an unusual high thermal stability. *J. Mol. Biol.* **2007**, *372*, 130–149. [CrossRef]
160. Yoneda, K.; Sakuraba, H.; Muraoka, I.; Oikawa, T.; Ohshima, T. Crystal structure of UDP-galactose 4-epimerase-like L-threonine dehydrogenase belonging to the intermediate short-chain dehydrogenase-reductase superfamily. *FEBS J.* **2010**, *277*, 5124–5132. [CrossRef]

161. Merlino, A.; Russo Krauss, I.; Castellano, I.; De Vendittis, E.; Rossi, B.; Conte, M.; Vergara, A.; Sica, F. Structure and flexibility in cold-adapted iron superoxide dismutases: The case of the enzyme isolated from *Pseudoalteromonas haloplanktis*. *J. Struct. Biol.* **2010**, *172*, 343–352. [CrossRef] [PubMed]
162. Zheng, Z.; Jiang, Y.H.; Miao, J.L.; Wang, Q.F.; Zhang, B.T.; Li, G.Y. Purification and characterization of a cold-active iron superoxide dismutase from a Psychrophilic Bacterium, *Marinomonas* sp. NJ522. *Biotechnol. Lett.* **2006**, *28*, 85–88. [CrossRef] [PubMed]
163. Wang, Q.F.; Wang, Y.F.; Hou, Y.H.; Shi, Y.L.; Han, H.; Miao, M.; Wu, Y.Y.; Liu, Y.P.; Yue, X.N.; Li, Y.J. Cloning, expression and biochemical characterization of recombinant superoxide dismutase from Antarctic psychrophilic bacterium *Pseudoalteromonas* sp. ANT506. *J. Basic Microbiol.* **2016**, *56*, 753–761. [CrossRef] [PubMed]
164. Na, J.; Im, H.; Lee, K. Expression and Purification of Recombinant Superoxide Dismutase (PaSOD) from Psychromonas arctica in *Escherichia coli*. *Bull. Korean Chem. Soc.* **2011**, *32*, 2405–2409. [CrossRef]
165. Kan, G.; Wen, H.; Wang, X.; Zhou, T.; Shi, C. Cloning and characterization of iron-superoxide dismutase in Antarctic yeast strain *Rhodotorula mucilaginosa* AN5. *J. Basic Microbiol.* **2017**, *57*, 680–690. [CrossRef] [PubMed]
166. Wang, W.; Sun, M.; Liu, W.; Zhang, B. Purification and characterization of a psychrophilic catalase from Antarctic *Bacillus*. *Can. J. Microbiol.* **2008**, *54*, 823–828. [CrossRef] [PubMed]
167. Sarmiento, F.; Peralta, R.; Blamey, J.M. Cold and Hot Extremozymes: Industrial Relevance and Current Trends. *Front. Bioeng. Biotechnol.* **2015**, *3*, 148. [CrossRef] [PubMed]
168. Ji, M.; Barnwell, C.V.; Grunden, A.M. Characterization of recombinant glutathione reductase from the psychrophilic Antarctic bacterium *Colwellia psychrerythraea*. *Extremophiles* **2015**, *19*, 863–874. [CrossRef] [PubMed]
169. Wang, Y.; Han, H.; Cui, B.; Hou, Y.; Wang, Y.; Wang, Q. A glutathione peroxidase from Antarctic psychrotrophic bacterium *Pseudoalteromonas* sp. ANT506: Cloning and heterologous expression of the gene and characterization of recombinant enzyme. *Bioengineered* **2017**, *8*, 742–749. [CrossRef]
170. Cotugno, R.; Rosaria Ruocco, M.; Marco, S.; Falasca, P.; Evangelista, G.; Raimo, G.; Chambery, A.; Di Maro, A.; Masullo, M.; De Vendittis, E. Differential cold-adaptation among protein components of the thioredoxin system in the psychrophilic eubacterium *Pseudoalteromonas haloplanktis* TAC 125. *Mol. BioSyst.* **2009**, *5*, 519–528. [CrossRef]
171. Wang, Q.; Hou, Y.; Shi, Y.; Han, X.; Chen, Q.; Hu, Z.; Liu, Y.; Li, Y. Cloning, expression, purification, and characterization of glutaredoxin from Antarctic sea-ice bacterium *Pseudoalteromonas* sp. AN178. *BioMed Res. Int.* **2014**, *2014*, 246871. [CrossRef] [PubMed]
172. Wang, Y.; Hou, Y.; Wang, Y.; Lu, Z.; Song, C.; Xu, Y.; Wei, N.; Wang, Q. Cloning, expression and enzymatic characteristics of a 2-Cys peroxiredoxin from Antarctic sea-ice bacterium *Psychrobacter* sp. ANT206. *Int. J. Biol. Macromol.* **2019**, *129*, 1047–1055. [CrossRef] [PubMed]
173. Birolo, L.; Tutino, M.L.; Fontanella, B.; Gerday, C.; Mainolfi, K.; Pascarella, S.; Sannia, G.; Vinci, F.; Marino, G. Aspartate aminotransferase from the Antarctic bacterium *Pseudoalteromonas haloplanktis* TAC 125. Cloning, expression, properties, and molecular modelling. *Eur. J. Biochem.* **2000**, *267*, 2790–2802. [CrossRef] [PubMed]
174. Shi, Y.; Wang, Q.; Hou, Y.; Hong, Y.; Han, X.; Yi, J.; Qu, J.; Lu, Y. Molecular cloning, expression and enzymatic characterization of glutathione S-transferase from Antarctic sea-ice bacteria *Pseudoalteromonas* sp. ANT506. *Microbiol. Res.* **2014**, *169*, 179–184. [CrossRef] [PubMed]
175. Angelaccio, S.; Florio, R.; Consalvi, V.; Festa, G.; Pascarella, S. Serine hydroxymethyltransferase from the cold adapted microorganism Psychromonas ingrahamii: A low temperature active enzyme with broad substrate specificity. *Int. J. Mol. Sci.* **2012**, *13*, 1314–1326. [CrossRef] [PubMed]
176. Albino, A.; Marco, S.; Di Maro, A.; Chambery, A.; Masullo, M.; De Vendittis, E. Characterization of a cold-adapted glutathione synthetase from the psychrophile *Pseudoalteromonas haloplanktis*. *Mol. BioSyst.* **2012**, *8*, 2405–2414. [CrossRef]
177. Georlette, D.; Jonsson, Z.O.; Van Petegem, F.; Chessa, J.; Van Beeumen, J.; Hubscher, U.; Gerday, C. A DNA ligase from the psychrophile *Pseudoalteromonas haloplanktis* gives insights into the adaptation of proteins to low temperatures. *Eur. J. Biochem.* **2000**, *267*, 3502–3512. [CrossRef] [PubMed]
178. De Luca, V.; Vullo, D.; Del Prete, S.; Carginale, V.; Osman, S.M.; AlOthman, Z.; Supuran, C.T.; Capasso, C. Cloning, characterization and anion inhibition studies of a gamma-carbonic anhydrase from the Antarctic bacterium *Colwellia psychrerythraea*. *Bioorg. Med. Chem.* **2016**, *24*, 835–840. [CrossRef] [PubMed]

179. De Luca, V.; Vullo, D.; Del Prete, S.; Carginale, V.; Scozzafava, A.; Osman, S.M.; AlOthman, Z.; Supuran, C.T.; Capasso, C. Cloning, characterization and anion inhibition studies of a new gamma-carbonic anhydrase from the Antarctic bacterium *Pseudoalteromonas haloplanktis*. *Bioorg. Med. Chem.* **2015**, *23*, 4405–4409. [CrossRef]
180. Angeli, A.; Del Prete, S.; Osman, S.M.; AlOthman, Z.; Donald, W.A.; Capasso, C.; Supuran, C.T. Activation Studies of the gamma-Carbonic Anhydrases from the Antarctic Marine Bacteria *Pseudoalteromonas haloplanktis* and *Colwellia psychrerythraea* with Amino Acids and Amines. *Mar. Drugs* **2019**, *17*, 238. [CrossRef]
181. Truong, L.V.; Tuyen, H.; Helmke, E.; Binh, L.T.; Schweder, T. Cloning of two pectate lyase genes from the marine Antarctic bacterium *Pseudoalteromonas haloplanktis* strain ANT/505 and characterization of the enzymes. *Extremophiles* **2001**, *5*, 35–44. [CrossRef] [PubMed]
182. Do, H.; Kim, S.J.; Lee, C.W.; Kim, H.W.; Park, H.H.; Kim, H.M.; Park, H.; Park, H.; Lee, J.H. Crystal structure of UbiX, an aromatic acid decarboxylase from the psychrophilic bacterium *Colwellia psychrerythraea* that undergoes FMN-induced conformational changes. *Sci. Rep.* **2015**, *5*, 8196. [CrossRef]
183. Do, H.; Lee, C.W.; Han, S.J.; Lee, S.G.; Kim, H.J.; Park, H.; Lee, J.H. Purification, crystallization and preliminary X-ray crystallographic studies of FMN-bound and FMN-free forms of aromatic acid decarboxylase (CpsUbiX) from the psychrophilic bacterium *Colwellia psychrerythraea* 34H. *Acta Crystallogr. Sect. F Struct. Biol. Commun.* **2014**, *70*, 215–220. [CrossRef] [PubMed]
184. Do, H.; Yun, J.S.; Lee, C.W.; Choi, Y.J.; Kim, H.Y.; Kim, Y.J.; Park, H.; Chang, J.H.; Lee, J.H. Crystal Structure and Comparative Sequence Analysis of GmhA from *Colwellia psychrerythraea* Strain 34H Provides Insight into Functional Similarity with DiaA. *Mol. Cells* **2015**, *38*, 1086–1095. [CrossRef] [PubMed]
185. See Too, W.C.; Few, L.L. Cloning of triose phosphate isomerase gene from an antarctic psychrophilic *Pseudomonas* sp. by degenerate and splinkerette PCR. *World J. Microbiol. Biotechnol.* **2010**, *26*, 1251–1259. [CrossRef] [PubMed]
186. Rentier-Delrue, F.; Mande, S.C.; Moyens, S.; Terpstra, P.; Mainfroid, V.; Goraj, K.; Lion, M.; Hol, W.G.; Martial, J.A. Cloning and overexpression of the triosephosphate isomerase genes from psychrophilic and thermophilic bacteria. Structural comparison of the predicted protein sequences. *J. Mol. Biol.* **1993**, *229*, 85–93. [CrossRef] [PubMed]
187. D'Amico, S.; Marx, J.C.; Gerday, C.; Feller, G. Activity-stability relationships in extremophilic enzymes. *J. Biol. Chem.* **2003**, *278*, 7891–7896. [CrossRef] [PubMed]
188. Tutino, M.L.; Duilio, A.; Moretti, M.A.; Sannia, G.; Marino, G. A rolling-circle plasmid from *Psychrobacter* sp. TA144: Evidence for a novel rep subfamily. *Biochem. Biophys. Res. Commun.* **2000**, *274*, 488–495. [CrossRef] [PubMed]
189. Kazuoka, T.; Takigawa, S.; Arakawa, N.; Hizukuri, Y.; Muraoka, I.; Oikawa, T.; Soda, K. Novel psychrophilic and thermolabile L-threonine dehydrogenase from psychrophilic *Cytophaga* sp. strain KUC-1. *J. Bacteriol.* **2003**, *185*, 4483–4489. [CrossRef]
190. Tutino, M.L.; Birolo, L.; Fontanella, B.; Mainolfi, K.; Vinci, F.; Sannia, G.; Marino, G. Aspartate aminotransferase from *Moraxella* TAC125: An unusual psychrophilic enzyme. In *Cold-Adapted Organisms*; Springer: Berlin/Heidelberg, Germany, 1999.
191. Adrio, J.L.; Demain, A.L. Microbial enzymes: Tools for biotechnological processes. *Biomolecules* **2014**, *4*, 117–139. [CrossRef]
192. Speciale, G.; Thompson, A.J.; Davies, G.J.; Williams, S.J. Dissecting conformational contributions to glycosidase catalysis and inhibition. *Curr. Opin. Struct. Biol.* **2014**, *28*, 1–13. [CrossRef] [PubMed]
193. Lombard, V.; Golaconda Ramulu, H.; Drula, E.; Coutinho, P.M.; Henrissat, B. The carbohydrate-active enzymes database (CAZy) in 2013. *Nucleic Acids Res.* **2014**, *42*, D490–D495. [CrossRef] [PubMed]
194. Dalmaso, G.Z.; Ferreira, D.; Vermelho, A.B. Marine extremophiles: A source of hydrolases for biotechnological applications. *Mar. Drugs* **2015**, *13*, 1925–1965. [CrossRef] [PubMed]
195. Shukla, T.P.; Wierzbicki, L.E. Beta-galactosidase technology: A solution to the lactose problem. *CRC Crit. Rev. Food Technol.* **1975**, *5*, 325–356. [CrossRef]
196. Karan, R.; Capes, M.D.; DasSarma, P.; DasSarma, S. Cloning, overexpression, purification, and characterization of a polyextremophilic beta-galactosidase from the Antarctic haloarchaeon Halorubrum lacusprofundi. *BMC Biotechnol.* **2013**, *13*, 3. [CrossRef]
197. Xu, K.; Tang, X.; Gai, Y.; Mehmood, M.; Xiao, X.; Wang, F. Molecular characterization of cold-inducible beta-galactosidase from *Arthrobacter* sp. ON14 isolated from Antarctica. *J. Microbiol. Biotechnol.* **2011**, *21*, 236–242. [PubMed]

198. Bialkowska, A.M.; Cieslinski, H.; Nowakowska, K.M.; Kur, J.; Turkiewicz, M. A new beta-galactosidase with a low temperature optimum isolated from the Antarctic *Arthrobacter* sp. 20B: Gene cloning, purification and characterization. *Arch. Microbiol.* **2009**, *191*, 825–835. [CrossRef]
199. Makowski, K.; Bialkowska, A.; Szczesna-Antczak, M.; Kalinowska, H.; Kur, J.; Cieslinski, H.; Turkiewicz, M. Immobilized preparation of cold-adapted and halotolerant Antarctic beta-galactosidase as a highly stable catalyst in lactose hydrolysis. *FEMS Microbiol. Ecol.* **2007**, *59*, 535–542. [CrossRef]
200. Van de Voorde, I. Evaluation of the cold-active *Pseudoalteromonas haloplanktis* β-galactosidase enzyme for lactose hydrolysis in whey permeate as primary step of d-tagatose production. *Process. Biochem.* **2014**, *49*, 2134–2140. [CrossRef]
201. Asghar, S.; Lee, C.R.; Park, J.S.; Chi, W.J.; Kang, D.K.; Hong, S.K. Identification and biochemical characterization of a novel cold-adapted 1,3-alpha-3,6-anhydro-L-galactosidase, Ahg786, from Gayadomonas joobiniege G7. *Appl. Microbiol. Biotechnol.* **2018**, *102*, 8855–8866. [CrossRef]
202. Roohi, R.; Kuddus, M.; Saima, S. Cold-active detergent-stable extracellular α-amylase from *Bacillus cereus* GA6: Biochemical characteristics and its perspectives in laundry detergent formulation. *J. Biochem. Technol.* **2013**, *4*, 636–644.
203. Qin, Y.; Huang, Z.; Liu, Z. A novel cold-active and salt-tolerant alpha-amylase from marine bacterium Zunongwangia profunda: Molecular cloning, heterologous expression and biochemical characterization. *Extremophiles* **2014**, *18*, 271–281. [CrossRef]
204. Dornez, E.; Verjans, P.; Arnaut, F.; Delcour, J.A.; Courtin, C.M. Use of psychrophilic xylanases provides insight into the xylanase functionality in bread making. *J. Agric. Food Chem.* **2011**, *59*, 9553–9562. [CrossRef]
205. Collins, T.; Meuwis, M.A.; Stals, I.; Claeyssens, M.; Feller, G.; Gerday, C. A novel family 8 xylanase, functional and physicochemical characterization. *J. Biol. Chem.* **2002**, *277*, 35133–35139. [CrossRef]
206. Lopez-Otin, C.; Bond, J.S. Proteases: Multifunctional enzymes in life and disease. *J. Biol. Chem.* **2008**, *283*, 30433–30437. [CrossRef]
207. Li, Q.; Yi, L.; Marek, P.; Iverson, B.L. Commercial proteases: Present and future. *FEBS Lett.* **2013**, *587*, 1155–1163. [CrossRef]
208. Vojcic, L.; Pitzler, C.; Korfer, G.; Jakob, F.; Ronny, M.; Maurer, K.H.; Schwaneberg, U. Advances in protease engineering for laundry detergents. *New Biotechnol.* **2015**, *32*, 629–634. [CrossRef]
209. Elleuche, S.; Schafers, C.; Blank, S.; Schroder, C.; Antranikian, G. Exploration of extremophiles for high temperature biotechnological processes. *Curr. Opin. Microbiol.* **2015**, *25*, 113–119. [CrossRef]
210. Kuddus, M.; Ramteke, P.W. Recent developments in production and biotechnological applications of cold-active microbial proteases. *Crit. Rev. Microbiol.* **2012**, *38*, 330–338. [CrossRef]
211. Tindbaek, N.; Svendsen, A.; Oestergaard, P.R.; Draborg, H. Engineering a substrate-specific cold-adapted subtilisin. *Protein Eng. Des. Sel.* **2004**, *17*, 149–156. [CrossRef]
212. Bialkowska, A.M.; Krysiak, J.; Florczak, T.; Szulczewska, K.M.; Wanarska, M.; Turkiewicz, M. The psychrotrophic yeast Sporobolomyces roseus LOCK 1119 as a source of a highly active aspartic protease for the in vitro production of antioxidant peptides. *Biotechnol. Appl. Biochem.* **2018**, *65*, 726–738. [CrossRef]
213. Kim, H.D.; Kim, S.M.; Choi, J.I. Purification, Characterization, and Cloning of a Cold-Adapted Protease from Antarctic Janthinobacterium lividum. *J. Microbiol. Biotechnol.* **2018**, *28*, 448–453. [CrossRef]
214. Craik, C.S.; Page, M.J.; Madison, E.L. Proteases as therapeutics. *Biochem. J.* **2011**, *435*, 1–16. [CrossRef]
215. Fornbacke, M.; Clarsund, M. Cold-adapted proteases as an emerging class of therapeutics. *Infect. Dis. Ther.* **2013**, *2*, 15–26. [CrossRef]
216. Jaeger, K.E.; Eggert, T. Lipases for biotechnology. *Curr. Opin. Biotechnol.* **2002**, *13*, 390–397. [CrossRef]
217. Joseph, B.; Ramteke, P.W.; Thomas, G. Cold active microbial lipases: Some hot issues and recent developments. *Biotechnol. Adv.* **2008**, *26*, 457–470. [CrossRef]
218. Gotor-Fernández, V.; Brieva, R.; Gotor, V. Lipases: Useful biocatalysts for the preparation of pharmaceuticals. *J. Mol. Catal. B Enzym.* **2006**, *40*, 111–120. [CrossRef]
219. Gotor-Fernández, V.; Busto, E.; Gotor, V. Candida antarctica Lipase B: An Ideal Biocatalyst for the Preparation of Nitrogenated Organic Compounds. *Adv. Synth. Catal.* **2006**, *348*, 797–812. [CrossRef]
220. Maharana, A.K.; Singh, S.M. A cold and organic solvent tolerant lipase produced by Antarctic strain *Rhodotorula* sp. Y-23. *J. Basic Microbiol.* **2018**, *58*, 331–342. [CrossRef]

221. Ramle, Z.; Rahim, R.A. Psychrophilic Lipase from Arctic Bacterium. *Trop. Life Sci. Res.* **2016**, *27*, 151–157. [CrossRef]
222. Arifin, A.R.; Kim, S.J.; Yim, J.H.; Suwanto, A.; Kim, H.K. Isolation and biochemical characterization of Bacillus pumilus lipases from the Antarctic. *J Microbiol. Biotechnol.* **2013**, *23*, 661–667. [CrossRef]
223. Florczak, T.; Daroch, M.; Wilkinson, M.C.; Bialkowska, A.; Bates, A.D.; Turkiewicz, M.; Iwanejko, L.A. Purification, characterisation and expression in Saccharomyces cerevisiae of LipG7 an enantioselective, cold-adapted lipase from the Antarctic filamentous fungus Geomyces sp. P7 with unusual thermostability characteristics. *Enzyme Microb. Technol.* **2013**, *53*, 18–24. [CrossRef]
224. Kumar, V.; Sinha, A.K.; Makkar, H.P.; De Boeck, G.; Becker, K. Phytate and phytase in fish nutrition. *J. Anim. Physiol. Anim. Nutr.* **2012**, *96*, 335–364. [CrossRef]
225. Rebello, S.; Jose, L.; Sindhu, R.; Aneesh, E.M. Molecular advancements in the development of thermostable phytases. *Appl. Microbiol. Biotechnol.* **2017**, *101*, 2677–2689. [CrossRef]
226. Park, I.; Cho, J. The phytase from antarctic bacterial isolate, *Pseudomonas* sp. JPK1 as a potential tool for animal agriculture to reduce manure phosphorus excretion. *Afr. J. Agric. Res.* **2011**, *6*, 1398–1406.
227. Awazu, N.; Shodai, T.; Takakura, H.; Kitagawa, M.; Mukai, H.; Kato, I. Microorganism-Derived Psychrophilic Endonuclease. U.S. Patent 8,034,597, 11 October 2011.
228. Thallinger, B.; Prasetyo, E.N.; Nyanhongo, G.S.; Guebitz, G.M. Antimicrobial enzymes: An emerging strategy to fight microbes and microbial biofilms. *Biotechnol. J.* **2013**, *8*, 97–109. [CrossRef]
229. See-Too, W.S.; Convey, P.; Pearce, D.A.; Chan, K.G. Characterization of a novel N-acylhomoserine lactonase, AidP, from Antarctic *Planococcus* sp. *Microb. Cell Fact.* **2018**, *17*, 179. [CrossRef]
230. Medigue, C.; Krin, E.; Pascal, G.; Barbe, V.; Bernsel, A.; Bertin, P.N.; Cheung, F.; Cruveiller, S.; D'Amico, S.; Duilio, A.; et al. Coping with cold: The genome of the versatile marine Antarctica bacterium *Pseudoalteromonas haloplanktis* TAC125. *Genome Res.* **2005**, *15*, 1325–1335. [CrossRef]
231. Methe, B.A.; Nelson, K.E.; Deming, J.W.; Momen, B.; Melamud, E.; Zhang, X.; Moult, J.; Madupu, R.; Nelson, W.C.; Dodson, R.J.; et al. The psychrophilic lifestyle as revealed by the genome sequence of *Colwellia psychrerythraea* 34H through genomic and proteomic analyses. *Proc. Natl. Acad. Sci. USA* **2005**, *102*, 10913–10918. [CrossRef]
232. Marizcurrena, J.J.; Morel, M.A.; Brana, V.; Morales, D.; Martinez-Lopez, W.; Castro-Sowinski, S. Searching for novel photolyases in UVC-resistant Antarctic bacteria. *Extremophiles* **2017**, *21*, 409–418. [CrossRef]

marine drugs

MDPI

Review

Deep Hypersaline Anoxic Basins as Untapped Reservoir of Polyextremophilic Prokaryotes of Biotechnological Interest

Stefano Varrella [1], Michael Tangherlini [2] and Cinzia Corinaldesi [1,*]

[1] Department of Materials, Environmental Sciences and Urban Planning, Polytechnic University of Marche, 60131 Ancona, Italy; s.varrella@univpm.it

[2] Stazione Zoologica Anton Dohrn, Villa Comunale, 80121 Napoli, Italy; michael.tangherlini@szn.it

* Correspondence: c.corinaldesi@univpm.it

Received: 28 November 2019; Accepted: 28 January 2020; Published: 30 January 2020

Abstract: Deep-sea hypersaline anoxic basins (DHABs) are considered to be among the most extreme ecosystems on our planet, allowing only the life of polyextremophilic organisms. DHABs' prokaryotes exhibit extraordinary metabolic capabilities, representing a hot topic for microbiologists and biotechnologists. These are a source of enzymes and new secondary metabolites with valuable applications in different biotechnological fields. Here, we review the current knowledge on prokaryotic diversity in DHABs, highlighting the biotechnological applications of identified taxa and isolated species. The discovery of new species and molecules from these ecosystems is expanding our understanding of life limits and is expected to have a strong impact on biotechnological applications.

Keywords: marine prokaryotes; microbial diversity; polyextremophiles; deep hypersaline anoxic basins; blue biotechnologies; extremozymes; polyextremophiles; limits of life

---

1. Introduction

Deep-sea ecosystems (waters and seabeds of the ocean beneath 200 m depth) are the largest, most remote, and least explored biomes of the biosphere, comprising more than two-thirds of the oceanic volume [1–3]. They are characterized by absence of light, an average depth of approximately 4200 m, temperatures below 4 °C, and a hydrostatic pressure of about 40 MPa; taken together, these factors encompass some of the harshest environments on our planet, representing a challenge for the existence of life [2]. Over the last few decades, many deep-sea surveys have resulted in the discovery of highly diversified and peculiar habitats [2,4–6], including hydrothermal vents, cold seeps, mud volcanoes, and deep hypersaline anoxic basins, where life conditions are even more extreme [7]. Among these, deep hypersaline anoxic basins (DHABs) are defined as polyextreme ecosystems [8,9].

DHABs were discovered at the end of the last century on the seafloor in different deep-sea areas (at depths ranging from 630 m to 3580 m) around the globe (Figure 1), including the Mediterranean Sea [10,11], the Red Sea [12–14] and the Gulf of Mexico [15]. Intriguingly, the discovery of new DHABs is still ongoing, such as with the recent discovery of the new Thetis, Kyros, and Haephestus basins in the Mediterranean Sea [16–18]. To date, with the recent finding of these new DHABs, 35 basins have been discovered around the world. The Bannock, Tyro, Urania, L'Atalante, and Discovery basins are the deepest known DHABs, being far below the photic zone (3200–3500 m deep), and are located along the Mediterranean Ridge in the Eastern Mediterranean Sea, an accretionary complex subjected to continental collision [19]. Two of the most studied DHABs in the Red Sea are the Shaban and the Kebrit deeps. The Shaban Deep comprises four depressions at a depth of 1325 m, whereas the Kebrit Deep is a rounded basin of approximately 1 km in diameter found at a depth of 1549 m [20].

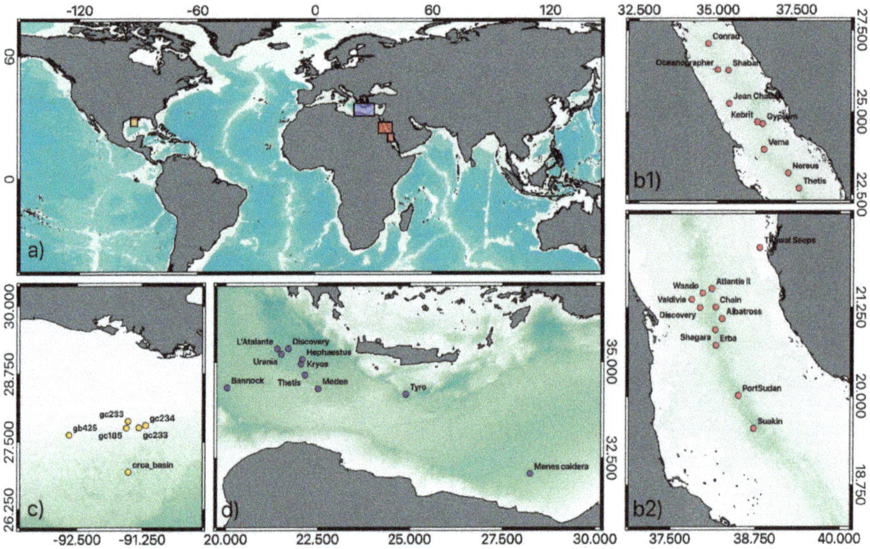

Figure 1. Global distribution of deep hypersaline anoxic basins (DHABs) (**a**). Locations and corresponding names of DHABs identified in the Red Sea (**b1–b2**), the Gulf of Mexico (**c**), and the Mediterranean Sea (**d**).

Different sampling strategies have been adopted to explore the general physical structure of DHABs. For instance, Mediterranean DHABs have been sampled through a rosette with Niskin bottles equipped with a conductivity, temperature, and depth (CTD) sensor and connected to a live camera to monitor the sampling operations [21–23]. Geochemical data of DHABs, such as those located in the Gulf of Mexico, have been collected through a brine-trapper, which was used to collect vertically water from different layers of the seawater–brine interface [24].

Despite the different geological features found in DHABs, most of them are derived from the re-dissolution of evaporitic minerals, like halite (NaCl-mineral) and kieserite ($MgSO_4$-mineral), after exposition to seawater due to tectonic activity [25,26]. This determines a salt-induced stratification of the water column (Figure 2), which drives the formation of a stable, dense, hypersaline brine lake with a variable thickness, ranging from one to tens of meters; this brine lake represents a polyextreme environment because its conditions hinder oxygen exchange, creating euxinic conditions, including high hydrostatic pressure, extremely low water activity and chaotropicity, and sharp oxy-, picno-, and chemoclines at the seawater–brine interface [21,23,27]. The salt concentration progressively increases over depth in the overlying halocline interface, reaching brines values up to 7–10 times higher than those existing in seawater [28].

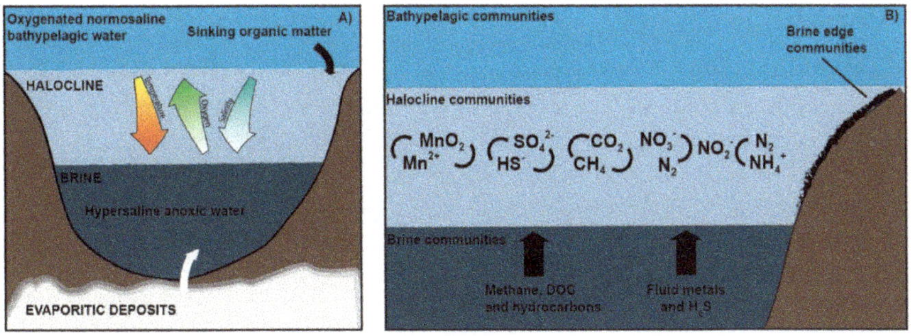

Figure 2. Simplified vertical section of a DHAB. The transition from the overlying seawater to the brine is commonly referred to as the halocline or brine–seawater interface, which is characterized by gradients of temperature, salinity, pH, and dissolved oxygen (**A**); the main biogeochemical processes taking place within the halocline are shown in (**B**). From left to right, the manganese cycle, the sulfate reduction and sulfide oxidation cycle, the methanogenesis and aerobic (anaerobic) methane oxidation cycle, and the anammox and denitrification cycle that occur in the halocline are shown [8,21,23,28–30]. DOC: Dissolved Organic Carbon.

Chemical and physical characteristics are specific to each DHAB and greatly vary depending on how the brine was formed along with the geographic localization (Table 1). The majority of the DHABs are thalassohaline (most of the dissolved ions are represented by those composing the overlaying seawater), whereas the Discovery, Kryos, and Hephaestus basins are athalassohaline and are characterized by high Mg^{2+} concentrations likely deriving from the dissolution of magnesium chloride salts (i.e., bischofite [18])

Table 1. Minimum and maximum values of the main physicochemical variables observed among DHABs.

Environmental Parameters	Ranges	DHABs	Location	References
Temperature	Min: 14 °C	La Medee	Mediterranean Sea	[31]
	Max: 68 °C	Atlantis II	Red Sea	[32]
Depth	Min 630 m	GC233	Gulf of Mexico	[33]
	Max: 3580 m	Discovery	Mediterranean Sea	[17]
Na^+	Min: 1751 mM	GC233	Gulf of Mexico	[24]
	Max 5300 mM	Tyro	Mediterranean Sea	[34]
Cl^-	Min: 2092 mM	GC233	Gulf of Mexico	[24]
	Max: 10,154.3 mM	Discovery	Mediterranean Sea	[17]
Mg^{2+}	Min: 8.7 mM	GB425	Gulf of Mexico	[24]
	Max: 5143 mM	Discovery	Mediterranean Sea	[17]
K^+	Min: 17.2 mM	Orca	Gulf of Mexico	[35]
	Max: 471 mM	La Medee	Mediterranean Sea	[31]
Ca^{2+}	Min: 1 mM	Discovery, Kyros	Mediterranean Sea	[17]
	Max: 150 mM	Atlantis II	Red Sea	[36]
SO_4^{2-}	Min: <1 mM	GB425; GC233	Gulf of Mexico	[24]
	Max: 333.1 mM	L'Atalante	Mediterranean Sea	[17]
Sulfide	Min: 0.002 mM	GC233	Gulf of Mexico	[24]
	Max: 16 mM	Urania	Mediterranean Sea	[16]

Overall, DHABs can be subdivided into four different systems: the seawater–brine interface, brines, the brine–sediment interface, and the sediments underlying the brines. Each of these features is characterized by specific conditions such as the steep halocline at the water–brine interface or the anoxic conditions of the sediments beneath the brines. In addition, the geochemical characteristics of each DHAB are mostly dependent on their geological evolution and origin. The high density of the brine prevents their mixing with the overlying oxygenated seawater, thus making the DHABs completely anoxic [16]. Their different hydrochemistry and physical separation for thousands of years has made these systems greatly interesting for scientists due to their potential similarity with extraterrestrial environments [18,34,37]. Despite their extreme conditions, many studies have provided evidence of a highly active prokaryotic community and of the presence of living metazoans, greatly extending our knowledge regarding the limits of organisms' adaptions to life [20,27,38–48]. These organisms require specific adaptations for withstanding numerous physicochemical stresses [49].

The complex structure and conditions of the DHABs, such as the presence of the steep halo- and oxyclines, have been found to influence the distribution, structure, and richness of the microbial communities living in these environments [19]. Many studies have been focused on the halocline, which entraps nutrients, sinking organic materials, minerals, and microbial cells, and creates environmental gradients of great interest not only for identifying and isolating novel organisms but also for clarifying their metabolic strategies employed for adapting to extreme conditions [19]. The variable accumulation of metals and nutrients, especially in the halocline, supports the presence of different ecological niches exploited by highly diverse microorganisms with peculiar features [38]. However, to date, our knowledge of how these organisms are affected and contribute to the geochemical properties of the DHABs is still limited.

The presence of life in these extreme environments has raised important questions about the molecular mechanisms that extremophiles have developed to overcome harsh conditions. Many studies have highlighted several peculiar adaptive strategies of halophilic microorganisms for maintaining stability and functionality of all their cellular components under such conditions [50,51]. Hence, microorganisms inhabiting extreme saline habitats not only have been considered useful subjects for ecological and evolutionary studies [50] but also hold an outstanding ability to produce bioactive molecules and enzymes, which can also be exploited for industrial and biotechnological purposes as well as for human wellness [52,53]. Considering the promising biotechnological potential of bacteria and archaea from DHABs due to their capability to live under extreme conditions, the present review provides an outline of the prokaryotic biodiversity in DHABs, highlighting their potential in producing enzymes and bioactive molecules for industrial, pharmaceutical, and environmental applications.

2. Prokaryotic Assemblages of DHABs

The specific characteristics and geochemical conditions of each DHAB have driven the development of different and highly-stratified communities. Brines and the seawater–brine interfaces, indeed, represent the most widely-studied domains within DHABs from both a taxonomic and ecological/functional point of view [21,23]. The halocline is a microbial "hotspot", harboring dense microbial populations that appear to be more metabolically active than those of the adjacent layers, with the presence of unique bacterial lineages having been found [21,22,44,54,55]. Several microbial lineages have been identified within DHAB brines. In particular, many members of the new Mediterranean Sea Brine Lake lineages (MSBL1–6) have been found extensively across hypersaline basins [56] from the Mediterranean to the Red Sea (despite their name), and include Archaea (e.g., MBSL1, which are sugar-fermenting organisms capable of autotrophic growth [23,56,57] and other major divisions of bacteria (MSBL2–6 [21,38]). Interestingly, the bacterial MSBL2 lineage has shown high similarity to the SB1 division found in the Shaban Deep brine pool, located in the Red Sea, which represents a novel halophilic lineage within bacteria, with no close cultivated relatives observed so far [28,38]. Similarly to the MBSL lineages, bacteria belonging to candidate division KB1 have been identified for the first time within the Kebrit Deep basin (Red Sea [20]) and subsequently have also been found in other DHABs of the Red Sea [58], as well as in other basins (e.g., the halocline of Mediterranean Sea brine pools and pools from the Gulf of Mexico [17,21,22,31,59]). Bacteria from this division can import and/or produce glycine betaine in response to osmotic stress [59]. The KB1 glycine betaine transport systems seem to aid not only in maintaining osmotic balance but also have a role in methane production [59]. Delta- and *Epsilonproteobacteria* are also widely distributed across DHABs. 16S rRNA gene libraries from the Bannock, Hephaestus, and L'Atalante basins (Mediterranean Sea) have provided evidence of the presence of sulfate-reducing *Deltaproteobacteria* (in particular belonging to the ANME-1 clade, responsible for the anaerobic oxidation of methane [16]) and sulfur-oxidizing Gamma- and *Epsilonproteobacteria* [21,22]. In the GC233 basin within the Gulf of Mexico, combining geochemical data and molecular analyses, different *Deltaproteobacteria* sulfate-reducers (related to *Desulfosarcinales, Desulfobacterium, Desulfobulbus*, and *Desulfocapsa*) and sulfide-oxidizing *Epsilonproteobacteria* have been found, leading to the hypothesizing of the presence of a sulfur-cycling microbial community [15,60].

Archaea associated with the ammonia-oxidizing *Thaumarchaeota* Marine Group I have also been found across several DHABs worldwide [18,21,22]. In particular, they have appeared to be the most representative prokaryotic members in different Red Sea DHABs, though with different contributions: in the Atlantis II and Discovery, 99% of archaeal operational taxonomic units (OTUs) were found to belong to the phylum *Thaumarchaeota*, whereas in the Erba basin the percentage was about 64% [30]. Members of this phylum are capable of fixing CO_2 and oxidizing methane, contributing to dark primary production [61]. Overall, the dominant thaumarchaeal lineage is closer to the genus Nitrosopumilus [62]. The adaptation of this genotype to the hostile brine–sediment interface environment can be possible not only by increasing intra-cellular salt concentrations [63] but also for the presence of "acidic tuned" membrane proteins which show optimal activity and stability at high salinity [64]. Furthermore, genomic analyses have revealed the presence of specific pathways for taking up a mixture of osmolytes and other genes encoding for the biosynthesis of ectoine/hydroxyectoine, which are not present in mesopelagic clades [30]. However, different DHAB geochemistry may shape other thaumarchaeal lineages. Genomic analyses have revealed a newly isolated methanogenic archeon from the sulfide-rich halocline of Kebrit, which holds adaptive traits (e.g., osmoprotection and oxidative stress response) for counteracting the harsh local conditions [65].

Apparently, as high salinity is one of the main features of DHABs, halophilic organisms have been found across all the basins, and most of the isolated halophilic strains also display interesting metabolic features. In particular, 33 halotolerant bacterial strains have been isolated from the halocline of the Urania, Bannock, Discovery, and L'Atalante basins [66]. For instance, *Halanaeroarchaeum sulfurireducens* M27-SA2 is a sulfur-reducing and acetate-oxidizing haloarcheon isolated from the Medee basin [67]. Moreover, several novel strains have been isolated from Red Sea DHABs, such as *Halorhabdus tiamatea* (a non-pigmented, fermenting member of the *Halobacteriaceae* [68]) and *Haloplasma contractile* (a highly unusual contractile bacterium belonging to the Haloplasmatales order, which can grow under 0.2–3.1 M NaCl conditions [69]. Two other strains of a novel species, *Marinobacter salsuginis* SD-14BT and SD-14C, have also been isolated from the halocline of the Shaban Deep [70].

In general, prokaryotic diversity and activity appear to be less marked in sediments under brines than in deep-sea control sediments [55]. This is likely due to the cumulative physico-chemical stressors that greatly limit the survival of microorganisms which could be better adapted to the extreme DHAB chemocline [27,55,71]. Proteobacteria, Actinobacteria, Deferribacteres, and Euryarchaeota have been found in sediments underlying either Discovery Deep or Atlantis II [72]. In the sediments of L'Atalante, OTUs belonging to the *Pseudoalteromonas, Halomonas*, and *Pseudomonas* genera have been observed to be the most represented within the abundant Gammaproteobacteria class, suggesting a mixed assemblage of halophilic and halotolerant microorganisms [55]. In addition, metatranscriptomic analyses have revealed that, in the sediments underlying the Urania basin, most transcripts are affiliated with rRNAs of the genera *Pseudomonas, Rhodobacter*, and *Clostridium*, and with sequences associated with mitomycin antibiotics typically produced by *Streptomyces* [71]. Prokaryotes inhabiting DHAB sediments are killed by viruses, which may represent the main mechanism of top-down control of prokaryotic dynamics in these ecosystems [42]. Since viruses are found to be well-preserved in DHAB sediments, they can shape prokaryotic assemblages [41]. Based on this information, it is possible to hypothesize that prokaryotes of DHABs can produce specific molecules against viral infections.

3. Biotechnological Potential of Prokaryotes Inhabiting DHABs

Generally, marine microorganisms represent an untapped source for the discovery and development of new biomolecules due to their rich biodiversity and genetic capacity to produce unique metabolites [73–75]. In this regard, it is well documented that many taxonomically novel marine species are promising sources of new bioactive compounds with noteworthy pharmaceutical activities, which can become sources of novel therapeutic agents [52,76]. In particular, marine extreme environments, like deep-sea and polar ecosystems or DHABs, have been revealed to be a rich source of secondary metabolites with novel structures and outstanding biological activities [28,52,77].

Due to the limited accessibility and remoteness of such extreme ecosystems and the need for sophisticated instruments for exploring and investigating them, they are still largely understudied and underexploited in comparison with terrestrial ecosystems.

Over the last few years, the advancement of technologies for deep-sea exploration [78] and "-omics" (e.g., environmental shotgun sequencing and metatranscriptomics) for the analysis of environmental strains of prokaryotes has revolutionized bioprospecting in extreme environments, thus increasing our knowledge of the genetic potential of microbial communities for the discovery of enzymes with a commercial value [79,80]. In addition, functional screening of extremophile metagenomes could represent a valuable approach to identify novel antibacterial and anticancer agents. In this regard, bioinformatic tools like the metabolite analysis shell (antiSMASH) have recently been used to detect from metagenomic samples collected from the Atlantis II, Discovery, and Kebrit DHABs promising specialized metabolism gene clusters (SMGCs) coding for products with reported antibacterial and anticancer effects, namely terpenes, peptides, polyketides, and phosphonates [81]. Two clones belonging to these libraries which exhibited antibacterial effects were screened by high-throughput sequencing (NGS) and bioinformatic analyses along with cytotoxicity assay (MTT) testing of the whole cell lysates against different cancer cell lines (MCF-7, U2OS, and 1BR-hTERT) [82]. Although culture-independent approaches have radically changed microbial bioprospecting in extreme environments, the development of biotechnological applications must be accompanied by the corresponding study of pure cultures. In this regard, despite the great biodiversity-highlighted trough metagenomics in DHABs, so far less than 100 bacterial strains (Figure 3, Table S1) have been isolated and cultured for testing their extracts in few biotechnological applications [66,83–85]. Bioinformatic analyses on the phylogeny of the 16s rDNA sequences of those cultured strains (carried out by aligning them on the SILVA database v132 on the ACT server [86]) showed that most of these prokaryotes are affiliated with Gammaproteobacteria and Bacilli; in addition, several sequences within the same database were found to be phylogenetically related to the cultured strains (Table S2), further suggesting that more prokaryotic strains with adaptations to polyextreme ecosystems with biotechnological potential might be found within the same clades of already-cultured strains. Novel sampling and cultivation methods should be developed as alternatives to overcome culture limitations, especially in extreme environments [87].

Since the beginning of the new millennium, a number of studies have indicated the beneficial roles of extremophilic marine prokaryotes, which are a relevant but still underexplored source of bioactive molecules of commercial significance [74,88,89]. Extremophiles undoubtedly show unique capabilities and adaptations which allow them to thrive in systems characterized by harsh environmental conditions [90]. In fact, polyextremophilic microorganisms utilize alternative metabolic pathways and adaptive mechanisms which have important applications in industrial and environmental fields [50]. Since these microorganisms live in a biologically competitive environment for space and nutrients, they have developed mechanisms of defence against competitors and predators for their own survival, synthesising secondary metabolites of great value in pharmaceutical and biotechnological applications [91,92]. The advances in genome sequencing of extremophilic microorganisms have allowed us to provide a comprehensive understanding of their applications [93–95]. Moreover, microbes with large genomes, usually inhabiting complex harsh environments, can produce a vast array of secondary metabolites [96,97].

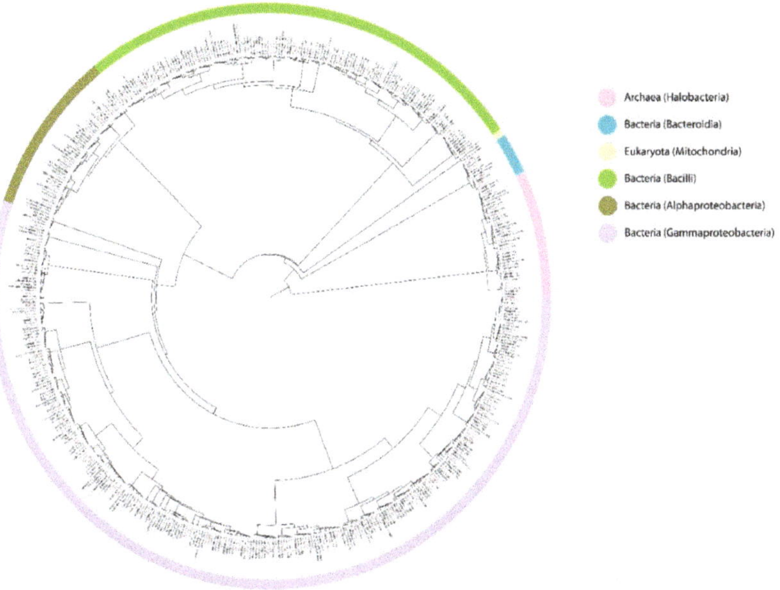

Figure 3. Phylogenetic tree of bacterial and archaeal strains isolated from DHABs. The tree was built using 16S rRNA gene sequences from [66,83–85] and phylogenetically close 16s rRNA sequences from the SILVA database v132.

3.1. DHABs as a Hidden Treasure for Biodiscovery of Pharmaceuticals

Over the last 50 years, the development of new multidrug-resistant pathogens, along with the consequent increase in infectious diseases, has become an important issue for human wellness [98]. Furthermore, anticancer chemotherapeutic resistance is recently becoming a biomedical challenge, arising either intrinsically or extrinsically, after therapy [99]. Thus, the need for the discovery and development of novel antimicrobial and chemotherapeutic drugs with new modes of action is nowadays becoming of fundamental importance [100,101]. Since most of the antibiotics currently available on the market have been extracted from terrestrial organisms or derived semisynthetically from fermentation products, the isolation of microorganisms from marine habitats represent an interesting possibility which can lead to the discovery of novel structures with antibiotic activity [102,103].

As such, the prokaryotic genera identified in DHABs isolated from different marine environmental sources, including extreme environments, represent an authentic treasure of many bioactive compounds useful for biomedical applications (Table 2).

Table 2. Bioactive molecules for pharmaceutical use produced by prokaryotes directly isolated from DHABs and promising bioactive molecules produced by prokaryotic taxa which have been identified in DHABs and isolated from other marine systems.

Marine Prokaryotes	Product	Bioactivity	Environmental Sources	Ref.
Alteromonas macleodii	Dithiolopyrrolone	Antibiotic and antitumor	Erba and Nereus DHABs	[84,104]
Alteromonas sp. B-10-31	Marinostatins B-1, C1, and C2	Serine protease inhibitor	Coastal seawater	[105]
Bacillus sp.	Macrolactins A–F	Cytotoxic, antimicrobial, antiviral	Deep sea	[106–109]
Bacillus halodurans	Enfuvirtide	Antiviral	Nereus DHAB	[84,110]
Bacillus MK-PNG-276A	Loloatins A–D	Antimicrobial	Great barrier reef	[111]
Bacillus sp.	Bogorol A	Antimicrobial	Seawater	[112]
Bacillus sp. CND-914	Halobacillin	Antitumor	Deep-sea sediments	[113]
Bacillus sp. MIX-62	Mixirins A–C	Antitumor		[114]
Bacteroidetes rapidithrix HC35	Ariakemicins A and B	Antimicrobial, cytotoxic	Sea mud	[115]
Erythrobacter sp.	Erythrazoles A and B Erythrolic acids A–E	Cytotoxic	Mangrove sediments	[116,117]
Halobacteroides lacunaris TB21	R-LPS	Immunomodulator	Thetis DHAB	[118]
Halomonas LOB-5	Loihichelins A–F	n.a.	Deep sea hydrothermal vents	[119]
Halomonas meridiana	n.a.	Antitumor	Nereus DHAB	[84]
Halomonas sp. GWS-BW-H8hM	3-(4′-Hydroxyphenyl)-4-phenylpyrrole-2,5-dicarboxylic acid (HPPD-1 and HPPD-2)	Cytotoxic	Seawater	[120]
Halomonas sp. GWS-BW-H8hM	2-Amino-6-hydroxyphenoxazin-3-one2-Amino-8-benzoyl-phenoxazin-3-one2-Amino-8-(4-hydroxybenzoyl)-6-hydroxyphenoxazin-3-one	Antimicrobial, cytotoxic	Seawater	[121]
Pseudoalteromonas carrageenovora IAM 12662	LPS	Antiviral	Erba DHAB	[84,122]
Pseudoalteromonas haloplanktis TAC125	Peptides	Antioxidant	Antarctic coastal sea water	[123]
Pseudoalteromonas mariniglutinosa	n.a.	Antitumor	Erba and Nereus DHABs	[84]
Pseudoalteromonas rava SANK 73390	Thiomarinols A–H and J	Antimicrobial	Seawater	[124,125]
Streptomyces aureoverticillatus (NPS001583)	Aureoverticillactam	Antitumor	Marine sediments	[126]
Streptomyces C42	Champacyclin	Antimicrobial	Deep sea	[127]
Streptomyces CNH-990	Marmycins A and B	Cytotoxic	Seawater	[128,129]
Streptomyces drozdowiczii SCSIO 10141	Marfomycins A, B, and E	Anti-infective	Deep sea	[130]
Streptomyces drozdowiczii NTK 97	Frigocyclinone	Antimicrobial	Antarctica	[131]
Streptomyces Merv 8102	Essramycin	Antimicrobial	Marine animals, plants, and sediments	[132]
Streptomyces niveus SCSIO 3406	Marfuraquinocins	Cytotoxic antimicrobial	Deep sea	[133]
Streptomyces scopuliridis SCSIO ZJ46	Desotamide B	Antimicrobial	Deep-sea sediments	[134]
Streptomyces sioyaensis SA-1758	Altemicidin	Cytotoxic, antimicrobial	Sea mud	[135]
Streptomyces sp. 12A35	Lobophorins H and I	Antimicrobial	Deep sea	[136]

Table 2. *Cont.*

Marine Prokaryotes	Product	Bioactivity	Environmental Sources	Ref.
Streptomyces sp. ART5	Articoside	Cytotoxic,	Arctic deep sea	[137]
Streptomyces sp. CNB-982	Cyclomarins A–C	anti-inflammatory	Marine sediments	[138, 139]
Streptomyces sp. CNQ-418	Marinopyrroles A–F	Antimicrobial, cytotoxic, anti-apoptotic	Deep-sea sediments	[140, 141]
Streptomyces sp. CNQ-85	Daryamides A–C (2E,4E)-7-Methylocta-2,4-dienoic acid amide 26	Antitumor, antifungal	Seawater	[142]
Streptomyces sp. CNR-698	Ammosamides A–D	Cytotoxic	Deep sea	[143–145]
Streptomyces sp. M045	Chinikomycins A and B	Antitumor	Seawater	[146]
Streptomyces sp. MDF-04-17-069	Tartrolon D	Cytotoxic	Marine sediments	[147]
Streptomyces sp. Mei37	Mansouramycins A–D	Antimicrobial, cytotoxic	Marine sediments	[148]
Streptomyces sp. NTK 935	Benzoxacystol	Antiproliferative	Deep sea	[149]
Streptomyces sp. SCSIO 03032	Spiroindimicins A–D	Antitumor	Deep sea	[150]
Streptomyces sp. SCSIO 11594	Dehydroxyaquayamycin, Marangucycline B	Antibacterial, antitumor	Deep sea	[151]
Streptomyces xiamenensis M1-94P	Xiamenmycin C and D	Anti-fibrotic	Deep-sea sediments	[152]
Streptomycete sp.	Piperazimycins A–C	Antitumor	Marine sediments	[153]
Zunongwangia profunda SM-A87	EPS	Antioxidant	Nereus DHAB	[154]

For instance, in Mediterranean DHABs transcripts related to *Streptomyces* have been identified, thus representing an important source of bioactive natural products with clinical or pharmaceutical applications [71,155]. Additionally, *Pseudoalteromonas flavipulchra* recently isolated from the Nereus halocline shows great antimicrobial activity which is associated with the different metabolites and/or enzymes that this species can produce [84,156,157].

An attractive example of the potential of extremophiles in the biomedical field has been provided by *Halobacteroides lacunaris* TB21, which was isolated from Thetis basin [118]. This polyextremophile organism produce a lipopolysaccharide (LPS) analog which can bind to the TLR4/MD-2 complex in HEK 293 hTLR4 cells, exerting an immunostimulant activity [118]. Additionally, *Pseudoalteromonas carrageenovora* isolated from Erba basin sediments is able to produce an LPS whose function is still undescribed [84,122]. This halophilic bacterium can also produce low molecular weight products from carrageenans, which have been reported to hold protective effects against the human immunodeficiency virus, the yellow fever virus, the herpes simplex viruses, the vaccine virus, and the pig fever virus [158]. Another interesting species isolated from the Nereus brine-pool–sea-water interface is *Bacillus halodurans,* which was engineered for the production of the anti-viral therapeutic peptide Enfuvirtide, marketed by Roche under the trademark Fuzeon®, which has given rise to possibilities for pharmaceutical applications [84,110]. In addition, *Zunongwangia profunda,* inhabiting the same interface, produces exopolysaccharides (EPS) with antioxidant properties [154].

Innovative research was carried out for screening the bioactivity of molecules extracted from the Atlantis II, Discovery, Kebrit, Nereus, and Erba DHABs [83,85]. Extracts from 36 isolates were tested on three different human cancer cell lines: HeLa, MCF-7, and DU145 [83,85]. In particular, many extracts from *Halomonas* strains have been found to induce apoptotic and cytotoxic effects. For example, *Halomonas meridiana* collected from Nereus halocline has been observed to prompt apoptosis of MCF-7 cells [85]. Recently, it was shown that the extract of *Pseudoalteromonas mariniglutinosa* collected from Erba and Nereus haloclines also inhibited the growth of MCF-7 cells [84]. *Halomonas* species can produce EPS which have been shown to have pro-apoptotic activity towards human T-leukemia cells and breast cancer MCF-7 cells [159,160]. Other bioactive extracts derived from *Chromohalobacter salexigens, Chromohalobacter israelensis, Halomonas meridiana,* and *Idiomarina loihiensis* have been found to be able to induce more than 70% mortality in HeLa cancer cells through different caspase-mediated apoptotic pathways [83].

Intriguingly, three extracts belonging to the genus *Salinivibrio* have been found to specifically blocked the growth of fibrosarcoma cells (HT-1080), opening up interesting perspectives for the discovery of new bioactive compounds produced by this genus [84]. The extracts of *Halomonas hamiltonii* and *Alcanivorax dieselolei* have been observed to inhibit the proliferation of BT20 cells, whereas the *Alteromonas macleodii* extracts collected from Nereus and Erba halocline were found to inhibit the cell growth of HCT [84]. *Alteromonas species* are also well known for producing dithiolopyrrolone, a potent antibiotic approved by the Food and Drug Administration and commercialized as Bactroban® (GlaxoSmithKline) [104]. These studies emphasize the wide diversity of brine pool microorganisms capable of producing bioactive molecules, highlighting the incredible potential of DHABs as a source of novel molecules exploitable in the pharmacological industry.

3.2. DHABs as a Reservoir of Polyextreme Enzymes

Today's society is moving toward "white" (i.e., industrial) biotechnology, which is growing for its efficiency from environmental and commercial points of view [161]. For example, natural enzyme catalysis has been utilized for application in a broader range of industrial settings, representing a valuable alternative to its chemical catalysts [162–164]. It is expected that 40% of the industrial application of chemical reactions that require organic solvents harmful to the environment will be replaced by enzymatic catalysis by 2030 [165]. The continuous demand for natural new enzymes that are biocompatible and non-toxic and which have high activity over a wide range of conditions, including temperature, salinity, pH, and metal concentrations, has been scaled up within pharmaceutical, food, and beverage industrial processes [166]. Hence, extremophilic microorganisms represent important sources of stable and valuable enzymes which are used as biocatalysts in industrial and biotechnological processes [53]. Enzymes from these organisms, which are called "extremozymes" due to their special features, can catalyze chemical reactions under conditions which inhibit or denature the non-extreme forms [167], including high salinity, acidic or basic pH, and high temperatures [168]. Thus, through the use of genetic engineering and/or by bioprospecting of extreme environments it is possible to discover and develop new extremozymes that can be suitable for many industrial processes [164]. Extremophilic bacteria and archaea produce enzymes which can be employed in industrial reactions using either directly living organisms or purified molecules, expanding the ranges of optimal enzyme performance and thus enabling biocatalysis under the enzymatically unfavourable conditions found in industrial processes [169]. Hence, the peculiar characteristics of extremophiles belonging to prokaryotic domains living in DHABs can represent a new source for exploitable enzymes for their capacity to operate under extreme conditions [170,171]. In fact, many of these molecules (e.g., aldehyde dehydrogenase, proteases, cellulases, esterases, ferredoxin oxidoreductase, agarase, amylases, κ-Carragenases, ketoreductases, and cyclodextrin glycosyltransferase) have been commercialized and have applications in different biotechnological areas with considerable benefits for many kinds of industries (Table 3). In particular, they are currently being employed in "red" biotechnology (i.e., biotechnology applied to pharmaceutical and medical fields). Other enzymes such as cellulase, chitinase, esterase, mercuric reductase, and β-glucosidases are exploited in "grey" (i.e., environmental) biotechnology while lipase is used in "blue" biotechnology, being applied to aquatic organisms and β-glucosidases and xylanase in biofuel production.

Table 3. DHAB microbiome as a source of polyextremozymes. The bacterial and archaeal species marked with an asterisk have been isolated from DHABs, whereas the other genera are potentially producers of extremozymes because these have identified from DHABs (but not cultured thus, being isolated from marine and/or other extreme environments).

Enzyme	Biological Source	Specific Adaptations	Function and/or Applications	Ref.
Aldehyde dehydrogenase (EC 1.2.1.3–7)	*Bacillus halodurans* from Nereus interface; Atlantis II Red Sea brine pool; Cytophaga sp. KUC-1 from Antarctic seawater and *Halobacterium salinarum*	Slight halophile; thermo- and psychrophilic	Biotransformation of a large number of drugs and other xenobiotics generates aldehydes as intermediates or as products resulting from oxidative deaminations	[172–175]
Protease (EC 3.4.21–25)	*Salinivibrio costicola** and *Pseudoalteromonas ruthenica** from Erba DHAB. *Bacillus circulans* BM15 and *PseudoAlteromonas sp.* 129-1. *Bacillus sp.* NPST-AK1, *Halobacterium halobium* (ATCC 43214), *Bacillus licheniformis*, *Bacillus halophilus*, *Pseudoalteromonas strain* EB27, *Halomonas meridiana* DSM 5425, *Bacillus sp.* (Ve2-20-91 (HM047794)), and *Bacillus caseinilyticus*	Haloalkaliphilic and thermotolerant alkaline	Protein hydrolysis finds a broad variety of potential applications in diverse biotechnological processes such as in the feed, food, pharmacology (anticancer and antihemolytic activity) and cosmetic (keratin-based preparation) industries, and cleaning processes (e.g., detergent additive)	[176–185]
Cellulase (EC 3.2.1.4)	Cytophaga hutchinsonii, Halorhabdus tiamatea from Shaban DHAB, *Bacillus sp.* SR22 from seawater, *Bacillus sp.*, *Vibrio sp.*, *Rhodococcus sp.*, *Clostridium* and *Streptomyces* from mangrove Halorhabdus utahensis from Great Salt Lake	Halo-alkali tolerant and thermotolerant	Breakdown of cellulose-producing polysaccharides; potential application in the food, animal feed, beer and wine, textile and laundry, and pulp and paper industries, agriculture, biofuel, pharmaceutical industries, and waste management	[186–191]
Chitinase (EC 3.2.1.14), chitin deacetylase (EC 3.5.1.41)	*Bacillus thuringiensis* HBK-51 from soil. *PseudoAlteromonas sp.* DC14, *Vibrio cholerae*, *Vibrio parahaemolyticus*, and *Arthrobacter sp.* AW19M34-1 from seawater	Halo-alkali tolerant and thermotolerant	Hydrolysis of chitin and hence N-acetyl chitobiose production which in turn can be useful in fermentation research and biomedicine. There have also been applications in the cosmetic and pharmaceutic fields	[192–194]
Esterase (EC 3.1.1.1)	*Zunongwangia profunda** from Atlantis II and Nereus interface and brine pools. *Alcanivorax dieselolei* B5(T) from Erba interface. *Bacillus cereus* AGP-03 from hot spring. *Archaeoglobus fulgidus*	Thermo-halotolerant and metal resistant; cold-active and organic solvent-tolerant	Leather manufacturing, flavor development in the dairy industry, oil biodegradation, and the synthesis of pharmaceuticals and chemicals	[195–200]
Ferredoxin oxidoreductase (EC 1.2.7.1)	*Halorhabdus tiamatea* SARL4BT* from Shaban DHAB. *Desulfovibrio sp.* from Atlantis II DHAB. Methanosarcina barkeri	Low-oxygen tolerant	Oxidation/reduction processes which are applied in the asymmetric oxyfunctionalization of steroids and other pharmaceuticals, synthesis and modification of polymers, oxidative degradation of pollutants, oxyfunctionalization of hydrocarbons, and the construction of biosensors for diverse clinical applications	[189,201,202]

Table 3. *Cont.*

Enzyme	Biological Source	Specific Adaptations	Function and/or Applications	Ref.
Lipase (EC 3.1.1.3)	Idiomarina sp. W33, Halo*Bacillus sp.*, and *Archaeoglobus fulgidus*. *Marinobacter alkaliphilus* ABN-IAUF-1. *Bacillus sp.*, *Arthrobacter sp.*, *Pseudomonas sp.*, and *Psychrobacter sp.* from Antarctic marine sediments. Oceano *Bacillus sp.* PUMB02 from seawater	Halo- alkalitolerant and hyperthermophilic	Hydrolysis of acylglycerols to release fatty acids and lower acylglycerols or glycerol. Lipase enzymes are exploited in the food, beverage, detergent, biofuel production, animal feed, textiles, leather, paper processing, and cosmetic industries	[203–208]
Mercuric reductase (EC 1.16.1.1)	Atlantis II deep-sea brine. *Chromohalobacter israelensis** from Erba and Atlantis II DHABs. *Bacillus firmus** from Discovery DHAB	Extreme halophilic and thermophilic	This enzyme can convert toxic mercury ions into relatively inert elemental mercury. It is very useful in waste-water treatments	[209,210]
Nitrilase (EC 3.5.5.1)	Red Sea Atlantis II brine	Thermostable and heavy metal tolerant	Nitrilase can hydrolyze a single cyano group in dinitriles or polynitriles, yelding cyanocarboxilic acids, which are used in different kinds of industries, including the food and pharmacology industries; also used for bioremediative purposes	[211]
Pullulanase (EC 3.2.1.41)	*Bacillus sp.* and *Streptomyces sp.*	Alkaliphilic	Utilized to hydrolyze the α-1,6 glucosidic linkages in starch, enabling a complete and efficient conversion of the branched polysaccharides into small fermentable sugars during the saccharification process	[212]
Xylanase (EC 3.2.1.8) and β-Xylosidase (EC 3.2.1.37)	*Staphylococcus sp.*, *Arthrobacter sp.*, *Streptomyces* sp., and *Vibrio sp.* XY-214 from seawater. Oceanospirillum linum CL8 and *Halorhabdus utahensis* from Great Salt Lake. *Halorhabdus tiamatea* SARL4BT* from Shaban DHAB. *Pseudoalteromonas mariniglutinosa** from Erba and Nereus DHAB. *Marinimicrobium haloxylanilyticum** from Kebrit DHAB. *Zunongwangia profunda** from Nereus and Atlantis II DHABs. *Halomonas meridiana** from Bannock, Erba, and Nereus DHABs. *Bacillus halodurans** from Nereus interface	Alkali-halotolerant and psychrophilic	Commercial exploitation in the areas of the food, feed, and paper and pulp industries; also used to increase sugar recovery from agricultural residues for biofuel production	[189,213–218]
α-agarase (EC 3.2.1.158) and β-agarase (EC 3.2.1.81)	*Alteromonas macleodii** from Erba, Discovery, and Nereus DHABs. *Alteromonas sp.* GNUM-1, *Alteromonas agarlyticus*, *Alteromonas sp.* strain C-1, *Vibrio sp.* PO-303, *Altermonas sp.* SY37-12, and Cytophaga flevensis from seawater and marine sediments	Moderate halophile	Degradation of agar-degrading bacteria used as oriental food; wide applications in the food industry, cosmetics, and medical fields, and as a tool enzyme for biological, physiological, and cytological studies	[219–221]

Table 3. *Cont.*

Enzyme	Biological Source	Specific Adaptations	Function and/or Applications	Ref.
α-amylase (EC 3.2.1.1)	*PontiBacillus chungwhensis** from Discovery DHAB. Halomonas meridiana* from Nereus, Erba, and Bannock DHABs. *Zunongwangia profunda** from Atlantis II and Nereus DHABs. *Cytophaga sp. HaloBacillus sp.*, *Bacillus sp.* GM8901, *Bacillus sp.* TSCVKK, and *Methanococcus jannaschii. Halobacterium sp.* from hypersaline environment. *Alteromonas haloplanctis* from Antarctic seawater	Moderate halophile and alkali- tolerant; hyperthermophilic	α-amylase has implications in the food, pharmaceutical, and chemical industries; multifunctional amylase exhibits transglycosylation and hydrolysis activities to produce isomaltooligosaccharides, maltooligosaccharides and glucose	[222–232]
β-glucosidases (EC 3.2.1.21)	*Halorhabdus tiamatea* SARL4BT* from Shaban DHAB. *Alteromonas sp.* L82 from the Mariana Trench. Cytophaga hutchinsonii	Low-oxygen tolerant, cold-adapted, and salt-tolerant	β-glucosidases convert cellobiose and short cellodextrins into glucose. β-glucosidases are widely used in the production of biofuels and ethanol from cellulosic agricultural wastes, in the production of wine, and in the flavor industry. They can cleave phenolic and phytoestrogen glucosides from fruits and vegetables for extracting medicinally important compounds and enhancing the quality of beverages	[189,191,233,234]
κ-Carragenases (EC 3.2.1.83)	*Pseudoalteromonas carrageenovora** from Erba sediments. *Bacillus sp. Alteronomonas sp.*, Cytophaga sp., and *PseudoAlteromonas sp. Pseudomonas sp.*, *Vibrio sp.* NJ-2, and *Vibrio parahaemolyticus* from seawater	Alkali-halotolerant	Production of oligosaccharides with potential applications in the biomedical field, in bioethanol production, in the textile industry, and as a detergent additive	[235–237]
Cyclodextrin glycosyltransferase (EC 2.4.1.19)	Bacillus lehensis* from Discovery DHAB	Alkali-halotolerant	Cyclodextrins produced by this enzyme have broad, non-toxic applications in the pharmaceutical, cosmetic, and food industries	[66,238]

For instance, the production of novel thermoactive and alkali-tolerant α-amylases has been documented for many prokaryotic species such as *Pontibacillus chungwhensis, Halomonas meridiana*, and *Zunongwangia profunda* isolated taxa from DHABs. This group of enzymes has a very wide spectrum of industrial application, including in the sugar production, animal nutrition, baking, brewing, and distilling industries, in the production of digestive aids, in the pharmaceutical industries, and in the production of biofuel [239]. Amylases are consistently the most important among the enzymes of industrial interest and are forecasted to reach US$ 6.2 billion by 2020 [240]. For this reason, there is noteworthy attention paid to extremophilic α-amylases that have activity and stability characteristics suitable for the harsh conditions, including extreme salinity (2–4 M NaCl) and elevated temperature (80°C), demanded by industrial activities [241].

Interestingly, nitrilases have also been identified in DHABs, and are employed as commercial biocatalysts for the synthesis of plastics, paints, and fibers in the chemical industries and are also employed in the pharmaceutical industries for the manufacturing of (S)-ibuprofen, a widely used non-steroidal anti-inflammatory drug [242]. Moreover, nitrilases can detoxify cyanide present within wastes and degrade herbicides, representing an enzyme of extreme importance in bioremediation [243]. Biotransformation using native organisms as catalysts tends to be insufficient because the amount of nitrilases present as total cellular proteins is very low, and the reaction rate is slow and unstable [244]. Thus, the nitrilase recently identified by metagenomes mining in the Atlantis II DHAB could represent a valuable alternative not only for its thermal stability and tolerance to heavy metals compared to closely related nitrilases but also for the great number of microorganisms which could possess and produce these enzymes [211]. Another example of utilising sequence-based and activity-based metagenomics in mining for potential industrial biocatalysts is the esterase EstATII collected from the Atlantis II basin in the Red Sea, which displays a combination of extremophilic properties [197]. This enzyme is thermophilic (optimum temperature 65 °C) and halotolerant (for up to 4.5M NaCl) and maintains significant activity in the presence of a wide variety of toxic heavy metals, making it a potentially useful biocatalyst [197]. In agreement with this study, O.16 esterase was identified in the Urania basin which shoswed remarkable polyextremophilic properties (i.e., 180× enhanced activity at 2 to 4 M NaCl and functioning at 40 MPa [198]). This enzyme also displayed increased activity when dissolved in 70% ethanol or n-propanol and extraordinarily high enantioselectivity in hydrolysis and transesterification of compounds important in the pharmaceutical, cosmetic, and food industries [198,245]. Thus, DHABs seem to be a suitable habitat for mining esterases which are potentially useful for industrial biotransformation, considering the great size of the lipolytic enzyme market, which is valued at the billion-dollar mark in the world's market [246].

A study conducted on bacterial strains isolated from haloclines of Urania, Bannock, Discovery, and L'Atalante showed that *Bacillus horneckiae* gave highly stereoselective reduction for racemic propyl ester of anti-2- oxotricyclo[2.2.1.0]heptan-7-carboxylic acid (R,S)-1, a key intermediate of the synthesis of D-cloprostenol (chemical analog of prostaglandin [66]). Another isolate of *Halomonas aquamarina* was found to enantioselectively hydrolyze this molecule, indicating the potential of DHAB extremophile microbiome and marine-derived esterases and ketoreductases in stereoselective biocatalysis [66]. The same authors also isolated *Bacillus lehensis* from Discovery DHABs which harness an alkali-tolerant cyclodextrin glycosyltransferase and are able to produce non-toxic products for the pharmaceutical, cosmetic, and food industries.

Overall, DHABs seem to be a suitable habitat for mining novel biocatalyst enzymes which are potentially useful for industrial biotransformations, encouraging further scientific challenges and research for fully realising the potential of DHAB extremozymes.

3.3. DHAB-Derived Prokaryotes: Promising Candidates for Enhanced Bioremediation of Oil Hydrocarbons

Petroleum hydrocarbons are among the most widespread pollutants on our planet and are becoming a severe problem because of their causing harmful damage to the environment and human health [247,248]. Oil pollution can occur in the environment following either catastrophic accidents (shipping disasters or pipeline failures) or natural oil seepages and biota [249]. Such contaminants can exert carcinogenic, neurotoxic, and mutagenic effects when organisms are exposed to them, significantly impacting the environment [250–252]. For these reasons, many innovative technologies have been developed for the clean-up of oil-polluted areas [247]. One of the most reliable of these is certainly bioremediation, which exploits the metabolic capabilities of microorganisms to break down recalcitrant hydrocarbons into harmless by-products, thus minimising the impact on the environment [253]. It is a more environmentally friendly alternative when compared with classical remediation techniques, which allow the reduction from the environment of a vast array of pollutants [254].

Most petroleum hydrocarbons encountered in the environment can be degraded or metabolized by indigenous bacteria which have developed specific pathways for sustaining their energetic and carbon requirements for living and blooming in the presence of these contaminants [255,256]. Indeed, many studies have focused their attention on hydrocarbon-degrading bacteria in oil-rich environments, including oil spill areas and oil reservoirs [257], and have demonstrated that their abundance is closely related to the respective types of petroleum hydrocarbons and surrounding environmental factors [258–261]. Despite this, many other normal and extreme microorganisms have been isolated and employed as biodegraders for dealing with petroleum hydrocarbons, representing a promising biotechnological alternative for achieving oil-hydrocarbon degradation [9,262]. Because of the particular physiological characteristics of microorganisms isolated from extreme environments, including DHABs, prokaryotes can be employed for enhanced bioremediation of oil hydrocarbons, especially in hypersaline environments [263,264]. For instance, members of the genera *Alcanivorax* and *Marinobacter,* which have been isolated respectively from Erba halocline and Shaban Deep [70,84], are essential marine hydrocarbonoclastic bacteria present in the active phase of oil spills, playing a significant role in the natural remediation of oil-polluted marine environments all over the world [265–267]. Their number increases very quickly after oil spills, although it declines only a few weeks later (see [268] as well as references therein). The outstanding bioremediation capacity of *A. dieselolei* has also been supported by sequencing the genome of the strain KS-293 isolated from surface seawater [269]. Its genome consistently contains multiple genes and enzymes involved in pathways associated with hydrocarbon degradation (linear and branched alkanes) and shows high similarity with *A. dieselolei* strain B5 [270–272]. This strain has been observed to preserve cell integrity under pressures of up to 10 MPa cultured with n-dodecane as a sole carbon source, downregulating 95% of its genes [273,274]. Additionally, Sass et al., 2008 demonstrated that the strain DS-1, closely related to *Bacillus aquimaris,* isolated from the Discovery DHAB, could grow with n-alkanes (n-dodecane and n-hexadecane) in the presence of 12–20% NaCl [275]. Furthermore, *Salinisphaera shabanensis* and *Marinobacter salsuginis* have been isolated from the Shaban Deep, displaying a high capacity to assimilate aliphatic hydrocarbons [70,276]. *S. shabanensis* can be cultured at a wide range of salinity and temperatures (0.2–4.8 M NaCl and 5–42 °C), on a vast array of substrates including n-alkanes (dodecane). *M. salsuginis* is a heterotrophic, facultative anaerobic bacterium capable of fermentation and nitrate reduction [70].

Moreover, other bacteria belonging to the genus *Marinobacteria* and isolated from seawater and Nereus halocline have shown to be efficient for bioremediation purposes for degrading hydrocarbons, including polycyclic aromatic hydrocarbons (PAHs), as revealed by the complete genome sequence of *Marinobacter flavimaris* SW-145 [277–280]. Other strains belonging to the genera *Vibrio, Pseudomonas, Arthrobacter Pseudoalteromonas, Idiomarina, Halomonas,* and *Thalassospira* identified in different DHABs have been collected and cultured from marine sediments and are able to grow on PAHs including naphthalene, dibenzothiophene, pyrene, and phenanthrene [21,39,267,281,282].

Even though many oil hydrocarbons can be easily degraded in low salinity marine habitats [267], very little is known about their fate in moderate and in hypersaline environments where microbial activity is enormously inhibited [263,283]. To this purpose, some archaea belonging to the class of *Halobacteria* identified in many DHABs hold great promise and have considerable potential to bioremediate hydrocarbons in high salty environments such as nearshore oil production sites, salt marshes, sabkhas, and other coastal flats, including industrial wastewaters [264,284].

Haloarchaea of the class Halobacteria identified in many DHABs located both in the Mediterranean and the Red Sea [17,44,56,189] can produce PAH-degrading enzymes, which may be exploited to remove aromatic hydrocarbons from the polluted environments safely [285]. In the hypersaline coastal areas of Kuwait, hydrocarbonoclastic haloarchaea, together with *M. flavimaris,* a diazotrophic strain able to grow under 1 M–3.5 M NaCl conditions, have effectively contributed to oil bioremediation [286].

Although more archaeal strains have been isolated, our information on the physiological, biochemical, and genomic basis of hydrocarbon degradation by members of the *Halobacteria* is still extremely scant [263,287]. Such information is crucial for designing novel and more efficient technologies employing haloarchaea for the remediation of contaminated high salinity environments.

4. Conclusions and Future Directions

Polyextremophilic bacteria and archaea are an extraordinary reservoir of novel enzymes and bioactive molecules which can provide important benefits for different biotechnological applications, ranging from medicine to environmental fields. So far, studies on DHABs are limited, and we urgently need to expand data on microbial diversity and ecology of these extreme ecosystems. The uniqueness of these habitats is able to select for highly specialized organisms which show extreme adaptions at morphological, physiological, biochemical, and genetic levels, hinting at a bright future for "blue" biotechnology. In this extensive literature review we have observed that polyextremophiles maintain several high metabolic similarities to other non-extreme prokaryotes. This important issue, which remains to be further investigated, could open new research perspectives on the production of the biomolecules' portfolio of marine microorganisms. Such explorations are expected to provide huge rewards not only in terms of the impact on existing industries for the discovery of new products with beneficial or useful properties, but also in the "blue" economy. This scenario is also perfectly framed within the Sustainable Development Goals of the United Nations, which aims to identify actual solutions for disease outbreaks, climate change, and environmental degradation in order to have safer, cleaner, and more efficient industrial manufacturing processes in order to improve human health and wellbeing from a sustainable development perspective.

Nowadays, "blue" biotechnologies are taking advantage of increasing numbers of "-omics" tools and high-throughput screenings for unveiling the chemical diversity of the extreme environments present in the oceans. These tools are facilitating the identification of prokaryotic metabolic adaptations, which can lead to the production of novel molecules and thus can be exploited for the development of new biotechnologies. To date, novel uncultured species identified in DHABs of the genera *Streptomyces*, *Pseuodalteromonas*, and *Bacillus* seem to hold great potential in producing new bioactive molecules. Among the culturable species identified in DHABs, *Chromohalobacter israelensis, Zunongwangia profunda, Marinobacter flavimaris, Alcanivorax dieselolei, Halomonas meridiana, Alteromonas macleodii,* and *Bacillus halodurans* are promising species for biotechnological applications. Further innovative technologies and studies applied to DHABs will be essential to carry out in-depth investigations and to disentangle microbial assemblages, functions, and metabolites of biotechnological interest from these peculiar systems. Thus, the actual development of DHAB-derived biotechnologies will depend on technological and methodological advancements and the ability of scientists to promote research projects for the study of these ecosystems.

Supplementary Materials: The following information is available online at http://www.mdpi.com/1660-3397/18/2/91/s1, Table S1: Prokaryotic strains isolated from DHABs, Table S2: Prokaryotic strains isolated from DHABs and their closest relatives obtained from phylogenetic analyses.

Author Contributions: C.C. conceived the study. S.V. conducted literature analysis and M.T. performed bioinformatic analyses on the available data. C.C., S.V., and M.T. contributed to data interpretation. S.V., C.C., and M.T. wrote the manuscript. All authors have read and agreed to the published version of the manuscript.

Funding: This research was funded by University Scientific Research, the Italian Ministry for Education, University, and Research (MIUR).

Conflicts of Interest: The authors declare that they have no conflict of interest.

References

1. Danovaro, R.; Corinaldesi, C.; Dell'Anno, A.; Snelgrove, P.V.R. The deep-sea under global change. *Curr. Biol.* **2017**, *27*, R461–R465. [CrossRef] [PubMed]
2. Danovaro, R.; Snelgrove, P.V.R.; Tyler, P. Challenging the paradigms of deep-sea ecology. *Trends Ecol. Evol.* **2014**, *29*, 465–475. [CrossRef] [PubMed]
3. Herring, P.J. *The biology of the deep ocean*; Oxford University Press: New York, NY, USA, 2001; pp. 1–25.
4. Bartlett, D.H. Microbial Life in the Trenches. *Mar. Technol. Soc. J.* **2009**, *43*, 128–131. [CrossRef]
5. Jørgensen, B.B.; Boetius, A. Feast and famine - Microbial life in the deep-sea bed. *Nat. Rev. Microbiol.* **2007**, *5*, 770–781. [CrossRef]
6. Ramirez-Llodra, E.; Brandt, A.; Danovaro, R.; De Mol, B.; Escobar, E.; German, C.R.; Levin, L.A.; Martinez Arbizu, P.; Menot, L.; Buhl-Mortensen, P.; et al. Deep, diverse and definitely different: Unique attributes of the world's largest ecosystem. *Biogeosciences* **2010**, *7*, 2851–2899. [CrossRef]
7. Merino, N.; Aronson, H.S.; Bojanova, D.P.; Feyhl-Buska, J.; Wong, M.L.; Zhang, S.; Giovannelli, D. Living at the extremes: Extremophiles and the limits of life in a planetary context. *Front. Microbiol.* **2019**, *10*, 1–25. [CrossRef]
8. Merlino, G.; Barozzi, A.; Michoud, G.; Ngugi, D.K.; Daffonchio, D. Microbial ecology of deep-sea hypersaline anoxic basins. *FEMS Microbiol. Ecol.* **2018**, *94*, 1–15. [CrossRef]
9. Barone, G.; Varrella, S.; Tangherlini, M.; Rastelli, E.; Dell'Anno, A.; Danovaro, R.; Corinaldesi, C. Marine Fungi: Biotechnological Perspectives from Deep-Hypersaline Anoxic Basins. *Diversity* **2019**, *11*, 113. [CrossRef]
10. Jongsma, D.; Fortuin, A.R.; Huson, W.; Troelstra, S.R.; Klaver, G.T.; Peters, J.M.; Van Harten, D.; De Lange, G.J.; Ten Haven, L. Discovery of an anoxic basin within the strabo trench, eastern mediterranean. *Nature* **1983**, *305*, 795–797. [CrossRef]
11. Camerlenghi, A. Anoxic basins of the eastern Mediterranean: Geological framework. *Mar. Chem.* **1990**, *31*, 1–19. [CrossRef]
12. Hartmann, M.; Scholten, J.C.; Stoffers, P.; Wehner, F. Hydrographic structure of brine-filled deeps in the Red Sea - new results from the Shaban, Kebrit, Atlantis II, and Discovery Deep. *Mar. Geol.* **1998**, *144*, 311–330. [CrossRef]
13. Pautot, G.; Guennoc, P.; Coutelle, A.; Lyberis, N. Discovery of a large brine deep in the northern Red Sea. *Nature* **1984**, *310*, 133–136. [CrossRef]
14. Backer, H.; Schoell, M. New Deeps with Brines and Metalliferous Sediments in the Red Sea. *Nat. Phys. Sci.* **1972**, *240*, 153–158. [CrossRef]
15. Shokes, R.F.; Trabant, P.K.; Presley, B.J.; Reid, D.F. Anoxic, hypersaline basin in the northern Gulf of Mexico. *Science* **1977**, *4297*, 1443–1446. [CrossRef] [PubMed]
16. La Cono, V.; Smedile, F.; Bortoluzzi, G.; Arcadi, E.; Maimone, G.; Messina, E.; Borghini, M.; Oliveri, E.; Mazzola, S.; L'Haridon, S.; et al. Unveiling microbial life in new deep-sea hypersaline Lake Thetis. Part I: Prokaryotes and environmental settings. *Environ. Microbiol.* **2011**, *13*, 2250–2268. [CrossRef] [PubMed]
17. Yakimov, M.M.; La Cono, V.; Spada, G.L.; Bortoluzzi, G.; Messina, E.; Smedile, F.; Arcadi, E.; Borghini, M.; Ferrer, M.; Schmitt-Kopplin, P.; et al. Microbial community of the deep-sea brine Lake Kryos seawater-brine interface is active below the chaotropicity limit of life as revealed by recovery of mRNA. *Environ. Microbiol.* **2015**, *17*, 364–382. [CrossRef]
18. La Cono, V.; Bortoluzzi, G.; Messina, E.; La Spada, G.; Smedile, F.; Giuliano, L.; Borghini, M.; Stumpp, C.; Schmitt-Kopplin, P.; Harir, M.; et al. The discovery of Lake Hephaestus, the youngest athalassohaline deep-sea formation on Earth. *Sci. Rep.* **2019**, *9*, 1679. [CrossRef]
19. Mapelli, F.; Barozzi, A.; Michoud, G.; Merlino, G.; Crotti, E.; Borin, S.; Daffonchio, D. An updated view of the microbial diversity in deep hypersaline anoxic basins. In *Adaption of Microbial Life to Environmental Extremes*; Stan-Lotter, H., Fendrihan, S., Eds.; Springer International Publishing: Cham, Switzerland, 2017; pp. 23–40. ISBN 9783319483276.
20. Eder, W.; Ludwig, W.; Huber, R. Novel 16S rRNA gene sequences retrieved from highly saline brine sediments of Kebrit Deep, Red Sea. *Arch. Microbiol.* **1999**, *172*, 213–218. [CrossRef]
21. Daffonchio, D.; Borin, S.; Brusa, T.; Brusetti, L.; van der Wielen, P.W.J.J.; Bolhuis, H.; Yakimov, M.M.; D'Auria, G.; Giuliano, L.; Marty, D.; et al. Stratified prokaryote network in the oxic–anoxic transition of a deep-sea halocline. *Nature* **2006**, *440*, 203–207. [CrossRef]

22. Yakimov, M.M.; La Cono, V.; Denaro, R.; D'Auria, G.; Decembrini, F.; Timmis, K.N.; Golyshin, P.N.; Giuliano, L. Primary producing prokaryotic communities of brine, interface and seawater above the halocline of deep anoxic lake L'Atalante, Eastern Mediterranean Sea. *ISME J.* **2007**, *1*, 743–755. [CrossRef]
23. Borin, S.; Brusetti, L.; Mapelli, F.; D'Auria, G.; Brusa, T.; Marzorati, M.; Rizzi, A.; Yakimov, M.; Marty, D.; De Lange, G.J.; et al. Sulfur cycling and methanogenesis primarily drive microbial colonization of the highly sulfidic Urania deep hypersaline basin. *Proc. Natl. Acad. Sci. USA* **2009**, *106*, 9151–9156. [CrossRef] [PubMed]
24. Joye, S.B.; MacDonald, I.R.; Montoya, J.P.; Peccini, M. Geophysical and geochemical signatures of Gulf of Mexico seafloor brines. *Biogeosciences* **2005**, *2*, 295–309. [CrossRef]
25. Cita, M.B. Exhumation of Messinian evaporites in the deep-sea and creation of deep anoxic brine-filled collapsed basins. *Sediment. Geol.* **2006**, *188–189*, 357–378. [CrossRef]
26. Hsü, K.J.; Cita, M.B.; Ryan, W.B.F. The origin of the Mediterranean evaporites. *Initial Reports Deep Sea Drill. Proj.* **1973**, *13*, 1203–1231.
27. van der Wielen, P.W.J.J.; Bolhuis, H.; Borin, S.; Daffonchio, D.; Corselli, C.; Giuliano, L.; D'Auria, G.; de Lange, G.J.; Huebner, A.; Varnavas, S.P.; et al. The enigma of prokaryotic life in deep hypersaline anoxic basins. *Science* **2005**, *307*, 121–123. [CrossRef]
28. Barozzi, A.; Mapelli, F.; Michoud, G.; Crotti, E.; Merlino, G.; Molinari, F.; Borin, S.; Daffonchio, D. Microbial Diversity and Biotechnological Potential of Microorganisms Thriving in the Deep-Sea Brine Pools. In *Extremophiles From Biology to Biotechnology*; Durvasula, R., Rao, D.S., Eds.; CRC Press: Boca Raton, FL, USA; Taylor & Francis, a CRC title, part of the Taylor & Francis imprint, a member of the Taylor & Francis Group, the academic division of T&F Informa plc: Boca Raton, FL, USA, 2018; pp. 19–32. ISBN 9781498774925.
29. Swift, S.A.; Bower, A.S.; Schmitt, R.W. Vertical, horizontal, and temporal changes in temperature in the Atlantis II and Discovery hot brine pools, Red Sea. *Deep. Res. Part I Oceanogr. Res. Pap.* **2012**, *64*. [CrossRef]
30. Ngugi, D.K.; Blom, J.; Alam, I.; Rashid, M.; Ba-Alawi, W.; Zhang, G.; Hikmawan, T.; Guan, Y.; Antunes, A.; Siam, R.; et al. Comparative genomics reveals adaptations of a halotolerant thaumarchaeon in the interfaces of brine pools in the Red Sea. *ISME J.* **2015**, *9*, 396–411. [CrossRef]
31. Yakimov, M.M.; La Cono, V.; Slepak, V.Z.; La Spada, G.; Arcadi, E.; Messina, E.; Borghini, M.; Monticelli, L.S.; Rojo, D.; Barbas, C.; et al. Microbial life in the Lake Medee, the largest deep-sea salt-saturated formation. *Sci. Rep.* **2013**, *3*, 1–9. [CrossRef]
32. Karbe, L. Hot Brines and the Deep Sea Environment. In *Red Sea*; Edwards, A.J., Head, S.J., Eds.; Elsevier: Oxford, UK, 1987; pp. 70–89.
33. MacDonald, I.R.; Guinasso, N.L.; Reilly, J.F.; Brooks, J.M.; Callender, W.R.; Gabrielle, S.G. Gulf of Mexico hydrocarbon seep communities: VI. Patterns in community structure and habitat. *Geo-Marine Lett.* **1990**, *10*, 244–252. [CrossRef]
34. De Lange, G.J.; Middelburg, J.J.; Van der Weijden, C.H.; Catalano, G.; Luther, G.W.; Hydes, D.J.; Woittiez, J.R.W.; Klinkhammer, G.P. Composition of anoxic hypersaline brines in the Tyro and Bannock Basins, eastern Mediterranean. *Mar. Chem.* **1990**, *31*, 63–88. [CrossRef]
35. Van Cappellen, P.; Viollier, E.; Roychoudhury, A.; Clark, L.; Ingall, E.; Lowe, K.; Dichristina, T. Biogeochemical cycles of manganese and iron at the oxic-anoxic transition of a stratified marine basin (Orca Basin, Gulf of Mexico). *Environ. Sci. Technol.* **1998**, *32*, 2931–2939. [CrossRef]
36. Schmidt, M.; Al-Farawati, R.; Botz, R. Geochemical Classification of Brine-Filled Red Sea Deeps. In *The Red Sea*; Rasullan, N.M.A., Stewart, C.F., Eds.; Springer Berlin Heidelberg: Cham, Switzerland, 2015; pp. 219–233.
37. Stock, A.; Filker, S.; Yakimov, M.; Stoeck, T. Deep Hypersaline Anoxic Basins as Model Systems for Environmental Selection of Microbial Plankton. In *Polyextremophiles Life Under Multiple Forms of Stress Life Under Multiple Forms of Stress*; Springer Netherlands: Dordrecht, The Netherlands, 2013; pp. 499–515.
38. Eder, W.; Schmidt, M.; Koch, M.; Garbe-Schönberg, D.; Huber, R. Prokaryotic phylogenetic diversity and corresponding geochemical data of the brine-seawater interface of the Shaban Deep, Red Sea. *Environ. Microbiol.* **2002**, *4*, 758–763. [CrossRef] [PubMed]
39. Sass, A.M.; Sass, H.; Coolen, M.J.L.; Cypionka, H.; Overmann, J. Microbial Communities in the Chemocline of a Hypersaline Deep-Sea Basin (Urania Basin, Mediterranean Sea). *Appl. Environ. Microbiol.* **2001**, *67*, 5392–5402. [CrossRef] [PubMed]
40. van der Wielen, P.W.J.J.; Heijs, S.K. Sulfate-reducing prokaryotic communities in two deep hypersaline anoxic basins in the Eastern Mediterranean deep sea. *Environ. Microbiol.* **2007**, *9*, 1335–1340. [CrossRef]

41. Danovaro, R.; Corinaldesi, C.; Dell'Anno, A.; Fabiano, M.; Corselli, C. Viruses, prokaryotes and DNA in the sediments of a deep-hypersaline anoxic basin (DHAB) of the Mediterranean Sea. *Environ. Microbiol.* **2005**, *7*, 586–592. [CrossRef]
42. Corinaldesi, C.; Tangherlini, M.; Luna, G.M.; Dell'Anno, A. Extracellular DNA can preserve the genetic signatures of present and past viral infection events in deep hypersaline anoxic basins. *Proc. R. Soc. B Biol. Sci.* **2014**, *281*, 1–10. [CrossRef]
43. Danovaro, R.; Gambi, C.; Dell'Anno, A.; Corinaldesi, C.; Pusceddu, A.; Neves, R.C.; Kristensen, R.M. The challenge of proving the existence of metazoan life in permanently anoxic deep-sea sediments. *BMC Biol.* **2016**, *14*, 1–7. [CrossRef]
44. Pachiadaki, M.G.; Yakimov, M.M.; Lacono, V.; Leadbetter, E.; Edgcomb, V. Unveiling microbial activities along the halocline of Thetis, a deep-sea hypersaline anoxic basin. *ISME J.* **2014**, *8*, 2478–2489. [CrossRef]
45. Edgcomb, V.P.; Orsi, W.; Breiner, H.W.; Stock, A.; Filker, S.; Yakimov, M.M.; Stoeck, T. Novel active kinetoplastids associated with hypersaline anoxic basins in the Eastern Mediterranean deep-sea. *Deep. Res. Part I Oceanogr. Res. Pap.* **2011**, *58*, 1040–1048. [CrossRef]
46. Alexander, E.; Stock, A.; Breiner, H.W.; Behnke, A.; Bunge, J.; Yakimov, M.M.; Stoeck, T. Microbial eukaryotes in the hypersaline anoxic L'Atalante deep-sea basin. *Environ. Microbiol.* **2009**, *11*, 360–381. [CrossRef]
47. Danovaro, R.; Dell'Anno, A.; Pusceddu, A.; Gambi, C.; Heiner, I.; Kristensen, R.M. The first metazoa living in permanently anoxic conditions. *BMC Biol.* **2010**, *8*, 30. [CrossRef] [PubMed]
48. Eder, W.; Jahnke, L.L.; Schmidt, M.; Huber, R. Microbial Diversity of the Brine-Seawater Interface of the Kebrit Deep, Red Sea, Studied via 16S rRNA Gene Sequences and Cultivation Methods. *Appl. Environ. Microbiol.* **2001**, *67*, 3077–3085. [CrossRef] [PubMed]
49. Cavalazzi, B.; Barbieri, R.; Gómez, F.; Capaccioni, B.; Olsson-Francis, K.; Pondrelli, M.; Rossi, A.P.; Hickman-Lewis, K.; Agangi, A.; Gasparotto, G.; et al. The Dallol Geothermal Area, Northern Afar (Ethiopia)—An Exceptional Planetary Field Analog on Earth. *Astrobiology* **2019**, *19*, 553–578. [CrossRef] [PubMed]
50. Poli, A.; Finore, I.; Romano, I.; Gioiello, A.; Lama, L.; Nicolaus, B. Microbial Diversity in Extreme Marine Habitats and Their Biomolecules. *Microorganisms* **2017**, *5*, 25. [CrossRef]
51. Gunde-Cimerman, N.; Plemenitaš, A.; Oren, A. Strategies of adaptation of microorganisms of the three domains of life to high salt concentrations. *FEMS Microbiol. Rev.* **2018**, *42*, 353–375. [CrossRef]
52. Giddings, L.-A.; Newman, D.J. Bioactive Compounds from Extremophiles. In *Bioactive Compounds from Extremophiles*; Springer: Cham, Switzerland, 2015; pp. 1–44.
53. Coker, J.A. Extremophiles and biotechnology: Current uses and prospects. *F1000Research* **2016**, *5*, 396–403. [CrossRef]
54. Sorokin, D.Y.; Kublanov, I.V.; Gavrilov, S.N.; Rojo, D.; Roman, P.; Golyshin, P.N.; Slepak, V.Z.; Smedile, F.; Ferrer, M.; Messina, E.; et al. Elemental sulfur and acetate can support life of a novel strictly anaerobic haloarchaeon. *ISME J.* **2016**, *10*, 240–252. [CrossRef]
55. Kormas, K.A.; Pachiadaki, M.G.; Karayanni, H.; Leadbetter, E.R.; Bernhard, J.M.; Edgcomb, V.P. Inter-comparison of the potentially active prokaryotic communities in the halocline sediments of Mediterranean deep-sea hypersaline basins. *Extremophiles* **2015**, *19*, 949–960. [CrossRef]
56. Mwirichia, R.; Alam, I.; Rashid, M.; Vinu, M.; Ba-Alawi, W.; Anthony Kamau, A.; Kamanda Ngugi, D.; Goker, M.; Klenk, H.P.; Bajic, V.; et al. Metabolic traits of an uncultured archaeal lineage-MSBL1-from brine pools of the Red Sea. *Sci. Rep.* **2016**, *6*, 1–14. [CrossRef]
57. La Cono, V.; Arcadi, E.; Spada, G.; Barreca, D.; Laganà, G.; Bellocco, E.; Catalfamo, M.; Smedile, F.; Messina, E.; Giuliano, L.; et al. A Three-Component Microbial Consortium from Deep-Sea Salt-Saturated Anoxic Lake Thetis Links Anaerobic Glycine Betaine Degradation with Methanogenesis. *Microorganisms* **2015**, *3*, 500–517. [CrossRef]
58. Guan, Y.; Hikmawan, T.; Antunes, A.; Ngugi, D.; Stingl, U. Diversity of methanogens and sulfate-reducing bacteria in the interfaces of five deep-sea anoxic brines of the Red Sea. *Res. Microbiol.* **2015**, *166*, 688–699. [CrossRef] [PubMed]
59. Nigro, L.M.; Hyde, A.S.; MacGregor, B.J.; Teske, A. Phylogeography, Salinity Adaptations and Metabolic Potential of the Candidate Division KB1 Bacteria Based on a Partial Single Cell Genome. *Front. Microbiol.* **2016**, *7*, 1–9. [CrossRef] [PubMed]

60. Joye, S.B.; Samarkin, V.A.; Orcutt, B.N.; MacDonald, I.R.; Hinrichs, K.U.; Elvert, M.; Teske, A.P.; Lloyd, K.G.; Lever, M.A.; Montoya, J.P.; et al. Metabolic variability in seafloor brines revealed by carbon and sulphur dynamics. *Nat. Geosci.* **2009**, *2*, 349–354. [CrossRef]
61. Stahl, D.A.; de la Torre, J.R. Physiology and Diversity of Ammonia-Oxidizing Archaea. *Annu. Rev. Microbiol.* **2012**, *66*, 83–101. [CrossRef]
62. Könneke, M.; Bernhard, A.E.; de la Torre, J.R.; Walker, C.B.; Waterbury, J.B.; Stahl, D.A. Isolation of an autotrophic ammonia-oxidizing marine archaeon. *Nature* **2005**, *437*, 543–546. [CrossRef]
63. Oren, A. Molecular ecology of extremely halophilic Archaea and Bacteria. *FEMS Microbiol. Ecol.* **2002**, *39*, 1–7. [CrossRef]
64. Oren, A. Life at High Salt Concentrations. In *The Prokaryotes*; Rosenberg, E., DeLong, E.F., Lory, S., Stackebrandt, E., Thompson, F., Eds.; Springer Berlin Heidelberg: Berlin, Germany, 2013; pp. 421–440.
65. Guan, Y.; Ngugi, D.K.; Vinu, M.; Blom, J.; Alam, I.; Guillot, S.; Ferry, J.G.; Stingl, U. Comparative Genomics of the Genus *Methanohalophilus*, Including a Newly Isolated Strain From Kebrit Deep in the Red Sea. *Front. Microbiol.* **2019**, *10*, 1–11. [CrossRef]
66. De Vitis, V.; Guidi, B.; Contente, M.L.; Granato, T.; Conti, P.; Molinari, F.; Crotti, E.; Mapelli, F.; Borin, S.; Daffonchio, D.; et al. Marine Microorganisms as Source of Stereoselective Esterases and Ketoreductases: Kinetic Resolution of a Prostaglandin Intermediate. *Mar. Biotechnol.* **2015**, *17*, 144–152. [CrossRef]
67. Messina, E.; Sorokin, D.Y.; Kublanov, I.V.; Toshchakov, S.; Lopatina, A.; Arcadi, E.; Smedile, F.; La Spada, G.; La Cono, V.; Yakimov, M.M. Complete genome sequence of "Halanaeroarchaeum sulfurireducens" M27-SA2, a sulfur-reducing and acetate-oxidizing haloarchaeon from the deep-sea hypersaline anoxic lake Medee. *Stand. Genomic Sci.* **2016**, *11*, 1–15. [CrossRef]
68. Antunes, A.; Taborda, M.; Huber, R.; Moissl, C.; Nobre, M.F.; da Costa, M.S. *Halorhabdus tiamatea* sp. nov., a non-pigmented extremely halophilic archaeon from a deep-sea hypersaline anoxic basin of the Red Sea, and emended description of the genus *Halorhabdus*. *Int. J. Syst. Evol. Microbiol.* **2008**, *58*, 215–220. [CrossRef]
69. Antunes, A.; Rainey, F.A.; Wanner, G.; Taborda, M.; Pätzold, J.; Nobre, M.F.; da Costa, M.S.; Huber, R. A New Lineage of Halophilic, Wall-Less, Contractile Bacteria from a Brine-Filled Deep of the Red Sea. *J. Bacteriol.* **2008**, *190*, 3580–3587. [CrossRef] [PubMed]
70. Antunes, A.; Francça, L.; Rainey, F.A.; Huber, R.; Fernanda Nobre, M.; Edwards, K.J.; da Costa, M.S. *Marinobacter salsuginis* sp. nov., isolated from the brine-seawater interface of the Shaban Deep, Red Sea. *Int. J. Syst. Evol. Microbiol.* **2007**, *57*, 1035–1040. [CrossRef] [PubMed]
71. Edgcomb, V.P.; Pachiadaki, M.G.; Mara, P.; Kormas, K.A.; Leadbetter, E.R.; Bernhard, J.M. Gene expression profiling of microbial activities and interactions in sediments under haloclines of E. Mediterranean deep hypersaline anoxic basins. *ISME J.* **2016**, *10*, 2643–2657. [CrossRef] [PubMed]
72. Siam, R.; Mustafa, G.A.; Sharaf, H.; Moustafa, A.; Ramadan, A.R.; Antunes, A.; Bajic, V.B.; Stingl, U.; Marsis, N.G.R.; Coolen, M.J.L.; et al. Unique Prokaryotic Consortia in Geochemically Distinct Sediments from Red Sea Atlantis II and Discovery Deep Brine Pools. *PLoS ONE* **2012**, *7*, e42872. [CrossRef] [PubMed]
73. Tortorella, E.; Tedesco, P.; Esposito, F.P.; January, G.G.; Fani, R.; Jaspars, M.; De Pascale, D.; Palma Esposito, F.; January, G.G.; Fani, R.; et al. Antibiotics from deep-sea microorganisms: Current discoveries and perspectives. *Mar. Drugs* **2018**, *16*, 355. [CrossRef]
74. Corinaldesi, C.; Barone, G.; Marcellini, F.; Dell'Anno, A.; Danovaro, R. Marine microbial-derived molecules and their potential use in cosmeceutical and cosmetic products. *Mar. Drugs* **2017**, *15*, 118. [CrossRef]
75. Lo Giudice, A.; Rizzo, C. Bacteria Associated with Marine Benthic Invertebrates from Polar Environments: Unexplored Frontiers for Biodiscovery? *Diversity* **2018**, *10*, 80. [CrossRef]
76. Andryukov, B.; Mikhailov, V.; Besednova, N. The Biotechnological Potential of Secondary Metabolites from Marine Bacteria. *J. Mar. Sci. Eng.* **2019**, *7*, 176. [CrossRef]
77. Núñez-Montero, K.; Barrientos, L. Advances in Antarctic Research for Antimicrobial Discovery: A Comprehensive Narrative Review of Bacteria from Antarctic Environments as Potential Sources of Novel Antibiotic Compounds Against Human Pathogens and Microorganisms of Industrial Importance. *Antibiotics* **2018**, *7*, 90. [CrossRef]
78. Corinaldesi, C. New perspectives in benthic deep-sea microbial ecology. *Front. Mar. Sci.* **2015**, *2*, 1–12. [CrossRef]
79. Kim, S.K. *Handbook of Marine biotechnology*; Springer-Verlag Berlin Heidelberg: Berlin, Germany, 2015; pp. 307–326. ISBN 9783642539718.

80. Ferrer, M.; Martínez-Martínez, M.; Bargiela, R.; Streit, W.R.; Golyshina, O.V.; Golyshin, P.N. Estimating the success of enzyme bioprospecting through metagenomics: Current status and future trends. *Microb. Biotechnol.* **2016**, *9*, 22–34. [CrossRef] [PubMed]
81. Ziko, L.; Adel, M.; Malash, M.N.; Siam, R. Insights into red sea brine pool specialized metabolism gene clusters encoding potential metabolites for biotechnological applications and extremophile survival. *Mar. Drugs* **2019**, *17*, 273. [CrossRef] [PubMed]
82. Ziko, L.; Saqr, A.-H.A.; Ouf, A.; Gimpel, M.; Aziz, R.K.; Neubauer, P.; Siam, R. Antibacterial and anticancer activities of orphan biosynthetic gene clusters from Atlantis II Red Sea brine pool. *Microb. Cell Fact.* **2019**, *18*, 56. [CrossRef] [PubMed]
83. Sagar, S.; Esau, L.; Holtermann, K.; Hikmawan, T.; Zhang, G.; Stingl, U.; Bajic, V.B.; Kaur, M. Induction of apoptosis in cancer cell lines by the Red Sea brine pool bacterial extracts. *BMC Complement. Altern. Med.* **2013**, *13*, 344. [CrossRef]
84. Esau, L.; Zhang, G.; Sagar, S.; Stingl, U.; Bajic, V.B.; Kaur, M. Mining the deep Red-Sea brine pool microbial community for anticancer therapeutics. *BMC Complement. Altern. Med.* **2019**, *19*. [CrossRef]
85. Sagar, S.; Esau, L.; Hikmawan, T.; Antunes, A.; Holtermann, K.; Stingl, U.; Bajic, V.B.; Kaur, M. Cytotoxic and apoptotic evaluations of marine bacteria isolated from brine-seawater interface of the Red Sea. *BMC Complement. Altern. Med.* **2013**, *13*, 1–8. [CrossRef]
86. Pruesse, E.; Peplies, J.; Glöckner, F.O. SINA: Accurate high-throughput multiple sequence alignment of ribosomal RNA genes. *Bioinformatics* **2012**, *28*, 1823–1829. [CrossRef]
87. Lewis, K.; Epstein, S.; D'Onofrio, A.; Ling, L.L. Uncultured microorganisms as a source of secondary metabolites. *J. Antibiot.* **2010**, *63*, 468–476. [CrossRef]
88. Ksouri, R.; Ksouri, W.M.; Jallali, I.; Debez, A.; Magné, C.; Hiroko, I.; Abdelly, C. Medicinal halophytes: Potent source of health promoting biomolecules with medical, nutraceutical and food applications. *Crit. Rev. Biotechnol.* **2012**, *32*, 289–326. [CrossRef]
89. Raddadi, N.; Cherif, A.; Daffonchio, D.; Neifar, M.; Fava, F. Biotechnological applications of extremophiles, extremozymes and extremolytes. *Appl. Microbiol. Biotechnol.* **2015**, *99*, 7907–7913. [CrossRef]
90. Singh, O.V. *Extremophiles*; Singh, O.V., Ed.; John Wiley & Sons, Inc.: Hoboken, NJ, USA, 2012; pp. 1–429. ISBN 9781118394144.
91. Rampelotto, P.H.; Trincone, A. *Grand Challenges in Marine Biotechnology*; Springer International Publishing: Cham, Switzerland, 2016; pp. 1–260. ISBN 978-3-319-69075-9.
92. Babu, P.; Chandel, A.K.; Singh, O.V. *Extremophiles and Their Applications in Medical Processes*; SpringerBriefs in Microbiology: Cham, Switzerland, 2015; pp. 1–54. ISBN 978-3-319-12807-8.
93. Shin, D.S.; Pratt, A.J.; Tainer, J.A. Archaeal genome guardians give insights into eukaryotic DNA replication and damage response proteins. *Archaea* **2014**, *2014*, 206735. [CrossRef] [PubMed]
94. Majhi, M.C.; Behera, A.K.; Kulshreshtha, N.M.; Mahmooduzafar, D.; Kumar, R.; Kumar, A. ExtremeDB: A Unified Web Repository of Extremophilic Archaea and Bacteria. *PLoS ONE* **2013**, *8*. [CrossRef] [PubMed]
95. Cárdenas, J.P.; Valdés, J.; Quatrini, R.; Duarte, F.; Holmes, D.S. Lessons from the genomes of extremely acidophilic bacteria and archaea with special emphasis on bioleaching microorganisms. *Appl. Microbiol. Biotechnol.* **2010**, *88*, 605–620. [CrossRef] [PubMed]
96. Land, M.; Hauser, L.; Jun, S.R.; Nookaew, I.; Leuze, M.R.; Ahn, T.H.; Karpinets, T.; Lund, O.; Kora, G.; Wassenaar, T.; et al. Insights from 20 years of bacterial genome sequencing. *Funct. Integr. Genomics* **2015**, *15*, 141–161. [CrossRef] [PubMed]
97. Baltz, R.H. Molecular beacons to identify gifted microbes for genome mining. *J. Antibiot.* **2017**, *70*, 639–646. [CrossRef] [PubMed]
98. Brown, E.D.; Wright, G.D. Antibacterial drug discovery in the resistance era. *Nature* **2016**, *529*, 336–343. [CrossRef]
99. Holohan, C.; Van Schaeybroeck, S.; Longley, D.B.; Johnston, P.G. Cancer drug resistance: An evolving paradigm. *Nat. Rev. Cancer* **2013**, *13*, 714–726. [CrossRef]
100. Ventola, C.L. The antibiotic resistance crisis: Part 1: Causes and threats. *P T* **2015**, *40*, 277–283.
101. Housman, G.; Byler, S.; Heerboth, S.; Lapinska, K.; Longacre, M.; Snyder, N.; Sarkar, S. Drug resistance in cancer: An overview. *Cancers* **2014**, *6*, 1769–1792. [CrossRef]

102. Trindade, M.; van Zyl, L.J.; Navarro-Fernández, J.; Elrazak, A.A. Targeted metagenomics as a tool to tap into marine natural product diversity for the discovery and production of drug candidates. *Front. Microbiol.* **2015**, *6*, 1–14. [CrossRef]
103. Malve, H. Exploring the ocean for new drug developments: Marine pharmacology. *J. Pharm. Bioallied Sci.* **2016**, *8*, 83–91. [CrossRef] [PubMed]
104. Li, B.; Wever, W.J.; Walsh, C.T.; Bowers, A.A. Dithiolopyrrolones: Biosynthesis, synthesis, and activity of a unique class of disulfide-containing antibiotics. *Nat. Prod. Rep.* **2014**, *31*, 905–923. [CrossRef] [PubMed]
105. Imada, C.; Maeda, M.; Hara, S.; Taga, N.; Simidu, U. Purification and characterization of subtilisin inhibitors 'Marinostatin' produced by marine *Alteromonas* sp. *J. Appl. Bacteriol.* **1986**, *60*, 469–476. [CrossRef]
106. Gustafson, K.; Roman, M.; Fenical, W. The Macrolactins, a Novel Class of Antiviral and Cytotoxic Macrolides from a Deep-Sea Marine Bacterium. *J. Am. Chem. Soc.* **1989**, *111*, 7519–7524. [CrossRef]
107. Nagao, T.; Adachi, K.; Sakai, M.; Nishijima, M.; Sano, H. Novel macrolactins as antibiotic lactones from a marine bacterium. *J. Antibiot.* **2001**, *54*, 333–339. [CrossRef]
108. Jaruchoktaweechai, C.; Suwanborirux, K.; Tanasupawatt, S.; Kittakoop, P.; Menasveta, P. New macrolactins from a marine *Bacillus* sp. Sc026. *J. Nat. Prod.* **2000**, *63*, 984–986. [CrossRef]
109. Xue, C.; Tian, L.; Xu, M.; Deng, Z.; Lin, W. A new 24-membered lactone and a new polyene δ-lactone from the marine bacterium *Bacillus marinus*. *J. Antibiot.* **2008**, *61*, 668–674. [CrossRef]
110. Berger, E.; Crampton, M.C.; Nxumalo, N.P.; Louw, M.E. Extracellular secretion of a recombinant therapeutic peptide by *Bacillus halodurans* utilizing a modified flagellin type III secretion system. *Microb. Cell Fact.* **2011**, *10*. [CrossRef]
111. Gerard, J.M.; Haden, P.; Kelly, M.T.; Andersen, R.J. Loloatins A-D, cyclic decapeptide antibiotics produced in culture by a tropical marine bacterium. *J. Nat. Prod.* **1999**, *62*, 80–85. [CrossRef]
112. Rahman, H.; Austin, B.; Mitchell, W.J.; Morris, P.C.; Jamieson, D.J.; Adams, D.R.; Spragg, A.M.; Schweizer, M. Novel anti-infective compounds from marine bacteria. *Mar. Drugs* **2010**, *8*, 498–518. [CrossRef]
113. Mondol, M.A.M.; Shin, H.J.; Islam, M.T. Diversity of secondary metabolites from marine *Bacillus* species: Chemistry and biological activity. *Mar. Drugs* **2013**, *11*, 2846–2872. [CrossRef] [PubMed]
114. Zhang, H.L.; Hua, H.M.; Pei, Y.H.; Yao, X.S. Three New Cytotoxic Cyclic Acylpeptides from Marine *Bacillus* sp. *Chem. Pharm. Bull.* **2004**, *52*, 1029–1030. [CrossRef] [PubMed]
115. Oku, N.; Adachi, K.; Matsuda, S.; Kasai, H.; Takatsuki, A.; Shizuri, Y. Ariakemicins A and B, novel polyketide-peptide antibiotics from a marine gliding bacterium of the genus *Rapidithrix*. *Org. Lett.* **2008**, *10*, 2481–2484. [CrossRef] [PubMed]
116. Hu, Y.; MacMillan, J.B. Erythrazoles A-B, cytotoxic benzothiazoles from a marine-derived *Erythrobacter* sp. *Org. Lett.* **2011**, *13*, 6580–6583. [CrossRef] [PubMed]
117. Hu, Y.; Legako, A.G.; Espindola, A.P.D.M.; MacMillan, J.B. Erythrolic acids A-E, meroterpenoids from a marine-derived *Erythrobacter* sp. *J. Org. Chem.* **2012**, *77*, 3401–3407. [CrossRef] [PubMed]
118. Di Lorenzo, F.; Palmigiano, A.; Paciello, I.; Pallach, M.; Garozzo, D.; Bernardini, M.-L.L.; Cono, V.L.; Yakimov, M.M.; Molinaro, A.; Silipo, A.; et al. The deep-sea polyextremophile *Halobacteroides lacunaris* TB21 rough-type LPS: Structure and inhibitory activity towards toxic LPS. *Mar. Drugs* **2017**, *15*, 201. [CrossRef]
119. Homann, V.V.; Sandy, M.; Tincu, J.A.; Templeton, A.S.; Tebo, B.M.; Butler, A. Loihichelins A-F, a suite of amphiphilic siderophores produced by the marine bacterium *Halomonas* LOB-5. *J. Nat. Prod.* **2009**, *72*, 884–888. [CrossRef]
120. Wang, L.; Große, T.; Stevens, H.; Brinkhoff, T.; Simon, M.; Liang, L.; Bitzer, J.; Bach, G.; Zeeck, A.; Tokuda, H.; et al. Bioactive hydroxyphenylpyrrole-dicarboxylic acids from a new marine *Halomonas* sp.: Production and structure elucidation. *Appl. Microbiol. Biotechnol.* **2006**, *72*, 816–822. [CrossRef]
121. Bitzer, J.; Große, T.; Wang, L.; Lang, S.; Beil, W.; Zeeck, A. New aminophenoxazinones from a marine *Halomonas* sp.: Fermentation, structure elucidation, and biological activity. *J. Antibiot.* **2006**, *59*, 86–92. [CrossRef]
122. Silipo, A.; Lanzetta, R.; Parrilli, M.; Sturiale, L.; Garozzo, D.; Nazarenko, E.L.; Gorshkova, R.P.; Ivanova, E.P.; Molinaro, A. The complete structure of the core carbohydrate backbone from the LPS of marine halophilic bacterium *Pseudoalteromonas carrageenovora* type strain IAM 12662T. *Carbohydr. Res.* **2005**, *340*, 1475–1482. [CrossRef]
123. Mitova, M.; Tutino, M.L.; Infusini, G.; Marino, G.; De Rosa, S. Exocellular peptides from antarctic psychrophile *Pseudoalteromonas haloplanktis*. *Mar. Biotechnol.* **2005**, *7*, 523–531. [CrossRef] [PubMed]

124. Shiozawa, H.; Shimada, A.; Takahashi, S. Thiomarinols D, E, F and G, new hybrid antimicrobial antibiotics produced by a marine bacterium. Isolated, structure, and antimicrobial activity. *J. Antibiot.* **1997**, *50*, 449–452. [CrossRef] [PubMed]
125. Shiozawa, H.; Kagasaki, T.; Takahashi, S.; Kinoshita, T.; Haruyama, H.; Domon, H.; Utsuib, Y.; Kodama, K. Thiomarinol, a new hybrid antimicrobial antibiotic produced by a marine bacterium fermentation, isolation, structure, and antimicrobial activity. *J. Antibiot.* **1993**, *46*, 1834–1842. [CrossRef] [PubMed]
126. Mitchell, S.S.; Nicholson, B.; Teisan, S.; Lam, K.S.; Potts, B.C.M. Aureoverticillactam, a novel 22-atom macrocyclic lactam from the marine actinomycete *Streptomyces aureoverticillatus*. *J. Nat. Prod.* **2004**, *67*, 1400–1402. [CrossRef]
127. Pesic, A.; Baumann, H.I.; Kleinschmidt, K.; Ensle, P.; Wiese, J.; Süssmuth, R.D.; Imhoff, J.F. Champacyclin, a new cyclic octapeptide from *Streptomyces* strain C42 isolated from the Baltic Sea. *Mar. Drugs* **2013**, *11*, 4834–4857. [CrossRef]
128. Kasanah, N.; Triyanto, T. Bioactivities of Halometabolites from Marine Actinobacteria. *Biomolecules* **2019**, *9*, 225. [CrossRef]
129. Martin, G.D.A.; Tan, L.T.; Jensen, P.R.; Dimayuga, R.E.; Fairchild, C.R.; Raventos-Suarez, C.; Fenical, W. Marmycins A and B, cytotoxic pentacyclic C-glycosides from a marine sediment-derived actinomycete related to the genus *Streptomyces*. *J. Nat. Prod.* **2007**, *70*, 1406–1409. [CrossRef]
130. Zhou, X.; Huang, H.; Li, J.; Song, Y.; Jiang, R.; Liu, J.; Zhang, S.; Hua, Y.; Ju, J. New anti-infective cycloheptadepsipeptide congeners and absolute stereochemistry from the deep sea-derived *Streptomyces drozdowiczii* SCSIO 10141. *Tetrahedron* **2014**, *70*, 7795–7801. [CrossRef]
131. Bruntner, C.; Binder, T.; Pathom-Aree, W.; Goodfellow, M.; Bull, A.T.; Potterat, O.; Puder, C.; Hörer, S.; Schmid, A.; Bolek, W.; et al. Frigocyclinone, a novel angucyclinone antibiotic produced by a *Streptomyces griseus* strain from Antarctica. *J. Antibiot.* **2005**, *58*, 346–349. [CrossRef]
132. El-Gendy, M.M.A.; Shaaban, M.; Shaaban, K.A.; El-Bondkly, A.M.; Laatsch, H. Essramycin: A first triazolopyrimidine antibiotic isolated from nature. *J. Antibiot.* **2008**, *61*, 149–157. [CrossRef]
133. Song, Y.; Huang, H.; Chen, Y.; Ding, J.; Zhang, Y.; Sun, A.; Zhang, W.; Ju, J. Cytotoxic and antibacterial marfuraquinocins from the deep south china sea-derived *Streptomyces niveus* scsio 3406. *J. Nat. Prod.* **2013**, *76*, 2263–2268. [CrossRef] [PubMed]
134. Song, Y.; Li, Q.; Liu, X.; Chen, Y.; Zhang, Y.; Sun, A.; Zhang, W.; Zhang, J.; Ju, J. Cyclic hexapeptides from the deep South China sea-derived *Streptomyces* scopuliridis SCSIO ZJ46 active against pathogenic gram-positive bacteria. *J. Nat. Prod.* **2014**, *77*, 1937–1941. [CrossRef] [PubMed]
135. Takahashi, A.; Kurasawa, S.; Ikeda, D.; Okami, Y.; Takeuchi, T. Altemicidin, a new acaricidal and antitumor substance. I. Taxonomy, fermentation, isolation and physico-chemical and biological properties. *J. Antibiot.* **1989**, *42*, 1556–1561. [CrossRef] [PubMed]
136. Pan, H.Q.; Zhang, S.Y.; Wang, N.; Li, Z.L.; Hua, H.M.; Hu, J.C.; Wang, S.J. New spirotetronate antibiotics, lobophorins H and I, from a South China Sea-derived *Streptomyces* sp. 12A35. *Mar. Drugs* **2013**, *11*, 3891–3901. [CrossRef]
137. Moon, K.; Ahn, C.H.; Shin, Y.; Won, T.H.; Ko, K.; Lee, S.K.; Oh, K.B.; Shin, J.; Nam, S.I.; Oh, D.C. New Benzoxazine Secondary Metabolites from an Arctic Actinomycete. *Mar. Drugs* **2014**, *12*, 2526–5238. [CrossRef]
138. Schultz, A.W.; Oh, D.C.; Carney, J.R.; Williamson, R.T.; Udwary, D.W.; Jensen, P.R.; Gould, S.J.; Fenical, W.; Moore, B.S. Biosynthesis and structures of cyclomarins and cyclomarazines, prenylated cyclic peptides of marine actinobacterial origin. *J. Am. Chem. Soc.* **2008**, *130*, 4507–4516. [CrossRef]
139. Renner, M.K.; Shen, Y.C.; Cheng, X.C.; Jensen, P.R.; Frankmoelle, W.; Kauffman, C.A.; Fenical, W.; Lobkovsky, E.; Clardy, J. Cyclomarins A-C, new antiinflammatory cyclic peptides produced by a marine bacterium (*Streptomyces* sp.). *J. Am. Chem. Soc.* **1999**, *121*, 11273–11276. [CrossRef]
140. Hughes, C.C.; Prieto-Davo, A.; Jensen, P.R.; Fenical, W. The marinopyrroles, antibiotics of an unprecedented structure class from a marine *Streptomyces* sp. *Org. Lett.* **2008**, *10*, 629–631. [CrossRef]
141. Hughes, C.C.; Kauffman, C.A.; Jensen, P.R.; Fenical, W. Structures, Reactivities, and Antibiotic Properties of the Marinopyrroles A–F. *J. Org. Chem.* **2010**, *75*, 3240–3250. [CrossRef]
142. Asolkar, R.N.; Jensen, P.R.; Kauffman, C.A.; Fenical, W. Daryamides A-C, weakly cytotoxic polyketides from a marine-derived actinomycete of the genus *Streptomyces* strain CNQ-085. *J. Nat. Prod.* **2006**, *69*, 1756–1759. [CrossRef]

143. Hughes, C.C.; MacMillan, J.B.; Gaudêncio, S.P.; Jensen, P.R.; Fenical, W. The ammosamides: Structures of cell cycle modulators from a marine-derived *Streptomyces* species. *Angew. Chemi. Int. Ed.* **2009**, *48*, 725–727. [CrossRef]
144. Hughes, C.C.; Fenical, W. Total synthesis of the ammosamides. *J. Am. Chem. Soc.* **2010**, *132*, 2528–2529. [CrossRef] [PubMed]
145. Pan, E.; Jamison, M.; Yousufuddin, M.; MacMillan, J.B. Ammosamide D, an oxidatively ring opened ammosamide analog from a marine-derived *Streptomyces variabilis*. *Org. Lett.* **2012**, *14*, 2390–2393. [CrossRef] [PubMed]
146. Li, F.; Maskey, R.P.; Qin, S.; Sattler, I.; Fiebig, H.H.; Maier, A.; Zeeck, A.; Laatsch, H. Chinikomycins A and B: Isolation, structure elucidation, and biological activity of novel antibiotics from a marine *Streptomyces* sp. isolate M045. *J. Nat. Prod.* **2005**, *68*, 349–353. [CrossRef] [PubMed]
147. Pérez, M.; Crespo, C.; Schleissner, C.; Rodríguez, P.; Zúñiga, P.; Reyes, F. Tartrolon D, a cytotoxic macrodiolide from the marine-derived actinomycete *Streptomyces* sp. MDG-04-17-069. *J. Nat. Prod.* **2009**, *72*, 2192–2194. [CrossRef] [PubMed]
148. Hawas, U.W.; Shaaban, M.; Shaaban, K.A.; Speitling, M.; Maier, A.; Kelter, G.; Fiebig, H.H.; Meiners, M.; Helmke, E.; Laatsch, H. Mansouramycins A-D, cytotoxic isoquinolinequinones from a marine Streptomycete. *J. Nat. Prod.* **2009**, *72*, 2120–2124. [CrossRef] [PubMed]
149. Nachtigall, J.; Schneider, K.; Bruntner, C.; Bull, A.T.; Goodfellow, M.; Zinecker, H.; Imhoff, J.F.; Nicholson, G.; Irran, E.; Süssmuth, R.D.; et al. Benzoxacystol, a benzoxazine-type enzyme inhibitor from the deep-sea strain *Streptomyces* sp. NTK 935. *J. Antibiot.* **2011**, *64*, 453–457. [CrossRef]
150. Zhang, W.; Liu, Z.; Li, S.; Yang, T.; Zhang, Q.; Ma, L.; Tian, X.; Zhang, H.; Huang, C.; Zhang, S.; et al. Spiroindimicins A-D: New bisindole alkaloids from a deep-sea-derived actinomycete. *Org. Lett.* **2012**, *14*, 3364–3367. [CrossRef]
151. Song, Y.; Liu, G.; Li, J.; Huang, H.; Zhang, X.; Zhang, H.; Ju, J. Cytotoxic and antibacterial angucycline- and prodigiosin-analogues from the deep-sea derived *Streptomyces* sp. SCSIO 11594. *Mar. Drugs* **2015**, *13*, 1304–1316. [CrossRef]
152. You, Z.Y.; Wang, Y.H.; Zhang, Z.G.; Xu, M.J.; Xie, S.J.; Han, T.S.; Feng, L.; Li, X.G.; Xu, J. Identification of two novel anti-fibrotic benzopyran compounds produced by engineered strains derived from *Streptomyces xiamenensis* M1-94P that originated from deep-sea sediments. *Mar. Drugs* **2013**, *11*, 4035–4049. [CrossRef]
153. Miller, E.D.; Kauffman, C.A.; Jensen, P.R.; Fenical, W. Piperazimycins: Cytotoxic hexadepsipeptides from a marine-derived bacterium of the genus *Streptomyces*. *J. Org. Chem.* **2007**, *72*, 323–330. [CrossRef] [PubMed]
154. Sun, M.-L.; Liu, S.-B.; Qiao, L.-P.; Chen, X.-L.; Pang, X.; Shi, M.; Zhang, X.-Y.; Qin, Q.-L.; Zhou, B.-C.; Zhang, Y.-Z.; et al. A novel exopolysaccharide from deep-sea bacterium *Zunongwangia profunda* SM-A87: Low-cost fermentation, moisture retention, and antioxidant activities. *Appl. Microbiol. Biotechnol.* **2014**, *98*, 7437–7445. [CrossRef] [PubMed]
155. Chater, K.F. Recent advances in understanding *Streptomyces*. *F1000Research* **2016**, *5*, 1–16. [CrossRef] [PubMed]
156. Hettiarachchi, S.A.; Lee, S.-J.; Lee, Y.; Kwon, Y.-K.; De Zoysa, M.; Moon, S.; Jo, E.; Kim, T.; Kang, D.-H.; Heo, S.-J.; et al. A rapid and efficient screening method for antibacterial compound-producing bacteria. *J. Microbiol. Biotechnol.* **2017**, *27*, 1441–1448. [PubMed]
157. Andreo-Vidal, A.; Sanchez-Amat, A.; Campillo-Brocal, J. The *Pseudoalteromonas luteoviolacea* L-amino Acid Oxidase with Antimicrobial Activity Is a Flavoenzyme. *Mar. Drugs* **2018**, *16*, 499. [CrossRef] [PubMed]
158. Kalitnik, A.A.; Byankina Barabanova, A.O.; Nagorskaya, V.P.; Reunov, A.V.; Glazunov, V.P.; Solov'eva, T.F.; Yermak, I.M. Low molecular weight derivatives of different carrageenan types and their antiviral activity. *J. Appl. Phycol.* **2013**, *25*, 65–72. [CrossRef]
159. Queiroz, E.A.I.F.; Fortes, Z.B.; da Cunha, M.A.A.; Sarilmiser, H.K.; Barbosa Dekker, A.M.; Öner, E.T.; Dekker, R.F.H.; Khaper, N. Levan promotes antiproliferative and pro-apoptotic effects in MCF-7 breast cancer cells mediated by oxidative stress. *Int. J. Biol. Macromol.* **2017**, *102*, 565–570. [CrossRef]
160. Ruiz-Ruiz, C.; Srivastava, G.K.; Carranza, D.; Mata, J.A.; Llamas, I.; Santamaría, M.; Quesada, E.; Molina, I.J. An exopolysaccharide produced by the novel halophilic bacterium *Halomonas stenophila* strain B100 selectively induces apoptosis in human T leukaemia cells. *Appl. Microbiol. Biotechnol.* **2011**, *89*, 345–355. [CrossRef]
161. Lorenz, P.; Eck, J. Metagenomics and industrial applications. *Nat. Rev. Microbiol.* **2005**, *3*, 510–516. [CrossRef]

162. Prasad, S.; Roy, I. Converting Enzymes into Tools of Industrial Importance. *Recent Pat. Biotechnol.* **2018**, *12*, 33–56. [CrossRef]
163. Bommarius, A.S.; Paye, M.F. Stabilizing biocatalysts. *Chem. Soc. Rev.* **2013**, *42*, 6534–6565. [CrossRef] [PubMed]
164. Madhavan, A.; Sindhu, R.; Binod, P.; Sukumaran, R.K.; Pandey, A. Strategies for design of improved biocatalysts for industrial applications. *Bioresour. Technol.* **2017**, *245*, 1304–1313. [CrossRef] [PubMed]
165. Martínez-Martínez, M.; Bargiela, R.; Ferrer, M. Metagenomics and the Search for Industrial Enzymes. In *Biotechnology of Microbial Enzymes: Production, Biocatalysis and Industrial Applications*; Brahmachari, G., Demain, A.L., Adrio, J.L., Eds.; Academic Press: Cambridge, MA, USA, 2016; pp. 1–608.
166. Chapman, J.; Ismail, A.; Dinu, C. Industrial Applications of Enzymes: Recent Advances, Techniques, and Outlooks. *Catalysts* **2018**, *8*, 238. [CrossRef]
167. Dumorné, K.; Córdova, D.C.; Astorga-Eló, M.; Renganathan, P. Extremozymes: A potential source for industrial applications. *J. Microbiol. Biotechnol.* **2017**, *27*, 649–659. [CrossRef] [PubMed]
168. Dalmaso, G.; Ferreira, D.; Vermelho, A. Marine Extremophiles: A Source of Hydrolases for Biotechnological Applications. *Mar. Drugs* **2015**, *13*, 1925–1965. [CrossRef] [PubMed]
169. Sarmiento, F.; Peralta, R.; Blamey, J.M. Cold and Hot Extremozymes: Industrial Relevance and Current Trends. *Front. Bioeng. Biotechnol.* **2015**, *3*, 1–15. [CrossRef]
170. Di Donato, P.; Buono, A.; Poli, A.; Finore, I.; Abbamondi, G.R.; Nicolaus, B.; Lama, L. Exploring marine environments for the identification of extremophiles and their enzymes for sustainable and green bioprocesses. *Sustainability* **2019**, *11*, 149. [CrossRef]
171. Bruno, S.; Coppola, D.; di Prisco, G.; Giordano, D.; Verde, C. Enzymes from Marine Polar Regions and Their Biotechnological Applications. *Mar. Drugs* **2019**, *17*, 544. [CrossRef]
172. Yamanaka, Y.; Kazuoka, T.; Yoshida, M.; Yamanaka, K.; Oikawa, T.; Soda, K. Thermostable aldehyde dehydrogenase from psychrophile, *Cytophaga* sp. KUC-1: Enzymological characteristics and functional properties. *Biochem. Biophys. Res. Commun.* **2002**, *298*, 632–637. [CrossRef]
173. Anburajan, L.; Meena, B.; Narendar Sivvaswamy, S. First report on molecular characterization of novel betaine aldehyde dehydrogenase from the halotolerant eubacteria, *Bacillus halodurans*. *Gene Reports* **2017**, *9*, 131–135. [CrossRef]
174. Kim, H.J.; Joo, W.A.; Cho, C.W.; Kim, C.W. Halophile aldehyde dehydrogenase from *Halobacterium salinarum*. *J. Proteome Res.* **2006**, *5*, 192–195. [CrossRef] [PubMed]
175. Akal, A.L.; Karan, R.; Hohl, A.; Alam, I.; Vogler, M.; Grötzinger, S.W.; Eppinger, J.; Rueping, M. A polyextremophilic alcohol dehydrogenase from the Atlantis II Deep Red Sea brine pool. *FEBS Open Bio* **2019**, *9*, 194–205. [CrossRef] [PubMed]
176. Borchert, E.; Knobloch, S.; Dwyer, E.; Flynn, S.; Jackson, S.A.; Jóhannsson, R.; Marteinsson, V.T.; O'Gara, F.; Dobson, A.D.W.W.; O'Gara, F.; et al. Biotechnological Potential of Cold Adapted *Pseudoalteromonas* spp. Isolated from 'Deep Sea' Sponges. *Mar. Drugs* **2017**, *15*, 184. [CrossRef] [PubMed]
177. Izotova, L.S.; Strongin, A.Y.; Chekulaeva, L.N.; Sterkin, V.E.; Ostoslavskaya, V.I.; Lyublinskaya, L.A.; Timokhina, E.A.; Stepanov, V.M. Purification and properties of serine protease from Halobacterium halobium. *J. Bacteriol.* **1983**, *155*, 826–830. [CrossRef] [PubMed]
178. Venugopal, M.; Saramma, A.V. An alkaline protease from *Bacillus circulans* BM15, newly isolated from a mangrove station: Characterization and application in laundry detergent formulations. *Indian J. Microbiol.* **2007**, *47*, 298–303. [CrossRef] [PubMed]
179. Wu, S.; Liu, G.; Zhang, D.; Li, C.; Sun, C. Purification and biochemical characterization of an alkaline protease from marine bacteria *Pseudoalteromonas* sp. 129-1. *J. Basic Microbiol.* **2015**, *55*, 1427–1434. [CrossRef]
180. Ibrahim, A.S.S.S.; Al-Salamah, A.A.; El-Badawi, Y.B.; El-Tayeb, M.A.; Antranikian, G. Detergent-, solvent- and salt-compatible thermoactive alkaline serine protease from halotolerant alkaliphilic *Bacillus* sp. NPST-AK15: Purification and characterization. *Extremophiles* **2015**, *19*, 961–971. [CrossRef]
181. Raval, V.H.; Pillai, S.; Rawal, C.M.; Singh, S.P. Biochemical and structural characterization of a detergent-stable serine alkaline protease from seawater haloalkaliphilic bacteria. *Process Biochem.* **2014**, *49*, 955–962. [CrossRef]
182. Mothe, T.; Sultanpuram, V.R. Production, purification and characterization of a thermotolerant alkaline serine protease from a novel species *Bacillus caseinilyticus*. *3 Biotech* **2016**, *6*, 1–10. [CrossRef]
183. Sanchez-Porro, C.; Martin, S.; Mellado, E.; Ventosa, A. Diversity of moderately halophilic bacteria producing extracellular hydrolytic enzymes. *J. Appl. Microbiol.* **2003**, *94*, 295–300. [CrossRef]

184. Sánchez-Porro, C.; Mellado, E.; Pugsley, A.P.; Francetic, O.; Ventosa, A. The haloprotease CPI produced by the moderately halophilic bacterium *Pseudoalteromonas ruthenica* is secreted by the type II secretion pathway. *Appl. Environ. Microbiol.* **2009**, *75*, 4197–4201. [CrossRef] [PubMed]
185. Lama, L.; Romano, I.; Calandrelli, V.; Nicolaus, B.; Gambacorta, A. Purification and characterization of a protease produced by an aerobic haloalkaliphilic species belonging to the *Salinivibrio* genus. *Res. Microbiol.* **2005**, *156*, 478–484. [CrossRef] [PubMed]
186. Behera, B.C.; Sethi, B.K.; Mishra, R.R.; Dutta, S.K.; Thatoi, H.N. Microbial cellulases—Diversity & biotechnology with reference to mangrove environment: A review. *J. Genet. Eng. Biotechnol.* **2017**, *15*, 197–210. [PubMed]
187. Maki, M.; Leung, K.T.; Qin, W. The prospects of cellulase-producing bacteria for the bioconversion of lignocellulosic biomass. *Int. J. Biol. Sci.* **2009**, *5*, 500–516. [CrossRef] [PubMed]
188. Dos Santos, Y.Q.; de Veras, B.O.; de França, A.F.J.; Gorlach-Lira, K.; Velasques, J.; Migliolo, L.; Dos Santos, E.A. A new salt-tolerant thermostable cellulase from a marine *bacillus* sp. Strain. *J. Microbiol. Biotechnol.* **2018**, *28*, 1078–1085. [CrossRef]
189. Werner, J.; Ferrer, M.; Michel, G.; Mann, A.J.; Huang, S.; Juarez, S.; Ciordia, S.; Albar, J.P.; Alcaide, M.; La Cono, V.; et al. *Halorhabdus tiamatea*: Proteogenomics and glycosidase activity measurements identify the first cultivated euryarchaeon from a deep-sea anoxic brine lake as potential polysaccharide degrader. *Environ. Microbiol.* **2014**, *16*, 2525–2537. [CrossRef]
190. Zhang, T.; Datta, S.; Eichler, J.; Ivanova, N.; Axen, S.D.; Kerfeld, C.A.; Chen, F.; Kyrpides, N.; Hugenholtz, P.; Cheng, J.F.; et al. Identification of a haloalkaliphilic and thermostable cellulase with improved ionic liquid tolerance. *Green Chem.* **2011**, *13*, 2083–2090. [CrossRef]
191. Zhang, C.; Wang, X.; Zhang, W.; Zhao, Y.; Lu, X. Expression and characterization of a glucose-tolerant β-1,4-glucosidase with wide substrate specificity from *Cytophaga hutchinsonii*. *Appl. Microbiol. Biotechnol.* **2017**, *101*, 1919–1926. [CrossRef]
192. Makhdoumi, A.; Dehghani-Joybari, Z.; Mashreghi, M.; Jamialahmadi, K.; Asoodeh, A. A novel halo-alkali-tolerant and thermo-tolerant chitinase from *Pseudoalteromonas* sp. DC14 isolated from the Caspian Sea. *Int. J. Environ. Sci. Technol.* **2015**, *12*, 3895–3904. [CrossRef]
193. Roman, D.L.; Roman, M.; Sletta, H.; Ostafe, V.; Isvoran, A. Assessment of the properties of chitin deacetylases showing different enzymatic action patterns. *J. Mol. Graph. Model.* **2019**, *88*, 41–48. [CrossRef]
194. Zhao, Y.; Park, R.D.; Muzzarelli, R.A.A. Chitin deacetylases: Properties and applications. *Mar. Drugs* **2010**, *8*, 24–46. [CrossRef] [PubMed]
195. Kim, S.B.; Lee, W.; Ryu, Y.W. Cloning and characterization of thermostable esterase from *Archaeoglobus fulgidus*. *J. Microbiol.* **2008**, *46*, 100–107. [CrossRef] [PubMed]
196. Ghati, A.; Paul, G. Purification and characterization of a thermo-halophilic, alkali-stable and extremely benzene tolerant esterase from a thermo-halo tolerant *Bacillus cereus* strain AGP-03, isolated from 'Bakreshwar' hot spring, India. *Process Biochem.* **2015**, *50*, 771–781. [CrossRef]
197. Mohamed, Y.M.; Ghazy, M.A.; Sayed, A.; Ouf, A.; El-Dorry, H.; Siam, R. Isolation and characterization of a heavy metal-resistant, thermophilic esterase from a Red Sea Brine Pool. *Sci. Rep.* **2013**, *3*, 3358. [CrossRef]
198. Ferrer, M.; Golyshina, O.V.; Chernikova, T.N.; Khachane, A.N.; Martins, V.A.P.; Santos, D.; Yakimov, M.M.; Timmis, K.N.; Golyshin, P.N. Microbial Enzymes Mined from the Urania Deep-Sea Hypersaline Anoxic Basin. *Chem. Biol.* **2005**, *12*, 895–904. [CrossRef] [PubMed]
199. Zhang, S.; Wu, G.; Liu, Z.; Shao, Z.; Liu, Z. Characterization of EstB, a novel cold-active and organic solvent-tolerant esterase from marine microorganism *Alcanivorax dieselolei* B-5(T). *Extremophiles* **2014**, *18*, 251–259. [CrossRef]
200. Rahman, M.A.; Culsum, U.; Tang, W.; Zhang, S.W.; Wu, G.; Liu, Z. Characterization of a novel cold active and salt tolerant esterase from *Zunongwangia profunda*. *Enzyme Microb. Technol.* **2016**, *85*, 1–11. [CrossRef]
201. Garczarek, F.; Dong, M.; Typke, D.; Witkowska, H.E.; Hazen, T.C.; Nogales, E.; Biggin, M.D.; Glaeser, R.M. Octomeric pyruvate-ferredoxin oxidoreductase from *Desulfovibrio vulgaris*. *J. Struct. Biol.* **2007**, *159*, 9–18. [CrossRef]
202. Bock, A.K.; Schönheit, P.; Teixeira, M. The iron-sulfur centers of the pyruvate:ferredoxin oxidoreductase from *Methanosarcina barkeri* (Fusaro). *FEBS Lett.* **1997**, *414*, 209–212.

203. Chen, C.K.M.; Lee, G.C.; Ko, T.P.; Guo, R.T.; Huang, L.M.; Liu, H.J.; Ho, Y.F.; Shaw, J.F.; Wang, A.H.J. Structure of the Alkalohyperthermophilic *Archaeoglobus fulgidus* Lipase Contains a Unique C-Terminal Domain Essential for Long-Chain Substrate Binding. *J. Mol. Biol.* **2009**, *390*, 672–685. [CrossRef]
204. Akbari, E.; Beheshti-Maal, K.; Nayeri, H. A novel halo-alkalo-tolerant bacterium, *Marinobacter alkaliphilus* ABN-IAUF-1, isolated from Persian Gulf suitable for alkaline lipase production. *Int. J. Environ. Sci. Technol.* **2018**, *15*, 1767–1776. [CrossRef]
205. Jeon, J.H.; Kim, J.-T.; Kim, Y.J.; Kim, H.-K.; Lee, H.S.; Kang, S.G.; Kim, S.-J.; Lee, J.-H. Cloning and characterization of a new cold-active lipase from a deep-sea sediment metagenome. *Appl. Microbiol. Biotechnol.* **2009**, *81*, 865–874. [CrossRef] [PubMed]
206. Loperena, L.; Soria, V.; Varela, H.; Lupo, S.; Bergalli, A.; Guigou, M.; Pellegrino, A.; Bernardo, A.; Calviño, A.; Rivas, F.; et al. Extracellular enzymes produced by microorganisms isolated from maritime Antarctica. *World J. Microbiol. Biotechnol.* **2012**, *28*, 2249–2256. [CrossRef] [PubMed]
207. Kiran, G.S.; Lipton, A.N.; Kennedy, J.; Dobson, A.D.W.; Selvin, J. A halotolerant thermostable lipase from the marine bacterium *Oceanobacillus* sp. PUMB02 with an ability to disrupt bacterial biofilms. *Bioeng. Bugs* **2014**, *5*, 305–318.
208. Ciok, A.; Dziewit, L. Exploring the genome of Arctic *Psychrobacter* sp. DAB_AL32B and construction of novel *Psychrobacter*-specific cloning vectors of an increased carrying capacity. *Arch. Microbiol.* **2019**, *201*, 559–569. [CrossRef] [PubMed]
209. Sayed, A.; Ghazy, M.A.; Ferreira, A.J.S.; Setubal, J.C.; Chambergo, F.S.; Ouf, A.; Adel, M.; Dawe, A.S.; Archer, J.A.C.; Bajic, V.B.; et al. A novel mercuric reductase from the unique deep brine environment of Atlantis II in the Red sea. *J. Biol. Chem.* **2014**, *289*, 1675–1687. [CrossRef]
210. Zhou, P.; Huo, Y.Y.; Xu, L.; Wu, Y.H.; Meng, F.X.; Wang, C.S.; Xu, X.W. Investigation of mercury tolerance in *Chromohalobacter israelensis* DSM 6768T and *Halomonas zincidurans* B6T by comparative genomics with *Halomonas xinjiangensis* TRM 0175T. *Mar. Genomics* **2014**, *19*, 15–16. [CrossRef]
211. Sonbol, S.A.; Ferreira, A.J.S.; Siam, R. Red Sea Atlantis II brine pool nitrilase with unique thermostability profile and heavy metal tolerance. *BMC Biotechnol.* **2016**, *16*, 1–13. [CrossRef]
212. Hii, S.L.; Tan, J.S.; Ling, T.C.; Ariff, A. Bin Pullulanase: Role in Starch Hydrolysis and Potential Industrial Applications. *Enzyme Res.* **2012**, *2012*, 1–14. [CrossRef]
213. Chakdar, H.; Kumar, M.; Pandiyan, K.; Singh, A.; Nanjappan, K.; Kashyap, P.L.; Srivastava, A.K. Bacterial xylanases: Biology to biotechnology. *3 Biotech* **2016**, *6*, 150. [CrossRef]
214. Araki, T.; Tani, S.; Maeda, K.; Hashikawa, S.; Nakagawa, H.; Morishita, T. Purification and Characterization of β-1,3-Xylanase from a Marine Bacterium, *Vibrio* sp. XY-214. *Biosci. Biotechnol. Biochem.* **1999**, *63*, 2017–2019. [CrossRef] [PubMed]
215. Wejse, P.L.; Ingvorsen, K.; Mortensen, K.K. Purification and characterisation of two extremely halotolerant xylanases from a novel halophilic bacterium. *Extremophiles* **2003**, *7*, 423–431. [CrossRef] [PubMed]
216. Kim, J.J.; Kwon, Y.K.; Kim, J.H.; Heo, S.J.; Lee, Y.; Lee, S.J.; Shim, W.B.; Jung, W.K.; Hyun, J.H.; Kwon, K.K.; et al. Effective microwell plate-based screening method for microbes producing cellulase and xylanase and its application. *J. Microbiol. Biotechnol.* **2014**, *24*, 1559–1565. [CrossRef] [PubMed]
217. Møller, M.F.; Kjeldsen, K.U.; Ingvorsen, K. *Marinimicrobium haloxylanilyticum* sp. nov., a new moderately halophilic, polysaccharide-degrading bacterium isolated from Great Salt Lake, Utah. *Antonie van Leeuwenhoek, Int. J. Gen. Mol. Microbiol.* **2010**, *98*, 553–565. [CrossRef]
218. Rattu, G.; Joshi, S.; Satyanarayana, T. Bifunctional recombinant cellulase–xylanase (rBhcell-xyl) from the polyextremophilic bacterium *Bacillus halodurans* TSLV1 and its utility in valorization of renewable agro-residues. *Extremophiles* **2016**, *20*, 831–842. [CrossRef]
219. Kim, J.; Hong, S.-K. Isolation and Characterization of an Agarase-Producing Bacterial Strain, *Alteromonas* sp. GNUM-1, from the West Sea, Korea. *J. Microbiol. Biotechnol.* **2012**, *22*, 1621–1628. [CrossRef]
220. Fu, X.T.; Kim, S.M. Agarase: Review of major sources, categories, purification method, enzyme characteristics and applications. *Mar. Drugs* **2010**, *8*, 200–218. [CrossRef]
221. Han, X.; Lin, B.; Ru, G.; Zhang, Z.; Liu, Y.; Hu, Z. Gene Cloning and Characterization of an α-Amylase from *Alteromonas macleodii* B7 for Enteromorpha Polysaccharide Degradation. *J. Microbiol. Biotechnol.* **2014**, *24*, 254–263. [CrossRef]

222. Sewalt, V.J.; Reyes, T.F.; Bui, Q. Safety evaluation of two α-amylase enzyme preparations derived from *Bacillus* licheniformis expressing an α-amylase gene from *Cytophaga* species. *Regul. Toxicol. Pharmacol.* **2018**, *98*, 140–150. [CrossRef]
223. Amoozegar, M.A.; Siroosi, M.; Atashgahi, S.; Smidt, H.; Ventosa, A. Systematics of haloarchaea and biotechnological potential of their hydrolytic enzymes. *Microbiology* **2017**, *163*, 623–645. [CrossRef]
224. Qin, Y.; Huang, Z.; Liu, Z. A novel cold-active and salt-tolerant α-amylase from marine bacterium *Zunongwangia profunda*: Molecular cloning, heterologous expression and biochemical characterization. *Extremophiles* **2014**, *18*, 271–281. [CrossRef] [PubMed]
225. Amoozegar, M.A.; Malekzadeh, F.; Malik, K.A. Production of amylase by newly isolated moderate halophile, *Halobacillus* sp. strain MA-2. *J. Microbiol. Methods* **2003**, *52*, 353–359. [CrossRef]
226. de Lourdes Moreno, M.; Pérez, D.; García, M.; Mellado, E.; De Lourdes Moreno, M.; Pérez, D.; García, M.T.; Mellado, E. Halophilic Bacteria as a Source of Novel Hydrolytic Enzymes. *Life* **2013**, *3*, 38–51. [CrossRef] [PubMed]
227. Kiran, K.; Koteswaraiah, P.; Chandra, T.S. Production of Halophilic α-Amylase by Immobilized Cells of Moderately Halophilic *Bacillus* sp. Strain TSCVKK. *Br. Microbiol. Res. J.* **2012**, *2*, 146–157. [CrossRef]
228. Uotsu-Tomita, R.; Tonozuka, T.; Sakai, H.; Sakano, Y. Novel glucoamylase-type enzymes from *Thermoactinomyces vulgaris* and *Methanococcus jannaschii* whose genes are found in the flanking region of the α-amylase genes. *Appl. Microbiol. Biotechnol.* **2001**, *56*, 465–473. [CrossRef]
229. Kim, J.W.; Flowers, L.O.; Whiteley, M.; Peeples, T.L. Biochemical confirmation and characterization of the family-57-like α-amylase of *Methanococcus jannaschii. Folia Microbiol.* **2001**, *46*, 467–473. [CrossRef]
230. Aghajari, N.; Feller, G.; Gerday, C.; Haser, R. Structures of the psychrophilic *Alteromonas haloplanctis* α-amylase give insights into cold adaptation at a molecular level. *Structure* **1998**, *6*, 1503–1516. [CrossRef]
231. Mageswari, A.; Subramanian, P.; Chandrasekaran, S.; Sivashanmugam, K.; Babu, S.; Gothandam, K.M. Optimization and immobilization of amylase obtained from halotolerant bacteria isolated from solar salterns. *J. Genet. Eng. Biotechnol.* **2012**, *10*, 201–208. [CrossRef]
232. Coronado, M.J.; Vargas, C.; Mellado, E.; Tegos, G.; Drainas, C.; Nieto, J.J.; Ventosa, A. The α-amylase gene amyH of the moderate halophile *Halomonas* meridiana: Cloning and molecular characterization. *Microbiology* **2000**, *146*, 861–868. [CrossRef]
233. Singh, G.; Verma, A.K.; Kumar, V. Catalytic properties, functional attributes and industrial applications of β-glucosidases. *3 Biotech* **2016**, *6*, 1–14. [CrossRef]
234. Sun, J.; Wang, W.; Yao, C.; Dai, F.; Zhu, X.; Liu, J.; Hao, J. Overexpression and characterization of a novel cold-adapted and salt-tolerant GH1 β-glucosidase from the marine bacterium *Alteromonas* sp. L82. *J. Microbiol.* **2018**, *56*, 656–664. [CrossRef] [PubMed]
235. Hebbale, D.; Bhargavi, R.; Ramachandra, T.V. Saccharification of macroalgal polysaccharides through prioritized cellulase producing bacteria. *Heliyon* **2019**, *5*, e01372. [CrossRef]
236. Zhu, B.; Ning, L. Purification and Characterization of a New *k*-Carrageenase from the Marine Bacterium *Vibrio* sp. NJ-2. *J. Microbiol. Biotechnol.* **2016**, *26*, 255–262. [CrossRef] [PubMed]
237. Xiao, A.; Zeng, J.; Li, J.; Zhu, Y.; Xiao, Q.; Ni, H. Molecular cloning, characterization, and heterologous expression of a new κ-carrageenase gene from *Pseudoalteromonas carrageenovora* ASY5. *J. Food Biochem.* **2018**, *42*. [CrossRef]
238. Blanco, K.C.; De Lima, C.J.B.; Monti, R.; Martins, J.; Bernardi, N.S.; Contiero, J. *Bacillus lehensis*—An alkali-tolerant bacterium isolated from cassava starch wastewater: Optimization of parameters for cyclodextrin glycosyltransferase production. *Ann. Microbiol.* **2012**, *62*, 329–337. [CrossRef]
239. Suriya, J.; Bharathiraja, S.; Krishnan, M.; Manivasagan, P.; Kim, S.-K. Marine Microbial Amylases. In *Advances in food and nutrition research*; Elsevier Inc. Academic Press: Cambridge, MA, USA, 2016; Volume 79, pp. 161–177. ISBN 978-0-12-804714-9.
240. Mehta, D.; Satyanarayana, T. Bacterial and archaeal α-amylases: Diversity and amelioration of the desirable characteristics for industrial applications. *Front. Microbiol.* **2016**, *7*. [CrossRef]
241. Jabbour, D.; Sorger, A.; Sahm, K.; Antranikian, G. A highly thermoactive and salt-tolerant α-amylase isolated from a pilot-plant biogas reactor. *Appl. Microbiol. Biotechnol.* **2013**, *97*, 2971–2978. [CrossRef]
242. Cowan, D.; Cramp, R.; Pereira, R.; Graham, D.; Almatawah, Q. Biochemistry and biotechnology of mesophilic and thermophilic nitrile metabolizing enzymes. *Extremophiles* **1998**, *2*, 207–216. [CrossRef]

243. Gupta, N.; Balomajumder, C.; Agarwal, V.K. Enzymatic mechanism and biochemistry for cyanide degradation: A review. *J. Hazard. Mater.* **2010**, *176*, 1–13. [CrossRef]
244. Nigam, V.K.; Arfi, T.; Kumar, V.; Shukla, P. Bioengineering of Nitrilases Towards Its Use as Green Catalyst: Applications and Perspectives. *Indian J. Microbiol.* **2017**, *57*, 131–138. [CrossRef]
245. Kuddus, M. Cold-active enzymes in food biotechnology: An updated mini review. *J. Appl. Biol. Biotechnol.* **2018**, *6*, 58–63.
246. Hasan, F.; Shah, A.A.; Hameed, A. Industrial applications of microbial lipases. *Enzyme Microb. Technol.* **2006**, *39*, 235–251. [CrossRef]
247. Mahjoubi, M.; Cappello, S.; Souissi, Y.; Jaouani, A.; Cherif, A. Microbial Bioremediation of Petroleum Hydrocarbon–Contaminated Marine Environments. In *Recent Insights in Petroleum Science and Engineering*; Zoveidavianpoor, M., Ed.; InTechOpen: London, UK, 2018; pp. 325–350.
248. Hassanshahian, M.; Cappello, S. Crude Oil Biodegradation in the Marine Environments. In *Biodegradation—Engineering and Technology*; Rolando Chamy, Ed.; InTechOpen: London, UK, 2013; pp. 101–135.
249. Floodgate, G.D. Biodegradation of hydrocarbons in the sea. In *Water Pollution Microbiology*; Mitchell, R., Ed.; Wiley-Interscience: New York, NY, USA, 1972; pp. 153–171.
250. Jarvis, I.W.H.; Dreij, K.; Mattsson, Å.; Jernström, B.; Stenius, U. Interactions between polycyclic aromatic hydrocarbons in complex mixtures and implications for cancer risk assessment. *Toxicology* **2014**, *321*, 27–39. [CrossRef] [PubMed]
251. Moreno, R.; Jover, L.; Diez, C.; Sardà, F.; Sanpera, C. Ten Years after the Prestige Oil Spill: Seabird Trophic Ecology as Indicator of Long-Term Effects on the Coastal Marine Ecosystem. *PLoS ONE* **2013**, *8*. [CrossRef]
252. Sikkema, J.; de Bont, J.A.; Poolman, B. Mechanisms of Membrane Toxicity of Hydrocarbons. *Microbiol. Rev.* **1995**, *59*, 201–222. [CrossRef]
253. Catania, V.; Santisi, S.; Signa, G.; Vizzini, S.; Mazzola, A.; Cappello, S.; Yakimov, M.M.; Quatrini, P. Intrinsic bioremediation potential of a chronically polluted marine coastal area. *Mar. Pollut. Bull.* **2015**, *99*, 138–149. [CrossRef]
254. Durval, I.J.B.; Resende, A.H.M.; Figueiredo, M.A.; Luna, J.M.; Rufino, R.D.; Sarubbo, L.A. Studies on Biosurfactants Produced using *Bacillus cereus* Isolated from Seawater with Biotechnological Potential for Marine Oil-Spill Bioremediation. *J. Surfactants Deterg.* **2018**, *22*, 349–363. [CrossRef]
255. Hazen, T.C.; Dubinsky, E.A.; DeSantis, T.Z.; Andersen, G.L.; Piceno, Y.M.; Singh, N.; Jansson, J.K.; Probst, A.; Borglin, S.E.; Fortney, J.L.; et al. Deep-sea oil plume enriches indigenous oil-degrading bacteria. *Science* **2010**, *330*, 204–208. [CrossRef]
256. Kleindienst, S.; Paul, J.H.; Joye, S.B. Using dispersants after oil spills: Impacts on the composition and activity of microbial communities. *Nat. Rev. Microbiol.* **2015**, *13*, 388–396. [CrossRef]
257. Speight, J.G.; El-Gendy, N.S. *Introduction to petroleum biotechnology*; Elsevier: Amsterdam, The Netherlands, 2017; ISBN 9780128051511.
258. Fuentes, S.; Méndez, V.; Aguila, P.; Seeger, M. Bioremediation of petroleum hydrocarbons: Catabolic genes, microbial communities, and applications. *Appl. Microbiol. Biotechnol.* **2014**, *98*, 4781–4794. [CrossRef]
259. Fuentes, S.; Barra, B.; Gregory Caporaso, J.; Seeger, M. From rare to dominant: A fine-tuned soil bacterial bloom during petroleum hydrocarbon bioremediation. *Appl. Environ. Microbiol.* **2016**, *82*, 888–896. [CrossRef] [PubMed]
260. Varjani, S.J.; Gnansounou, E. Microbial dynamics in petroleum oilfields and their relationship with physiological properties of petroleum oil reservoirs. *Bioresour. Technol.* **2017**, *245*, 1258–1265. [CrossRef] [PubMed]
261. Coulon, F.; McKew, B.A.; Osborn, A.M.; McGenity, T.J.; Timmis, K.N. Effects of temperature and biostimulation on oil-degrading microbial communities in temperate estuarine waters. *Environ. Microbiol.* **2007**, *9*, 177–186. [CrossRef] [PubMed]
262. Xu, X.; Liu, W.; Tian, S.; Wang, W.; Qi, Q.; Jiang, P.; Gao, X.; Li, F.; Li, H.; Yu, H. Petroleum Hydrocarbon-Degrading Bacteria for the Remediation of Oil Pollution Under Aerobic Conditions: A Perspective Analysis. *Front. Microbiol.* **2018**, *9*, 1–11. [CrossRef]
263. Fathepure, B.Z. Recent studies in microbial degradation of petroleum hydrocarbons in hypersaline environments. *Front. Microbiol.* **2014**, *5*. [CrossRef]
264. Oren, A. Aerobic Hydrocarbon-Degrading Archaea. In *Taxonomy, Genomics and Ecophysiology of Hydrocarbon-Degrading Microbes*; Springer International Publishing: Cham, Switzerland, 2017; pp. 1–12.

265. Gutierrez, T.; Singleton, D.R.; Berry, D.; Yang, T.; Aitken, M.D.; Teske, A. Hydrocarbon-degrading bacteria enriched by the Deepwater Horizon oil spill identified by cultivation and DNA-SIP. *ISME J.* **2013**, *7*, 2091–2104. [CrossRef]
266. Yakimov, M.M.; Timmis, K.N.; Golyshin, P.N. Obligate oil-degrading marine bacteria. *Curr. Opin. Biotechnol.* **2007**, *18*, 257–266. [CrossRef]
267. McGenity, T.J.; Folwell, B.D.; McKew, B.A.; Sanni, G.O. Marine crude-oil biodegradation: A central role for interspecies interactions. *Aquat. Biosyst.* **2012**, *8*, 10. [CrossRef]
268. Head, I.M.; Jones, D.M.; Röling, W.F.M. Marine microorganisms make a meal of oil. *Nat. Rev. Microbiol.* **2006**, *4*, 173–182. [CrossRef]
269. Barbato, M.; Mapelli, F.; Magagnini, M.; Chouaia, B.; Armeni, M.; Marasco, R.; Crotti, E.; Daffonchio, D.; Borin, S. Hydrocarbon pollutants shape bacterial community assembly of harbor sediments. *Mar. Pollut. Bull.* **2016**, *104*, 211–220. [CrossRef]
270. Barbato, M.; Mapelli, F.; Chouaia, B.; Crotti, E.; Daffonchio, D.; Borin, S. Draft genome sequence of the hydrocarbon-degrading bacterium *Alcanivorax dieselolei* KS-293 isolated from surface seawater in the Eastern Mediterranean Sea. *Genome Announc.* **2015**, 3. [CrossRef] [PubMed]
271. Wang, W.; Shao, Z. The long-chain alkane metabolism network of *Alcanivorax dieselolei*. *Nat. Commun.* **2014**, *5*. [CrossRef] [PubMed]
272. Li, A.; Shao, Z. Biochemical characterization of a haloalkane dehalogenase DadB from *Alcanivorax dieselolei* B-5. *PLoS ONE* **2014**, *9*. [CrossRef] [PubMed]
273. Scoma, A.; Barbato, M.; Hernandez-Sanabria, E.; Mapelli, F.; Daffonchio, D.; Borin, S.; Boon, N. Microbial oil-degradation under mild hydrostatic pressure (10 MPa): Which pathways are impacted in piezosensitive hydrocarbonoclastic bacteria? *Sci. Rep.* **2016**, *6*, 1–14. [CrossRef]
274. Barbato, M.; Scoma, A.; Mapelli, F.; De Smet, R.; Banat, I.M.; Daffonchio, D.; Boon, N.; Borin, S. Hydrocarbonoclastic alcanivorax isolates exhibit different physiological and expression responses to N-dodecane. *Front. Microbiol.* **2016**, *7*, 1–14. [CrossRef]
275. Sass, A.M.; McKew, B.A.; Sass, H.; Fichtel, J.; Timmis, K.N.; McGenity, T.J. Diversity of *Bacillus*-like organisms isolated from deep-sea hypersaline anoxic sediments. *Saline Systems* **2008**, *4*, 1–11. [CrossRef]
276. Antunes, A.; Eder, W.; Fareleira, P.; Santos, H.; Huber, R. *Salinisphaera shabanensis* gen. nov., sp. nov., a novel, moderately halophilic bacterium from the brine-seawater interface of the Shaban Deep, Red Sea. *Extremophiles* **2003**, *7*, 29–34. [CrossRef]
277. Palau, M.; Boujida, N.; Manresa, À.; Miñana-Galbis, D. Complete genome sequence of *Marinobacter flavimaris* LMG 23834T, which is potentially useful in bioremediation. *Genome Announc.* **2018**, *6*, 1–2. [CrossRef]
278. Marquez, M.C. Marinobacter hydrocarbonoclasticus Gauthier et al. 1992 and Marinobacter aquaeolei Nguyen et al. 1999 are heterotypic synonyms. *Int. J. Syst. Evol. Microbiol.* **2005**, *55*, 1349–1351. [CrossRef]
279. Handley, K.M.; Lloyd, J.R. Biogeochemical implications of the ubiquitous colonization of marine habitats and redox gradients by Marinobacter species. *Front. Microbiol.* **2013**, *4*, 1–10. [CrossRef]
280. Gomes, M.B.; Gonzales-Limache, E.E.; Sousa, S.T.P.; Dellagnezze, B.M.; Sartoratto, A.; Silva, L.C.F.; Gieg, L.L.M.; Valoni, E.; Souza, R.S.; Torres, A.P.R.; et al. Exploring the potential of halophilic bacteria from oil terminal environments for biosurfactant production and hydrocarbon degradation under high-salinity conditions. *Int. Biodeterior. Biodegradation* **2018**, *126*, 231–242. [CrossRef]
281. Kodama, Y.; Stiknowati, L.I.; Ueki, A.; Ueki, K.; Watanabe, K. Thalassospira tepidiphila sp. nov., a polycyclic aromatic hydrocarbon-degrading bacterium isolated from seawater. *Int. J. Syst. Evol. Microbiol.* **2008**, *58*, 711–715. [CrossRef] [PubMed]
282. Budiyanto, F.; Thukair, A.; Al-Momani, M.; Musa, M.M.; Nzila, A. Characterization of Halophilic Bacteria Capable of Efficiently Biodegrading the High-Molecular-Weight Polycyclic Aromatic Hydrocarbon Pyrene. *Environ. Eng. Sci.* **2018**, *35*, 616–626. [CrossRef]
283. Castillo-Carvajal, L.C.; Sanz-Martín, J.L.; Barragán-Huerta, B.E. Biodegradation of organic pollutants in saline wastewater by halophilic microorganisms: A review. *Environ. Sci. Pollut. Res.* **2014**, *21*, 9578–9588. [CrossRef] [PubMed]
284. Paniagua-Michel, J.; Babu, Z. Fathepure Microbial Consortia and Biodegradation of Petroleum Hydrocarbons in Marine Environments. In *Microbial Action on Hydrocarbons*; Kumar, V., Kumar, M., Prasad, R., Eds.; Springer Nature: Singapore, 2019; pp. 1–20.

285. Erdoğmuş, S.F.; Mutlu, B.; Korcan, S.E.; Güven, K.; Konuk, M. Aromatic hydrocarbon degradation by halophilic archaea isolated from ÇamaltI Saltern, Turkey. *Water. Air. Soil Pollut.* **2013**, *224*. [CrossRef]
286. Al-Mailem, D.M.; Eliyas, M.; Radwan, S.S. Oil-bioremediation potential of two hydrocarbonoclastic, diazotrophic *Marinobacter* strains from hypersaline areas along the Arabian Gulf coasts. *Extremophiles* **2013**, *17*, 463–470. [CrossRef] [PubMed]
287. Edbeib, M.F.; Wahab, R.A.; Huyop, F. Halophiles: Biology, adaptation, and their role in decontamination of hypersaline environments. *World J. Microbiol. Biotechnol.* **2016**, *32*, 1–23. [CrossRef]

marine drugs

MDPI

Article

A Cold-Adapted Chitinase-Producing Bacterium from Antarctica and Its Potential in Biocontrol of Plant Pathogenic Fungi

Kezhen Liu [1,2], Haitao Ding [2,*], Yong Yu [2] and Bo Chen [2,*]

[1] College of Marine Science, Shanghai Ocean University, Shanghai 201306, China; 18043425667@163.com
[2] MNR Key Laboratory for Polar Science, Polar Research Institute of China, Shanghai 200136, China; yuyong@pric.org.cn
* Correspondence: htding@outlook.com (H.D.); chenbo@pric.org.cn (B.C.); Tel.: +86-21-5871-8663 (H.D.); +86-21-5871-1026 (B.C.)

Received: 14 November 2019; Accepted: 5 December 2019; Published: 10 December 2019

Abstract: To obtain chitinase-producing microorganisms with high chitinolytic activity at low temperature, samples collected from Fildes Peninsula in Antarctica were used as sources for bioprospecting of chitinolytic microorganisms. A cold-adapted strain, designated as GWSMS-1, was isolated from marine sediment and further characterized as *Pseudomonas*. To improve the chitinase production, one-factor-at-a-time and orthogonal test approaches were adopted to optimize the medium components and culture conditions. The results showed that the highest chitinolytic activity (6.36 times higher than that before optimization) was obtained with 95.41 U L^{-1} with 15 g L^{-1} of glucose, 1 g L^{-1} of peptone, 15 g L^{-1} of colloid chitin and 0.25 g L^{-1} of magnesium ions contained in the medium, cultivated under pH 7.0 and a temperature of 20 °C. To better understand the application potential of this strain, the enzymatic properties and the antifungal activity of the crude chitinase secreted by the strain were further investigated. The crude enzyme showed the maximum catalytic activity at 35 °C and pH 4.5, and it also exhibited excellent low-temperature activity, which still displayed more than 50% of its maximal activity at 0 °C. Furthermore, the crude chitinase showed significant inhibition of fungi *Verticillium dahlia* CICC 2534 and *Fusarium oxysporum* f. sp. *cucumerinum* CICC 2532, which can cause cotton wilt and cucumber blight, respectively, suggesting that strain GWSMS-1 could be a competitive candidate for biological control in agriculture, especially at low temperature.

Keywords: Antarctica; chitinase; cold-adapted; optimization; antifungal; *Pseudomonas*

1. Introduction

Chitin is a polysaccharide consisting of β-*N*-acetyl-D-glucosamine (GlcNAc) units linked by β-1,4 glycosidic bonds [1]. Chitin is a major resource for the preparation of chitin oligosaccharides, chitosan oligosaccharides and other chitin derivatives, which have tremendous applicable values in the fields of medicine, food, health care and environmental protection [2]. Generally, chitin can be decomposed through physical, chemical or biological approaches [3]. Although physical and chemical methods have been used broadly, both of them have many invincible drawbacks such as low yield, high cost, poor product uniformity and environmental pollution, while a biological method possesses the advantages of mild reaction condition, good yield, high product uniformity and environmental friendliness, especially for the enzymatic method implemented by chitinase [4].

Chitinases, which are capable of hydrolyzing chitin to release GlcNAc and *N*-acetyl chitin oligosaccharides [5], have been found in many organisms, including bacteria [6], fungi [7], plants [8], insects [9] and even humans [10]. Chitinases and chitinase-producing microorganisms have received considerable attention due to their potential applications in biological control of fungal pathogens [11] and preparation of chitin derivatives [4] in recent years. Although plenty of chitinase-producing microorganisms have been discovered and characterized, such as *Sanguibacter antarcticus* KOPRI 21702 [12], *Basidiobolus ranarum* [13], *Bacillus pumilus* U5 [14], *Chitinolyticbacter meiyuanensis* SYBC-H1 [15], *Paenibacillus* sp. D1 [16], *Serratia Marcescens* XJ-01 [17], *Streptomyces* sp. ANU 6277 [18], *Lysinibacillus fusiformis* B-CM18 [19], *Streptomyces griseorubens* C9 [20], *Streptomyces pratensis* KLSL55 [21], *Humicola grisea* ITCC 10360.16 [22], *Cohnella* sp. A01 [23], *Serratia marcescens* JPP1 [24] and *Stenotrophomonas maltophilia* [25], their chitinolytic activities are still fairly low, especially at low and intermediate temperatures, which leads to the high cost and limited large-scale application of chitinases or chitinase-producing microorganisms. As a rule of thumb, cold-adapted enzymes usually display higher activity than their mesophilic and thermophilic counterparts at the same temperature [26]. Such enzymes can be more easily found in Antarctica, a natural resource pool of cold-adapted microorganisms [27].

To obtain chitinase-producing microorganisms with high chitinolytic activity, samples collected from Fildes Peninsula on King George Island of Antarctica were used as sources for bioprospecting of chitinolytic microorganisms. The production of chitinase of the selected strain was optimized by statistical design. Besides, enzymatic properties and antifungal potential of the extracellular chitinase secreted by the strain were also investigated in this study.

2. Results

2.1. Screening, Isolation and Identification of the Chitinase-Producing Bacterium

Strain GWSMS-1, isolating from marine sediment, produced a clear transparent zone on the colloidal chitin plate (Figure 1a), indicating that it is capable of secreting chitinase to hydrolyze the colloidal chitin around itself. The native-PAGE was conducted to further verify the chitinase activity of the secreted enzyme. As shown in Lane 2 of Figure 1b, a clear band was observed on the gel, implying the presence of chitinase in the crude enzyme secreted by strain GWSMS-1.

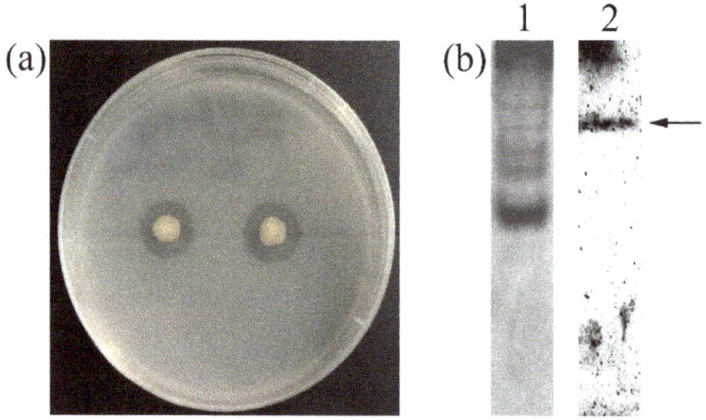

Figure 1. Screening and confirmation of the chitinase-producing bacterium. (**a**) Inoculation of strain GWSMS-1 on colloidal chitin plate. (**b**) Native-PAGE of concentrated crude chitinase secreted by strain GWSMS-1. In lane 1, the gel was stained by Coomassie Brilliant Blue R-250. In lane 2, the gel was stained by Calcofluor White M2R. The proposed chitinase was indicated by an arrow.

Strain GWSMS-1 was classified into genus *Pseudomonas* by molecular identification using 16S-rDNA sequencing. To understand the evolutionary relationship between *Pseudomonas* sp. GWSMS-1 and its phylogenetically related species, a 16S rDNA-based phylogenetic analysis was conducted using a total of thirty-one 16S rDNA gene sequences retrieved from EzBioCloud web server [28]. The 16S rDNA of strain GWSMS-1 showed the highest similarity (99.79%) with *Pseudomonas guineae* LMG 24016 [29], a psychrotolerant bacterium also isolated from Antarctica (Figure 2). Since these two strains occupied a distinct position in genus *Pseudomonas*, it is suggested that they might experience a similar evolutionary journey to adapt to the extreme environment of Antarctica.

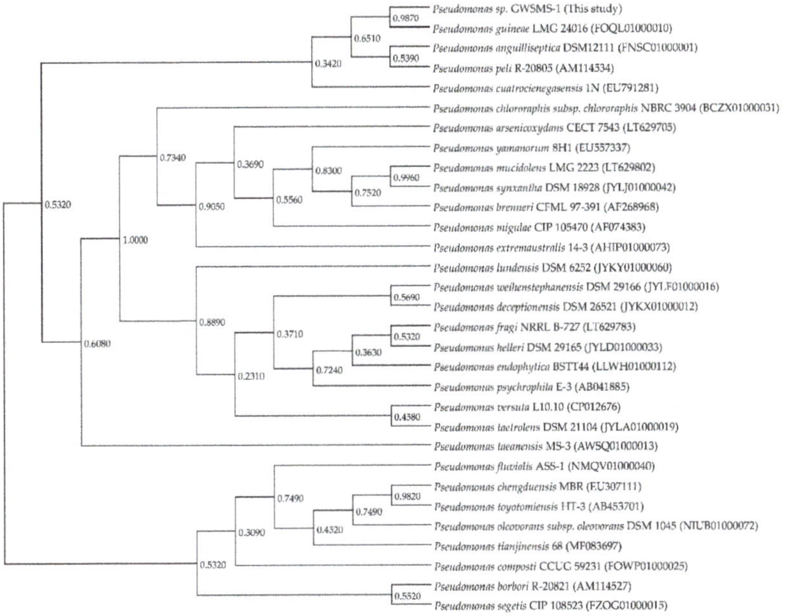

Figure 2. Phylogenetic analysis based on 16S rDNA sequences of *Pseudomonas* sp. GWSMS-1 and its phylogenetically related species. The GenBank accession number is provided following the species name.

2.2. One-Factor-at-a-Time Optimization

The change of chitinolytic activity of *Pseudomonas* sp. GWSMS-1 during the fermentation process was monitored to determine the fermentation time for chitinase production with the highest activity. As shown in Figure 3, the chitinolytic activity could be detected in the fermentation broth after 24 h of cultivation, and it achieved its maximum on the sixth day. It is worth mentioning that the chitinolytic activity (solid circle) increased with the increase in protein concentration (empty circle) in the first six days, but decreased sharply with increased consumption of chitin in later days. It is proposed that the chitinase of strain GWSMS-1 is an inducible enzyme, which could only be produced in the presence of chitin with high enough concentration. Therefore, fermentation broth cultivated for 6 days was used for measuring the chitinolytic activity in further study.

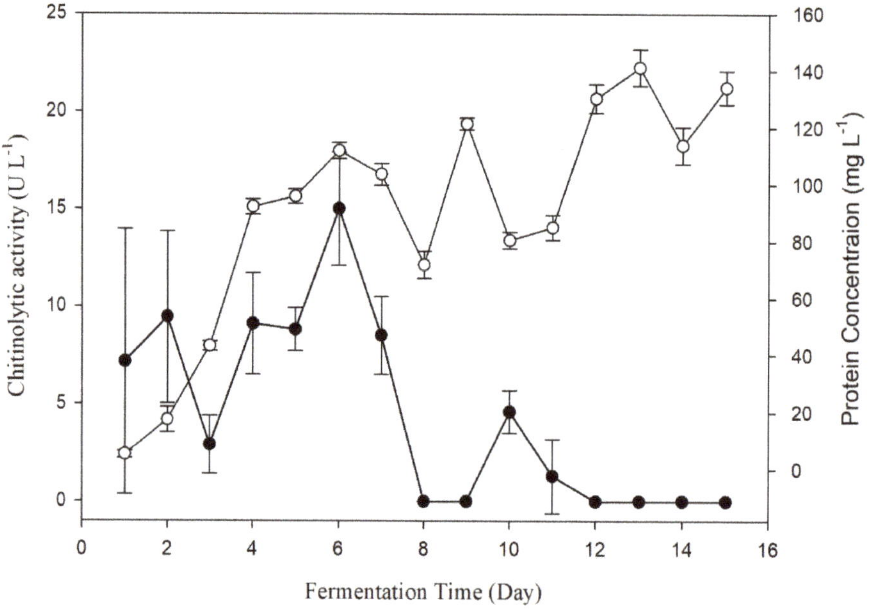

Figure 3. Changes in the chitinolytic activity of *Pseudomonas* sp. GWSMS-1 during the fermentation process. Chitinolytic activity and protein concentration are represented as solid and empty circles, respectively.

The results of carbon source selection showed that the carbon source exerted a significant influence on the chitinolytic activity, which was undetectable when glycerol was used as carbon source, while the strain produced the highest amount of chitinolytic activity when glucose was used as carbon source (Figure 4a) with a concentration of 10 g L^{-1} (Figure 4c). Nitrogen source test results displayed that the organic nitrogen sources had a better effect on chitinolytic activity than those of inorganic nitrogen sources (Figure 4b). The highest chitinolytic activity was determined from the fermentation broth when peptone was employed as the nitrogen source with a concentration of 2 g L^{-1} (Figure 4d). In addition, different chitin concentrations also affected the production of chitinase by *Pseudomonas* sp. GWSMS-1, and the highest apparent yield of the enzyme was observed when the chitin concentration was 10 g L^{-1} (Figure 4e). The fermentation condition optimization showed that the optimum temperature, pH and shaking speed for the production of chitinolytic enzymes were determined as 20 °C (Figure 4f), 7.0 (Figure 4g) and 100–150 rpm (Figure 4h), respectively.

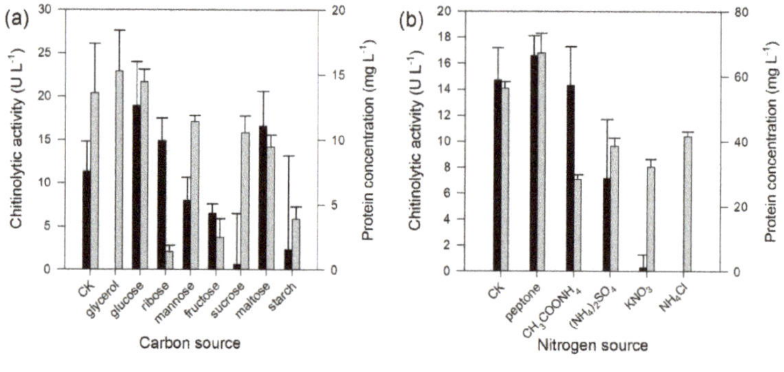

Figure 4. *Cont.*

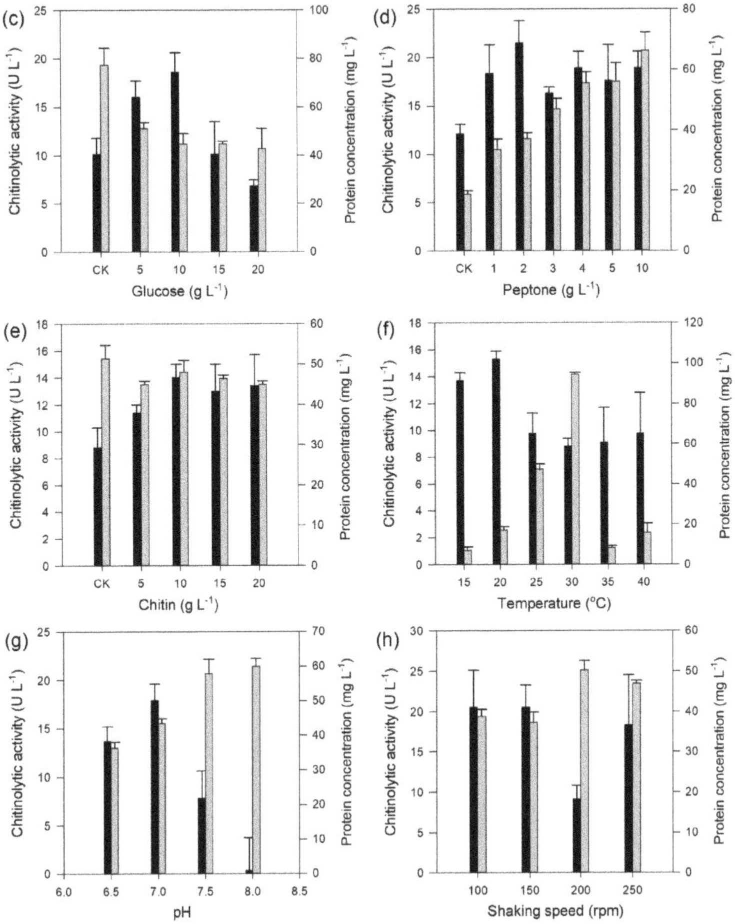

Figure 4. Chitinase production of *Pseudomonas* sp. GWSMS-1 optimized by the one-factor-at-a-time method. Effects of (**a**) carbon source, (**b**) nitrogen source, (**c**) glucose concentration, (**d**) peptone concentration, (**e**) chitin concentration, (**f**) temperature, (**g**) pH and (**h**) shaking speed on the chitinase production. Chitinolytic activity and protein concentration are represented as black and grey bars, respectively.

2.3. Orthogonal Design

With the aim of obtaining more chitinase secreted by strain GWSMS-1, the medium components were further optimized by orthogonal design. The results showed that the apparent highest chitinolytic activity of 72.16 U L^{-1} was obtained with the seventh combination (Table 1). Further analysis of the data implied that the desired highest activity would be achieved when the concentrations of glucose, peptone, colloid chitin and magnesium ions are 15 g L^{-1}, 1 g L^{-1}, 15 g L^{-1} and 1 mM, respectively. Subsequently, an additional experiment was performed to verify this combination, which was not included in the orthogonal test. Finally, the chitinolytic activity was determined as 95.41 U L^{-1} with the above combination, which was higher than the apparent highest activity (72.16 U L^{-1}) observed in the orthogonal test. In variance analysis, $F_{0.01} = 6.23$ is used as a reference value, and $F > 6.23$ means a significant effect of the factor. According to the variance analysis of the orthogonal test showed in

Table 2, all these four factors involved in the optimization showed significant effects on the yield of chitinase at the $p = 0.01$ level, and peptone and chitin were the most significant factors.

Table 1. Orthogonal design and the responding chitinolytic activity.

No.	(A) Glucose (g L^{-1})	(B) Peptone (g L^{-1})	(C) Chitin (g L^{-1})	(D) Mg^{2+} (mM)	Chitinolytic Activity (U L^{-1})
1	5	1	5	1	52.25 ± 3.73
2	5	2	10	5	16.17 ± 2.16
3	5	3	15	10	22.64 ± 6.26
4	10	1	10	10	18.66 ± 3.73
5	10	2	15	1	51.01 ± 2.15
6	10	3	5	5	7.46 ± 6.47
7	15	1	15	5	72.16 ± 7.77
8	15	2	5	10	37.32 ± 3.73
9	15	3	10	1	6.22 ± 2.16
K1	91.07	143.08	97.04	109.49	
K2	77.14	104.51	41.06	95.80	
K3	115.71	36.33	145.81	78.63	
k1	30.36	47.69	32.35	36.50	
k2	25.71	34.84	13.69	31.93	
k3	38.57	12.11	48.60	26.21	
Range	12.86	35.58	34.91	10.29	
Factor order		B > C > A > D			
Optimization combination	A3	B1	C3	D1	

Table 2. Analysis of Variance (ANOVA).

Source	Sum of Square	Degrees of Freedom	Mean Square	F-value	*p*-value
Glucose	762.85	2	381.42	17.42	<0.01
Peptone	5843.69	2	2921.84	133.43	<0.01
Chitin	5495.72	2	2747.86	125.49	<0.01
Mg^{2+}	478.03	2	239.02	10.92	<0.01
Error	394.16	18	21.90		
Total	39843.59	27			

Therefore, the final medium for chitinase production of *Pseudomonas* sp. GWSMS-1 was determined as follows (L^{-1}): glucose 15 g, peptone 1 g, colloidal chitin 15 g, $MgSO_4{\cdot}7H_2O$ 0.25 g, KH_2PO_4 0.3 g, $K_2HPO_4{\cdot}3H_2O$ 1 g.

2.4. Temperature and pH-Dependent Enzymatic Properties of Chitinase

The crude chitinase showed chitinolytic activity in a wide temperature range with the maximum catalytic activity at 35 °C. Furthermore, the enzyme also exhibited excellent low-temperature activity, which still displayed more than 50% of its maximal activity at 0 °C (Figure 5a). A generally accepted hypothesis is that high low-temperature activity of cold-adapted enzymes evolved to facilitate binding and conversion of the substrate at low temperatures, which is consistently accompanied by weak thermal stability on account of the intrinsic structural flexibility of the enzymes, which is supposed to be a result of evolutionary pressure [30]. The crude enzyme was only stable at low temperature and was rapidly inactivated with increasing temperature (Figure 5b). The crude chitinase had a high chitinolytic activity between pH 4.0–5.0, with an optimum catalytic activity at pH 4.5 (Figure 5c), indicating that the chitinase might be an acidic enzyme. The pH stability of the crude chitinase exhibited a similar pattern to that of the activity response to pH, which was stable in the pH range of 4.0 to 5.0 and rapidly deactivated under other pH values (Figure 5d).

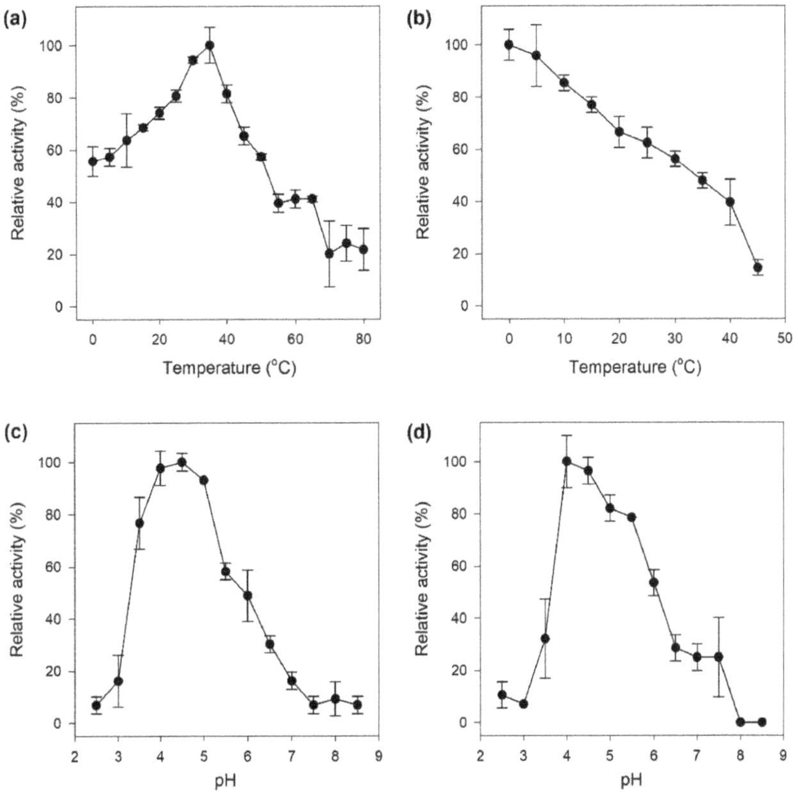

Figure 5. Enzymatic properties of the crude chitinase. (**a**) Optimal temperature; (**b**) temperature stability; (**c**) optimal pH; (**d**) pH stability.

2.5. Antifungal Activity

As a key component of fungal cell wall, chitin is essential for fungal pathogens to maintain their cell structure integrity. Considering that chitinase is capable of degrading chitin to decompose the fungal cell wall, it is indispensable to evaluate the antifungal potential of strain GWSMS-1. However, since strain GWSMS-1 is not one of GRAS (generally regarded as safe) strains, it cannot be applied to the medical field without any safety tests, whereas the requirement is less stringent for agricultural application. Therefore, five common phytopathogenic fungi were selected to evaluate the potential application in biocontrol of strain GWSMS-1. As shown in Figure 6, the crude enzymes significantly inhibited the phytopathogenic fungi *Verticillium dahlia* CICC 2534 and *Fusarium oxysporum* f. sp. *cucumerinum* CICC 2532 and slightly inhibited *Aspergillus niger* CICC 2039 and *Penicillium macrosclerotiorum* CICC 40649, even after incubation for 7 days, while not showing any inhibition toward *Alternaria brassicicola* CICC 2646 during the entire incubation.

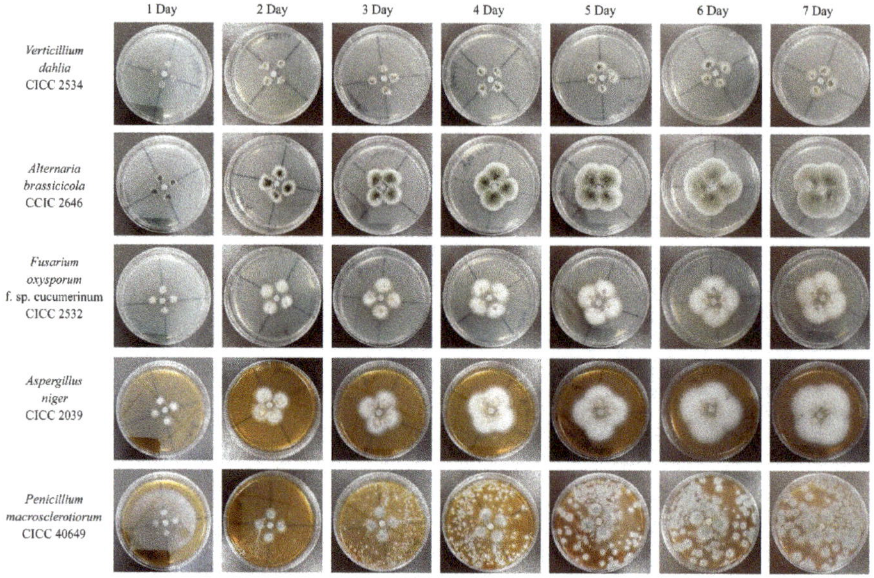

Figure 6. Antifungal activity of the chitinase secreted by *Pseudomonas* sp. GWSMS-1.

3. Discussion

In this study, a chitinase-producing strain GWSMS-1 was isolated from marine sediment near the China's Great Wall Station in Antarctica and characterized as a member of genus *Pseudomonas*. Statistical optimization of the chitinase production, the enzymatic properties and the antifungal activity of the chitinase was conducted for better evaluating the application potential of this strain.

Enzyme production is one of the most important limitations for the large-scale application of enzymes, which significantly affects the usage cost. Generally, the yield of an enzyme is optimized from two aspects: medium indigents and culture conditions. In this study, the optimum culture conditions, including temperature, pH and shaking speed, were determined as 20 °C, 7.0 and 150 rpm, respectively, which shared similar conditions except for temperature with other strains reported previously (Table 3). It is obvious that the optimum temperatures for the secretion of chitinase by different strains are associated with their optimum growth temperature. Dissolved oxygen level, represented by shaking speed, has little effect on chitinase production among different strains. Another noticeable difference in culture conditions among different chitinase-producing strains is the fermentation time, which ranged from 1 to 8 days (Table 3). Comparing with mesophilic microorganisms, *Pseudomonas* sp. GWSMS-1 has a relatively long fermentation time to achieve its maximum yield of chitinase as a cold-adapted microorganism. However, some mesophilic and thermophilic strains, such as *Streptomyces griseorubens* C9 [20], *Bacillus pumilus* U5 [14] and *Humicola grisea* ITCC 10360.16 [22], also showed similar fermentation periods to GWSMS-1, which might be due to their intrinsic regulation of metabolism. In the further study, strain GWSMS-1 could be genetically modified by metabolic engineering to reduce the fermentation time in order to make the fermentation process economical.

Table 3. Summary of the optimized liquid fermentation conditions of chitinase-producing microorganisms.

Strains	Source	Method	Component [a] ($g\ L^{-1}$)	Condition	Yield (Final/Initial)
Pseudomonas sp. GWSMS-1 (this study)	Sediments, Antarctic	OFAT OD	Colloidal chitin: 15.0 Glucose: 15.0 Peptone: 1.0 $MgSO_4·7H_2O$: 0.25 KH_2PO_4: 0.3 $K_2HPO_4·3H_2O$: 1.0	Temperature: 20 °C pH: 7.0 Rotary speed: 150 rpm Time: 6 days	6.36
Sanguibacter antarcticus KOPRI 21702 [12]	Sea sand, Antarctic	OFAT PBD RSM	Chitin: 2.0 Glycerol: 10.0 Peptone: 5.0 Yeast extract: 1.0 $Fe(C_6H_5O_7)$: 0.01 NaCl: 23.0 $MgCl_2$: 2.5 Na_2SO_4: 3.24 $CaCl_2$: 1.8 $NaHCO_3$: 0.16	Temperature: 25 °C pH: 6.5 DO: 30% Time: 3 days	7.5
Basidiobolus ranarum [13]	Frog excrement	RSM	Colloidal chitin: 15 Lactose: 1.25 Malt extract: 0.25 Peptone: 0.75	Temperature: 25 °C pH: 9.0 Rotary speed: 200 rpm Time: 5 days	7.71
Bacillus pumilus U5 [14]	Soil, Iran	PBD RSM	Chitin: 4.760 Yeast extract: 0.439 $MgSO_4·7H_2O$: 0.0055 $FeSO_4·7H_2O$: 0.019	Temperature: 30 °C pH: 6.5 Rotary speed: 150 rpm Time: 8 days	1.20
Chitinolyticbacter meiyuanensis SYBC-H1 [15]	Soil, China	PBD RSM	Chitin: 3.8 Inulin: 3.55 Urea: 3.1 $(NH_4)_2SO_4$: 0.64 $MgSO_4·7H_2O$: 0.5 $FeSO_4·7H_2O$: 0.02 KH_2PO_4: 0.7 K_2HPO_4: 0.3	Temperature: 30 °C pH: 7.0 Rotary speed: 200 rpmTime: 4 days	15.5
Paenibacillus sp. D1 [16]	Effluent, India	PBD RSM	Chitin: 3.75 Yeast extract: 0.6 5Urea: 0.33 $MgSO_4$: 0.30 K_2HPO_4: 1.17	Temperature: 30 °C pH: 7.2 Rotary speed: 180 rpm Time: 3 days	2.56

Table 3. *Cont.*

Strains	Source	Method	Component [a] (g L^{-1})	Condition	Yield (Final/ Initial)
Serratia Marcescens XJ-01 [17]	Fishing field, China	OFA TOD	Colloidal chitin: 7.5 $(NH_4)_2SO_4$: 5 $MgSO_4{\cdot}7H_2O$: 0.5 KH_2PO_4: 2.4 $K_2HPO_4{\cdot}3H_2O$: 0.6	Temperature: 32 °C pH: 8.0 Rotary speed: 180 rpm Time: 32 h	N.M. [c]
Streptomyces sp. ANU 6277 [18]	Soil, India	OFAT	Colloidal chitin: 10.0 Starch: 2.0 Yeast extract: 4.0 KH_2PO_4: 2 $MgSO_4{\cdot}7H_2O$: 1 $FeSO_4{\cdot}7H_2O$: 0.1	Temperature: 35 °C pH: 6.0 Time: 2.5 days	N.M.
Lysinibacillus fusiformis B-CM18 [19]	Chickpea rhizosphere	OFAT RSM	Colloidal chitin: 5.50 Starch: 0.55 Yeast extract: 0.55 NaCl: 4.5 NH_4Cl: 1.0 $CaCl_2$: 0.1 $MgSO_4$: 0.12 KH_2PO_4: 3.0 Na_2HPO_4: 6.0	Temperature: 32.5 °C pH: 7.0 Rotary speed: 150 rpm Time: 2–5 days	56.1
Streptomyces griseorubens C9 [20]	Soil, Algeria	PBD RSM	Colloidal chitin: 20.0 Yeast extract: 0.25 Data syrup: 4.7 K_2HPO_4/KH_2PO_4: 1.81	Temperature: 40 °C pH: natural Rotary speed: 150 rpm Time: 7 days	26.38
Streptomyces pratensis KLSL55 [21]	Soil, India	OFAT	Colloidal chitin: 15 Fructose: 12.5 KNO_3: 5 Mn^{2+}: 0.5	Temperature: 40 °C pH: 8.0 Rotary speed: 160 rpm Time: 2 days	14.3
Humicola grisea ITCC 10360.16 [22]	Desert soil, India	PBD RSM	Chitin: 7.49 Colloidal chitin: 4.91 Yeast extract: 5.5 KCl: 0.19 NH_4Cl: 1.0 $MgSO_4{\cdot}7H_2O$: 0.2 KH_2PO_4: 0.68 K_2HPO_4: 0.87	Temperature: 45 °C pH: 6.5 Rotary speed: 150 rpm Time: 8 days	1.43

Table 3. *Cont.*

Strains	Source	Method	Component [a] (g L^{-1})	Condition	Yield (Final/ Initial)
Cohnella sp. A01 [23]	Wastewater, Iran	OFAT OD	Colloidal Chitin: 15 NH_4NO_3: 5 KH_2PO_4: 0.7 NaCl: 1.7	Temperature: 60 °C pH: 6.5 Rotary speed: 180 rpm Time: 3 days	N.M.
Serratia marcescens JPP1 [24]	Peanut hulls, China	PBD RSM	Colloidal chitin: 12.7 Glucose: 7.34 Peptone: 5.0 $(NH_4)_2SO_4$: 1.32 $MgSO_4{\cdot}7H_2O$: 0.5 K_2HPO_4: 0.7	N.M.	2.1
Stenotrophomonas maltophilia [25]	Soil, India	PBD RSM	Colloidal chitin: 4.94 Maltose: 5.56 Yeast extract: 0.62 KH_2PO_4: 1.33 $MgSO_4{\cdot}7H_2O$: 0.65	N.M.	N.M.

OFAT, one-factor-at-a-time; OD, orthogonal design; PBD, Plackeet–Burmann Design; RSM, response surface methodology; N.M., not mentioned in the corresponding study. [a] The trace elements added into the medium were omitted.

Since only a few strains, such as *Thermococcus chitonophagus* [31], *Microbispora* sp. V2 [32] and *Metarrhizium anisopliae* [33], can utilize chitin as the sole carbon source, most of the chitinolytic microorganisms cannot produce chitinolytic enzymes with chitin as the sole carbon source. Therefore, it is necessary to add additional carbon sources that are feasible to utilize by these strains through co-metabolism (Table 3). The additional carbon source mainly provides energy for cell growth and proliferation as the primary matrix, while chitin is decomposed and utilized as the secondary matrix. In general, glucose is the best carbon source for enzyme production, and strain GWSMS-1 is no exception. However, other small molecules such as lactose and glycerol showed a better effect on chitinase secretion than glucose in some cases (Table 3). Unlike the variety of carbon source preferences of different strains, almost all the studies showed that the organic nitrogen source is better for enzyme production than the inorganic nitrogen source (Table 3), which inhibited the synthesis of chitinase during fermentation; organic nitrogen was better for strain GWSMS-1 as well.

The potential application in biocontrol of fungi of the cold-active chitinase secreted by strain GWSMS-1 was evaluated using five common plant pathogens. The crude chitinase showed significant inhibition on fungi *Verticillium dahlia* CICC 2534 and *Fusarium oxysporum* f. sp. *cucumerinum* CICC 2532 which can cause cotton wilt and cucumber blight, respectively, suggesting that strain GWSMS-1 would be a competitive candidate for the biological control in agriculture.

4. Materials and Methods

4.1. Chemicals, Agents and Media

Chitin, potassium ferricyanide and *N*-acetyl-D-glucosamine (NAG) were available from Sigma-Aldrich (St. Louis, MO, USA). All other chemicals of analytical grade were purchased from Sangon Biotech (Shanghai, China).

Colloidal chitin was prepared according to Souza et al. [34] as follows: five grams of chitin powder was added to 60 mL of concentrated HCl slowly and incubated overnight, with vigorous stirring at room temperature. The mixture was added to 200 mL precooling ethanol and incubated at room temperature overnight with vigorous stirring. The precipitate was harvested by centrifugation at 5000 *g* for 20 min at 4 °C. The colloidal chitin was washed with sterile distilled water to neutral and stored in the dark at 4 °C.

Potassium ferrocyanide solution was prepared by dissolving 0.5 g potassium ferrocyanide in 1 liter of 0.5 M Na_2CO_3 buffer and stored in a dark environment.

The initial liquid medium consisted of peptone (2 g L^{-1}), glucose (1 g L^{-1}), colloid chitin (5 g L^{-1}), $FeSO_4{\cdot}7H_2O$ (0.01 g L^{-1}), $MgSO_4{\cdot}7H_2O$ (0.5 g L^{-1}), KH_2PO_4 (0.3 g L^{-1}) and $K_2HPO_4{\cdot}3H_2O$ (0.917 g L^{-1}), while the solid medium contained agar at a concentration of 1.5%.

4.2. Screening and Characterization of Chitinase-Producing Microorganisms

Samples of seal and penguin feces, soil and marine sediment, collected from Fildes Peninsula (60°20′S–60°56′S, 44°05′W–46°25′W) in Antarctica, were used as sources for bioprospecting of chitinase-producing microorganisms. Strains which formed transparent zones on the colloidal chitin plate at 15 °C were selected for further study. The isolates were characterized by 16S rDNA sequencing. The 16S rDNA gene was amplified using genomic DNA as templates, with universal primer pairs 27F (5′-AGAGTTTGATCMTGGCTCAG-3′ (27F) and 1492R (5′-TACGGYTACCTTGTTACGACTT-3′).

The PCR products were ligated with the pMD19-T vector and transformed into *E. coli* DH5α competent cells for sequencing. The nucleotide sequence of the 16S rDNA gene was subject to BLAST server (http://www.ncbi.nlm.nih.gov/BLAST) to find homologous sequences. Multiple sequence alignment was conducted using the software Clustal X 2.0 [35]. The phylogenetic tree was constructed using the neighbor-joining method [36] in MEGA 6.0 [37], with a bootstrap test of 1000 replicates.

4.3. Preparation of Crude Chitinase

The fermentation broth was centrifuged at 8000× *g* for 10 min, and the supernatant was concentrated by using a 10 kDa ultrafiltration centrifuge tube. The eluate was then filtered through a 0.22 μm filter and stored at −20 °C for further experiments.

4.4. Native-PAGE and Active Staining of Chitinase

To obtain enough crude chitinase for native-PAGE, the crude chitinase was further concentrated as follows: the crude enzyme was mixed with appropriate amount of colloidal chitin and incubated at 4 °C for 2 h; the mixture was washed twice with 50 mM of Tris-HCl (pH 8.0), then the concentrated chitinase was eluted by using 50 mM of acetate buffer (pH 4.0) and dialyzed by using 50 mM of Tris-HCl (pH 8.0). The native-PAGE was performed using 4% stacking gel and 12% separating gel with 0.5% colloidal chitin added. The gel was stained by Coomassie Brilliant Blue R-250 and Calcofluor White M2R [38] to verify the chitinase activity of the crude enzyme.

4.5. Chitinase Activity Assay

Chitinase activity was determined by measuring the amount of NAG generated from colloidal chitin using a potassium ferrocyanide solution, according to Taiji et al. [39]. An appropriate amount of crude extracellular chitinase secreted by strain GWSMS-1 was mixed with colloidal chitin (1%, *m*/*v*) suspended in 50 mM phosphate buffer at pH 6.0. The mixture of enzyme and substrate was incubated at 30 °C for 2 h, then treated at 100 °C for 5 min to inactivate the enzyme. Subsequently, the reaction solution was centrifugated at 10,000× *g* for 5 min to remove the precipitate, and 0.05 mL of supernatant was mixed with 1.45 mL potassium ferrocyanide solution. The absorbance of the mixture at 420 nm was measured after treating at 100 °C for 15 min and cooling to room temperature. The NAG concentration was calculated based on the standard curve obtained under the same condition. One unit of chitinase activity was defined as the amount of enzyme required to produce 1 μmol of NAG per minute at 30 °C in a phosphate buffer at pH 6.0.

4.6. One-Factor-at-a-Time Optimization

To obtain maximum extracellular chitinase secreted by strain GWSMS-1, the one-factor-at-a-time method was adopted to optimize the medium composition including carbon and nitrogen sources, carbon, nitrogen and chitin concentration, as well as the culture conditions including fermentation time, temperature, pH and shaking speed (Table 4). All experiments were performed in triplicate.

Table 4. Factors and variables of one-factor-at-a-time optimization.

Factors	Variables
Time (days)	1, 2, 3, 4, 5, 6, 7, 8, 9, 10, 11, 12, 13, 14, 15
Carbon source	glycerol, glucose, ribose, mannose, fructose, sucrose, maltose, starch
Nitrogen source	peptone, CH_3COONH_4, $(NH_4)_2SO_4$, KNO_3, NH_4Cl
Glucose (g L^{-1})	5, 10, 15, 20
Peptone (g L^{-1})	1, 2, 3, 4, 5, 10
Chitin (g L^{-1})	5, 10, 15, 20
Temperature (°C)	15, 20, 25, 30, 35, 40
pH	5.0, 6.0, 6.5, 7.0, 7.5, 8.0, 9.0
Shaking speed (rpm)	100, 150, 200, 250

4.7. Orthogonal Design

Based on the results of the single factor test, the medium composition was further optimized by orthogonal design. The orthogonal test employed a four-factor and three-level orthogonal table L_9 (3^4) to optimize concentrations of glucose, peptone, chitin and magnesium ions (Table 5). All experiments were performed with three replicates.

Table 5. Levels of orthogonal design.

Levels	Glucose (g L^{-1})	Peptone (g L^{-1})	Chitin (g L^{-1})	Mg^{2+} (mM)
1	5	1	5	1
2	10	2	10	5
3	15	3	15	10

4.8. Temperature and pH-Dependent Enzymatic Properties of Crude Chitinase

Generally, the activity and stability of enzymes can be determined by pH denaturation and thermal denaturation [40]. The optimal temperature of the crude chitinase was determined by assaying the activity at different temperatures ranging from 0 to 80 °C with 5 °C intervals at pH 6.0. The thermal stability was determined by measuring the residual activity after treating the crude enzyme at different temperatures from 0 to 45 °C with 5 °C intervals at pH 6.0 for 30 min. The optimum pH for the crude chitinase was determined by measuring the activity in acetate buffer (pH 2.5–3.5), citric acid buffer (pH 4.0–5.5), phosphate buffer (pH 6.0–7.5), Tris-HCl buffer (pH 8.0–9.0) and glycine–NaOH buffer (pH 9.5–11.0) at 30 °C. The pH stability was assayed by measuring the residual activity after incubating the crude enzyme in the buffers mentioned above at 30 °C for 30 min.

4.9. Antifungal Activity Assay

The antifungal activity of the extracellular chitinase secreted by strain GWSMS-1 was investigated by hyphal extension inhibition. Hyphal extension inhibition assay was estimated by the paper disk method. Filter papers with a 6 mm diameter were immersed in the concentrated crude enzyme solution for 5 min. A piece of soaked filter paper was placed at the center of the petri dishes containing potato dextrose agar (PDA). The mycelium of the test fungi was inoculated around the filter paper and incubated at 20 °C for 7 days for the mycelia to grow. The heat-inactivated crude enzyme was used as a control. Fungi used in this study were purchased from China Center of Industrial Culture Collection (CICC) (Beijing China), including *Verticillium dahlia* CICC 2534, *Alternaria brassicicola* CICC 2646, *Fusarium oxysporum* f. sp. *cucumerinum* CICC 2532, *Aspergillus niger* CICC 2039 and *Penicillium macrosclerotiorum* CICC 40649.

5. Conclusions

In this study, a cold-adapted chitinase-producing strain GWSMS-1 was isolated from marine sediment and characterized as *Pseudomonas*. Strategy coupling of the one-factor-at-a-time and the orthogonal test was employed to optimize the chitinase production of the strain. The optimized production was about 6.36 times higher than that before optimization. Based on the biochemical characterization, the crude chitinase was determined as a typical cold-active enzyme, which exhibited excellent low-temperature activity at 0 °C. In addition, it also showed significant inhibition of two plant pathogens, suggesting that strain GWSMS-1 would be a competitive candidate for the biological control in agriculture, especially in high latitudes.

Author Contributions: H.D. and B.C. conceived and designed the experiments; K.L. performed the experiments; H.D., K.L., and Y.Y. analyzed the data; H.D., Y.Y. and B.C. contributed reagents/materials/analysis tools; H.D. and K.L. wrote the paper.

Funding: This research was funded by National Key R&D Program of China (2018YFC1406701, 2018YFC1406704), Youth Innovation Fund of Polar Science (201602) and Qingdao National Laboratory for Marine Science and Technology (QNLM2016ORP0310).

Conflicts of Interest: The authors declare no conflict of interest.

References

1. Moussian, B. Chitin: Structure, Chemistry and Biology. *Adv. Exp. Med. Biol.* **2019**, *1142*, 5–18. [PubMed]

2. Guan, G.; Azad, M.A.K.; Lin, Y.; Kim, S.W.; Tian, Y.; Liu, G.; Wang, H. Biological Effects and Applications of Chitosan and Chito-Oligosaccharides. *Front. Physiol.* **2019**, *10*, 516. [CrossRef] [PubMed]
3. Schmitz, C.; Auza, L.G.; Koberidze, D.; Rasche, S.; Fischer, R.; Bortesi, L. Conversion of Chitin to Defined Chitosan Oligomers: Current Status and Future Prospects. *Mar. Drugs* **2019**, *17*, 452. [CrossRef] [PubMed]
4. Jung, W.J.; Park, R.D. Bioproduction of chitooligosaccharides: Present and perspectives. *Mar. Drugs* **2014**, *12*, 5328–5356. [CrossRef] [PubMed]
5. Le, B.; Yang, S.H. Microbial chitinases: Properties, current state and biotechnological applications. *World J. Microbiol. Biotechnol.* **2019**, *35*, 144. [CrossRef] [PubMed]
6. Bhattacharya, D.; Nagpure, A.; Gupta, R.K. Bacterial chitinases: Properties and potential. *Crit. Rev. Biotechnol.* **2007**, *27*, 21–28. [CrossRef]
7. Hartl, L.; Zach, S.; Seidl-Seiboth, V. Fungal chitinases: Diversity, mechanistic properties and biotechnological potential. *Appl. Microbiol. Biotechnol.* **2012**, *93*, 533–543. [CrossRef]
8. Volpicella, M.; Leoni, C.; Fanizza, I.; Placido, A.; Pastorello, E.A.; Ceci, L.R. Overview of plant chitinases identified as food allergens. *J. Agric. Food Chem.* **2014**, *62*, 5734–5742. [CrossRef]
9. Arakane, Y.; Muthukrishnan, S. Insect chitinase and chitinase-like proteins. *Cell. Mol. Life Sci.* **2010**, *67*, 201–216. [CrossRef]
10. Kumar, A.; Zhang, K.Y.J. Human Chitinases: Structure, Function, and Inhibitor Discovery. *Adv. Exp. Med. Biol.* **2019**, *1142*, 221–251.
11. Neeraja, C.; Anil, K.; Purushotham, P.; Suma, K.; Sarma, P.; Moerschbacher, B.M.; Podile, A.R. Biotechnological approaches to develop bacterial chitinases as a bioshield against fungal diseases of plants. *Crit. Rev. Biotechnol.* **2010**, *30*, 231–241. [CrossRef] [PubMed]
12. Han, S.J.; Park, H.; Lee, S.G.; Lee, H.K.; Yim, J.H. Optimization of cold-active chitinase production from the Antarctic bacterium, Sanguibacter antarcticus KOPRI 21702. *Appl. Microbiol. Biotechnol.* **2011**, *89*, 613–621. [CrossRef] [PubMed]
13. Mishra, P.; Kshirsagar, P.R.; Nilegaonkar, S.S.; Singh, S.K. Statistical optimization of medium components for production of extracellular chitinase by Basidiobolus ranarum: A novel biocontrol agent against plant pathogenic fungi. *J. Basic Microbiol.* **2012**, *52*, 539–548. [CrossRef] [PubMed]
14. Tasharrofi, N.; Adrangi, S.; Fazeli, M.; Rastegar, H.; Khoshayand, M.R.; Faramarzi, M.A. Optimization of Chitinase Production by Bacillus pumilus Using Plackett-Burman Design and Response Surface Methodology. *Iran. J. Pharm. Res.* **2011**, *10*, 759–768.
15. Hao, Z.; Cai, Y.; Liao, X.; Zhang, X.; Fang, Z.; Zhang, D. Optimization of nutrition factors on chitinase production from a newly isolated Chitiolyticbacter meiyuanensis SYBC-H1. *Braz. J. Microbiol.* **2012**, *43*, 177–186. [CrossRef]
16. Singh, A.K.; Mehta, G.; Chhatpar, H.S. Optimization of medium constituents for improved chitinase production by Paenibacillus sp. D1 using statistical approach. *Lett. Appl. Microbiol.* **2009**, *49*, 708–714. [CrossRef]
17. Xia, J.L.; Xiong, J.; Zhang, R.Y.; Liu, K.K.; Huang, B.; Nie, Z.Y. Production of Chitinase and its Optimization from a Novel Isolate Serratia marcescens XJ-01. *Indian J. Microbiol.* **2011**, *51*, 301–306. [CrossRef]
18. Narayana, K.J.; Vijayalakshmi, M. Chitinase Production by Streptomyces sp. ANU 6277. *Braz. J. Microbiol.* **2009**, *40*, 725–733. [CrossRef]
19. Singh, R.K.; Kumar, D.P.; Solanki, M.K.; Singh, P.; Srivastva, A.K.; Kumar, S.; Kashyap, P.L.; Saxena, A.K.; Singhal, P.K.; Arora, D.K. Optimization of media components for chitinase production by chickpea rhizosphere associated Lysinibacillus fusiformis B-CM18. *J. Basic Microbiol.* **2013**, *53*, 451–460. [CrossRef]
20. Meriem, G.; Mahmoud, K. Optimization of chitinase production by a new Streptomyces griseorubens C9 isolate using response surface methodology. *Ann. Microbiol.* **2017**, *67*, 175–183. [CrossRef]
21. Shivalee, A.; Lingappa, K.; Mahesh, D. Influence of bioprocess variables on the production of extracellular chitinase under submerged fermentation by Streptomyces pratensis strain KLSL55. *J. Genet. Eng. Biotechnol.* **2018**, *16*, 421–426. [CrossRef] [PubMed]
22. Kumar, M.; Brar, A.; Vivekanand, V.; Pareek, N. Production of chitinase from thermophilic Humicola grisea and its application in production of bioactive chitooligosaccharides. *Int. J. Biol. Macromol.* **2017**, *104*, 1641–1647. [CrossRef] [PubMed]
23. Aliabadi, N.; Aminzadeh, S.; Karkhane, A.A.; Haghbeen, K. Thermostable chitinase from Cohnella sp. A01: Isolation and product optimization. *Braz. J. Microbiol.* **2016**, *47*, 931–940. [CrossRef] [PubMed]

24. Wang, K.; Yan, P.S.; Cao, L.X. Chitinase from a novel strain of Serratia marcescens JPP1 for biocontrol of aflatoxin: Molecular characterization and production optimization using response surface methodology. *BioMed Res. Int.* **2014**, *2014*, 482623.
25. Khan, M.A.; Hamid, R.; Ahmad, M.; Abdin, M.Z.; Javed, S. Optimization of culture media for enhanced chitinase production from a novel strain of Stenotrophomonas maltophilia using response surface methodology. *J. Microbiol. Biotechnol.* **2010**, *20*, 1597–1602. [CrossRef]
26. Siddiqui, K.S. Some like it hot, some like it cold: Temperature dependent biotechnological applications and improvements in extremophilic enzymes. *Biotechnol. Adv.* **2015**, *33*, 1912–1922. [CrossRef]
27. Bruno, S.; Coppola, D.; di Prisco, G.; Giordano, D.; Verde, C. Enzymes from Marine Polar Regions and Their Biotechnological Applications. *Mar. Drugs* **2019**, *17*, 544. [CrossRef]
28. Yoon, S.H.; Ha, S.M.; Kwon, S.; Lim, J.; Kim, Y.; Seo, H.; Chun, J. Introducing EzBioCloud: A taxonomically united database of 16S rRNA gene sequences and whole-genome assemblies. *Int. J. Syst. Evol. Microbiol.* **2017**, *67*, 1613–1617.
29. Bozal, N.; Montes, M.J.; Mercade, E. Pseudomonas guineae sp. nov., a novel psychrotolerant bacterium from an Antarctic environment. *Int. J. Syst. Evol. Microbiol.* **2007**, *57*, 2609–2612. [CrossRef]
30. Rabbani, G.; Ahmad, E.; Khan, M.V.; Ashraf, M.T.; Bhat, R.; Khan, R.H. Impact of structural stability of cold adapted Candida antarctica lipase B (CaLB): In relation to pH, chemical and thermal denaturation. *RSC Adv.* **2015**, *5*, 20115–20131. [CrossRef]
31. Andronopoulou, E.; Vorgias, C.E. Multiple components and induction mechanism of the chitinolytic system of the hyperthermophilic archaeon Thermococcus chitonophagus. *Appl. Microbiol. Biotechnol.* **2004**, *65*, 694–702. [CrossRef] [PubMed]
32. Nawani, N.N.; Kapadnis, B.P.; Das, A.D.; Rao, A.S.; Mahajan, S.K. Purification and characterization of a thermophilic and acidophilic chitinase from Microbispora sp. V2. *J. Appl. Microbiol.* **2002**, *93*, 965–975. [CrossRef] [PubMed]
33. St Leger, R.J.; Cooper, R.M.; Charnley, A.K. Cuticle-degrading Enzymes of Entomopathogenic Fungi: Regulation of Production of Chitinolytic Enzymes. *Microbiology* **1986**, *132*, 1509–1517. [CrossRef]
34. Souza, C.P.; Burbano-Rosero, E.M.; Almeida, B.C.; Martins, G.G.; Albertini, L.S.; Rivera, I.N.G. Culture medium for isolating chitinolytic bacteria from seawater and plankton. *World J. Microbiol. Biotechnol.* **2009**, *25*, 2079–2082. [CrossRef]
35. Larkin, M.A.; Blackshields, G.; Brown, N.P.; Chenna, R.; McGettigan, P.A.; McWilliam, H.; Valentin, F.; Wallace, I.M.; Wilm, A.; Lopez, R.; et al. Clustal W and Clustal X version 2.0. *Bioinformatics* **2007**, *23*, 2947–2948. [CrossRef]
36. Saitou, N.; Nei, M. The neighbor-joining method: A new method for reconstructing phylogenetic trees. *Mol. Biol. Evol.* **1987**, *4*, 406–425.
37. Tamura, K.; Stecher, G.; Peterson, D.; Filipski, A.; Kumar, S. MEGA6: Molecular Evolutionary Genetics Analysis version 6.0. *Mol. Biol. Evol.* **2013**, *30*, 2725–2729. [CrossRef]
38. Trudel, J.; Asselin, A. Detection of chitinase activity after polyacrylamide gel electrophoresis. *Anal. Biochem.* **1989**, *178*, 362–366. [CrossRef]
39. Imoto, T.; Yagishita, K. A Simple Activity Measurement of Lysozyme. *Agric. Biol. Chem.* **1971**, *35*, 1154–1156. [CrossRef]
40. Rabbani, G.; Ahmad, E.; Zaidi, N.; Fatima, S.; Khan, R.H. pH-Induced molten globule state of Rhizopus niveus lipase is more resistant against thermal and chemical denaturation than its native state. *Cell Biochem. Biophys.* **2012**, *62*, 487–499. [CrossRef]

marine drugs

Review

Properties and Applications of Extremozymes from Deep-Sea Extremophilic Microorganisms: A Mini Review

Min Jin [1,2], Yingbao Gai [1], Xun Guo [1], Yanping Hou [1] and Runying Zeng [1,2,*]

1 State Key Laboratory Breeding Base of Marine Genetic Resource, Third Institute of Oceanography, Ministry of Natural Resources, Xiamen 361000, China; jinmin@tio.org.cn (M.J.); Gaiyingbao@tio.org.cn (Y.G.); guoxun0528@163.com (X.G.); Houyanping@tio.org.cn (Y.H.)

2 Southern Marine Science and Engineering Guangdong Laboratory (Zhuhai), Zhuhai 519000, China

* Correspondence: zeng@tio.org.cn; Tel.: +86-592-2195323

Received: 29 October 2019; Accepted: 19 November 2019; Published: 21 November 2019

Abstract: The deep sea, which is defined as sea water below a depth of 1000 m, is one of the largest biomes on the Earth, and is recognised as an extreme environment due to its range of challenging physical parameters, such as pressure, salinity, temperature, chemicals and metals (such as hydrogen sulphide, copper and arsenic). For surviving in such extreme conditions, deep-sea extremophilic microorganisms employ a variety of adaptive strategies, such as the production of extremozymes, which exhibit outstanding thermal or cold adaptability, salt tolerance and/or pressure tolerance. Owing to their great stability, deep-sea extremozymes have numerous potential applications in a wide range of industries, such as the agricultural, food, chemical, pharmaceutical and biotechnological sectors. This enormous economic potential combined with recent advances in sampling and molecular and omics technologies has led to the emergence of research regarding deep-sea extremozymes and their primary applications in recent decades. In the present review, we introduced recent advances in research regarding deep-sea extremophiles and the enzymes they produce and discussed their potential industrial applications, with special emphasis on thermophilic, psychrophilic, halophilic and piezophilic enzymes.

Keywords: deep sea; extremophilic microorganisms; extremozyme; thermophilic enzyme; psychrophilic enzyme; halophilic enzyme; piezophilic enzyme

1. Deep-Sea Extremophilic Microorganisms: A Novel Source of Extremozymes

Nearly three-quarters of the Earth's surface area is covered by ocean, the average depth of which is 3800 m, implying that the vast majority of our planet comprises deep-sea environments. The deep sea is one of the most mysterious and unexplored environments on the Earth, and it supports diverse microbial communities that play important roles in biogeochemical cycles [1]. The deep sea is also recognised as an extreme environment, as it is characterised by the absence of sunlight and the presence of predominantly low temperatures and high hydrostatic pressures, and these environmental conditions become even more challenging in particular habitats, such as deep-sea hydrothermal vents with their extremely high temperatures of >400 °C, deep hypersaline anoxic basins (DHABs) with their extremely high salinities and abysses of up to 11 km depth with their extremely high pressures.

Deep-sea extremophiles are living organisms that can survive and proliferate in deep-sea environments that have extreme physical (pressure and temperature) and geochemical (pH, salinity and redox potential) conditions that are lethal to other organisms. The majority of deep-sea extremophiles belong to the prokaryotes, which are microorganisms in the domains of Archaea and Bacteria [2,3]. These extremophilic microorganisms are functionally diverse and widely distributed in taxonomy [4], and they are classified into thermophiles (55 °C to 121 °C), psychrophiles (−2 °C to 20 °C), halophiles (2–5 M NaCl or KCl), piezophiles (>500 atmospheres), alkalophiles (pH > 8), acidophiles (pH < 4) and metalophiles (high concentrations of metals, e.g., copper, zinc, cadmium and arsenic) according to the extreme environments in which they grow and the extreme conditions they can tolerate. Many deep-sea extremophiles tolerate more than one extreme condition, and thus are polyextremophiles [5]. These extreme conditions are generally harmful to the majority of organisms, but extremophilic microorganisms are able to survive and thrive in them due to their highly flexible metabolisms and the unique structural characteristics of their biomacromolecules [6,7].

In the past few decades, deep-sea extremophilic microorganisms have attracted the attention of researchers searching for novel bioactive substances such as enzymes that can be used in the major sectors of industry worldwide [8]. The diverse temperatures, salinities, pHs and pressures that are provided by nature in extreme deep-sea environments can be utilised to search for novel and potentially robust enzymes that are more suitable for industrial applications [9], and it has been found that the extremozymes that are produced by deep-sea extremophilic microorganisms have a wide variety of industrial applications due to their high activities and great stabilities under extreme conditions. Indeed, the stability and enzymatic activities of extremozymes make them valuable alternatives to ordinary biotechnological processes, bestowing them with considerable economic potential in the agricultural, feed, food, beverage, pharmaceutical, detergent, leather, textile, pulp and biomining industries [10].

Although a lot of enzymes have been identified to date worldwide, the majority of which have been evaluated for industrial applications, the enzyme market remains inadequate in meeting industrial demands [11] largely due to many of the enzymes that are presently available being unable to tolerate industrial conditions [12]. The industrial process demands biocatalysts that can resist a range of harsh conditions, including temperature, pH, salinity and pressure, while exhibiting high conversion rates and reproducibilities [13]. Furthermore, it is important that the enzymes that are used in technologies are compatible with ecological processes [14]. While only a few extremozymes are presently being produced and used at the industrial level, the development of novel industrial processes based on these enzymes is being promoted by advances in deep-sea extremophile and extremozyme research, the growing demand for novel biocatalysts in industries, breakthroughs in deep-sea sampling techniques and the rapid development of new molecular and omics technologies, such as metagenomics, proteomics, protein engineering, gene-directed evolution and synthetic biology [15]. Thus, the discovery of enzymes with novel enzymatic activities and improved stability remains a priority in enzyme research [10].

2. Strategies for Discovering Extremozymes in Deep-Sea Environments

The classic method that is used to discover novel extremozymes from deep-sea microorganisms is the cultivation of microorganisms followed by screening for the desired enzymes. However, while numerous extremozymes with promising properties for industrial applications have been isolated from deep-sea environments using this method, approximately 99.9% of those environmental microorganisms cannot be cultivated using traditional laboratory techniques [16], meaning that the discovery of many useful extremozymes would not be possible using this method alone. Metagenomic technologies have been developed to bypass the requirement for the isolation or cultivation of microorganisms, and they could prove to be a powerful tool for discovering novel genes and enzymes directly from uncultured microorganisms [17]; indeed, metagenomes have been successfully employed to search for extremozymes from deep-sea environments, overcoming the bottlenecks associated with the uncultivability of extremophiles [18].

Metagenomic analyses are based on the direct isolation of genomic DNA from environmental samples, and they are either sequence based (i.e., putative enzymes are obtained based on their conserved sequences) or function based (i.e., functional enzymes are obtained based on the expressed features such as a specific enzyme activity) [19]. In the sequence-based approach, the colony hybridisation technique is used for screening metagenomic clones using an oligonucleotide primer or probes for the target gene, and the desired gene may also be amplified by polymerase chain reaction

(PCR) using specific or degenerate primers and subsequently cloned into suitable expression vectors. Besides, the desired gene sequences can sometimes be directly retrived from metagenomics data after proper bioinformatic annotations, and then be synthesized de novo and codon-optimized if required. This sequence-based technique leads to the discovery of novel sequences that are similar to existing known sequences, and this provides the possibility of finding enzymes efficiently [20]. However, the ability to identify specific enzymes using this method depends on existing bioinformatic analyses, thus many novel or unknown activities can be overlooked [21].

The common function-based metagenomic strategies include enzyme activity-based screening performed in culture plates; for example, the use of the starch-iodine staining test for detecting amylase activity. Functional metagenomics has some advantages over the sequence-based approach because the identification of genes according to their functions rather than their sequences eliminates the possibility of incorrect annotations or obtaining similar sequences of gene products with different or multiple functions. Furthermore, functional screening is more suitable for identifying novel genes encoding novel enzymes because it does not rely on gene sequence information [22]. The primary disadvantage of this screening method is that gene expression may fail due to difficulties in promoter recognition, low translation efficiency, lack of specific cofactors in certain expression hosts, protein misfolding and post-translational modification defects of the desired proteins. However, all these issues can be solved using vectors with a wide host range that enables expression in a variety of hosts, vectors that are adapted to a large insert size and Rosetta strains of *Escherichia coli*, which contains transfer ribonucleic acid (tRNA) for rare amino acid codons [17,23]. Consequently, the function-based metagenomic approach is now the most frequently used technique for screening for novel extremozymes from the deep sea [24–27].

The application of enzymes in industrial processes sometimes fails due to the presence of undesirable properties and a lack of stability and robustness [28]. However, molecular approaches can be used to engineer natural proteins and develop more effective extremozymes with enhanced stabilities and activities for industrial purposes. The enhancement of the stability of enzymes can prove to be very beneficial because it would enable them to maintain high activity for prolonged periods of time under challenging physicochemical conditions, which would be a useful characteristic for numerous industrial processes. One method that can be used to stabilise proteins is protein engineering [29,30], which has become a powerful approach for altering or improving enzymatic characteristics in the past two decades. Protein engineering is divided into the following two methods: (1) directed evolution, where a random mutagenesis is applied to a protein [31]; and (2) rational protein design, where knowledge of the structure and function of the protein is exploited to modify its characteristics [32]. Both these methods have been successfully applied to increase the activity, selectivity and thermostability of proteins.

3. Properties and Applications of Extremozymes Isolated from Deep-Sea Extremophilic Microorganisms

Hundreds of industrial processes and products benefit from the use of enzymes that have been isolated from microorganisms. However, the majority of the enzymes that are presently on the market are produced using mesophilic enzymes, which are often inhibited under the extreme conditions of several industrial processes [10]. In addition, the stability of the biocatalyst is important for reducing costs because enzymes that are sufficiently stable to withstand the industrial conditions can be used for repeated cycles of the biocatalytic process, and hence aid in reducing expenditures. Thus, the exploration of deep-sea extremophilic microorganisms provides an opportunity for obtaining extremozymes that are stable under a variety of different conditions, which may be attractive in industrial processes. Furthermore, enzymes that catalyse reactions under non-physiological conditions and/or with non-natural substrates can also be found in deep-sea environments [33]. Consequently, deep-sea extremozymes have received increasing attention for their applications in various industrial processes owing to their adaptability to harsh physical and chemical conditions [11].

3.1. Deep-Sea Thermophilic Enzymes

Deep-sea thermophiles have been one of the most studied groups of extremophiles over the past four decades [34,35]. These microorganisms are able to grow at high temperatures of 41 °C–120 °C [36,37], therefore, they produce extremozymes with high-temperature resistance. These thermophilic enzymes use a variety of mechanisms to tolerate extreme temperatures, possessing electrostatic interactions and physical properties that allow them to maintain their activity. In general, thermophilic enzymes have similar three-dimensional structures to their mesophilic counterparts but have many more charged residues on their surfaces and different amino acid contents. In addition, thermophilic enzymes usually have shorter loops, thereby inhibiting nonspecific interactions that are induced by their increased flexibility at high temperatures [38,39]. Thermophilic enzymes also have increased number of bisulphide bonds formed between two cysteine residues, which enhances their structural rigidity and, thus, resistance to unfolding at high temperatures [40,41].

To date, thermophilic enzymes have attracted the most attention among the various types of extremozymes because enzymes that are adapted to higher temperatures have several important advantages to industrial processes. High temperatures not only significantly increase the solubility of many reagents, particularly polymeric substrates, but also reduce the risk of contamination, which would result in unfavourable complications. Moreover, high temperatures also promote faster reactions, maintain a low viscosity and increase solvent miscibility [42]. Thermophilic enzymes are usually capable of accepting proteolysis and extreme conditions, such as the presence of organic solvents, denaturing agents and high salinity, making them attractive in the biorefinery, paper and bleaching, and first- and second-generation biofuel industries [43]. A large number of enzymes from deep-sea thermophilic microorganisms have been characterised to date (Table 1) [35], and thermophilic proteases, lipases and polymer-degrading enzymes, in particular, have found their way into industrial applications [11].

Table 1. Representative thermophilic enzymes from deep-sea microorganisms.

Source	Habitat	Enzyme	Thermostability	References
Bacillus sp. JM7	deep-sea water	keratinase	50 °C (70%, 1 h)	[44]
Pyrococcus furiosus	deep-sea vents	prolidase	100 °C (100%, 12 h)	[45]
Geobacillus sp. EPT9	deep-sea vents	lipase	80 °C (44%, 1 h)	[46]
Geobacillus sp. 12AMOR1	deep-sea vents	monoacylglycerol lipase	70 °C (half-life 1 h)	[47]
Flammeovirga Sp. OC4	deep-sea water	β-Agarase	50 °C (35%, 144 h)	[48]
Flammeovirga pacifica	deep-sea water	β-Agarase	50 °C (100%, 10 h)	[49]
Microbulbifer strain JAMB-A7	deep-sea sediment	β-Agarase	50 °C (half-life 502 min)	[50]
Flammeovirga pacifica	deep-sea water	α-amylase	60 °C (81%, 20 min)	[51]
Geobacillus sp. 4j	deep-sea sediment	α-amylase	80 °C (half-life 4.25 h)	[52]
Fosmid library	deep-sea vents	cellulase	92 °C (half-life 2 h)	[24]
Flammeovirga pacifica	deep-sea water	arylsulfatase	50 °C (70%, 12 h)	[53]
Staphylothermus marinus	deep-sea vents	amylopullulanase	100 °C (half-life 50 min)	[54]
Geobacillus sp. MT-1	deep-sea vents	xylanase	65 °C (half-life 50 min)	[55]

The diversity of deep-sea thermophiles makes them valuable in the search for novel thermostable proteolytic enzymes [56,57], which are attractive for use in the detergent, food and feed industries. Jin et al. [44] reported the purification and characterisation of a thermostable and alkali-stable keratinase Ker02562 from *Bacillus* sp. JM7, which was isolated from the deep sea. This enzyme was shown to be stable at 50 °C and in extreme alkaline environments (pH 10–13) and so may have significant applications in the detergent industry, as the enzymes that are used in detergent additives need to be able to withstand temperatures of 40–60 °C and an alkaline pH (pH 9.0–11.0) [58]. Other thermophilic proteases with important industrial applications include thermolysin, which is used in the synthesis of dipeptides, DNA-processing enzymes and pretaq protease, which is used to clean up DNA before PCR amplification [59]. For example, the proline dipeptidase named prolidase, which was identified from the archaeon hyperthermophile *Pyrococcus furiosus* isolated from deep-sea vents and volcanic marine mud in Italy and specifically cleaves dipeptides with proline at the C-terminus and a nonpolar residue (Met, Phe, Val, Leu, Ala) at the amino terminus, is by far the most thermostable example of a prolidase known to date, with a temperature optimum above 100 °C and no loss of activity after 12 h at this temperature [45].

Industrial and biotechnological processes also require thermostable lipases for use in processes such as grease esterification, hydrolysis, transesterification, interesterification and organic biosynthesis. Zhu et al. [46] cloned and characterised a thermostable lipase from the deep-sea hydrothermal field thermophile *Geobacillus* sp. EPT9 and found that the recombinant lipase was optimally active at 55 °C and pH 8.5 and exhibited good thermostability, retaining 44% residual activity after incubation at 80 °C for 1 h. A thermostable monoacylglycerol lipase (GMGL) has also been identified from the thermophilic bacterium *Geobacillus* sp. 12AMOR1, which was isolated from a deep-sea hydrothermal vent site in the Arctic [47]. GMGL is active on monoacylglycerol substrate but not diacylglycerol or triacylglycerol, and recombinant GMGL shows the highest hydrolysis activity at 60 °C and pH 8.0 and has a half-life of 60 min at 70 °C. These thermostable lipases have considerable potential for applications in the food, detergent, cosmetics, perfumery, pharmaceutical, pulp and paper, and chemical industries [60].

Deep-sea thermostable polymer-degrading enzymes, such as agarases, amylases and cellulases, are another group of industrially important biocatalysts that have received much interest. Agarases catalyse agar hydrolysis and have been successfully utilised to produce agar-oligosaccharides, which possess a variety of biological and physiological functions that are beneficial to human health and thus have potential applications in the food and nutraceutical industries [14,61–63]. Since the gelling temperature of agar is approximately 40 °C, thermostable agarases are required for the efficient recovery of DNA from agar gel and are also advantageous for the industrial production of oligosaccharides from agar. Hou et al. reported the expression and characterisation of a novel thermostable and pH-stable β-agarase AgaP4383 from the deep-sea bacterium *Flammeovirga pacifica* WPAGA1 [49]. Phenotypic and genomic analyses revealed that *F. pacifica* WPAGA1 is capable of degrading and metabolising complex polysaccharides and can grow on the red alga *Gracilaria lemaneiformis* as a sole carbon source [64,65], and that AgaP4383 exhibits endolytic activity on agar degradation, producing neoagarotetraose and neoagarohexaose as the final products. AgaP4383 also exhibits good thermostability, with no loss of activity after incubation at 50 °C for 10 h [63]. Recently, a novel thermostable and pH-stable β-agarase Aga4436 was reported from another deep-sea bacterium in the genus *Flammeovirga*, *Flammeovirga* Sp. OC4, which also shows high activity and stability at high temperatures [48]. These favourable properties of AgaP4383 and Aga4436 could make them attractive for use in the food and biotechnology industries.

Thermostable amylolytic enzymes are one of the most interesting groups of enzymes for industrial processes, as they are important for the hydrolysis of starch at high temperatures, promoting the reactions and reducing the risk of contamination [66]. Several thermostable amylases have been reported from deep-sea microorganisms [51,52,67], some of which have been developed into products. For example, Fuelzyme®, a product from Verenium Corporation (San Diego, CA, USA), utilises an alpha-amylase from the thermophile *Thermococcus* sp., which was isolated from a deep-sea hydrothermal vent. Fuelzyme® operates in extremely high temperatures (>110 °C) and at an acidic pH (4.0–6.5), making it suitable for mash liquefaction during ethanol production, releasing dextrins and oligosaccharides with lower molecular weights and better solubilities [67]. However, Fuelzyme® and Spezyme® (DuPont-Genencor Science, Wilmington, DE, USA) are only presently used in the production of biofuel. It has been proposed that the combined use of these commercially available amylases and other *Bacillus* amylases will increase the efficiency of industrial starch processing and will be suitable for downstream applications [68].

Thermophilic enzymes are also widely used in industrial lignocellulolytic processes, with thermostable cellulases having applications in the food, animal feed, textile, and pulp and paper industries [7]. Functional screening of fosmid expression libraries derived from deep-sea hydrothermal vents identified an extreme cellulase that was active and thermostable at 92 °C. This enzyme showed endolytic activities against a variety of linear 1,4-β-glucans, such as phosphoric acid swollen cellulose, carboxymethyl cellulose, lichenan and β-glucan. Other industrial important thermostable polymer-degrading enzymes have also been identified and characterised from deep-sea environments, such as amylopullulanases, arylsulphatases and xylanases [53–55].

3.2. *Deep-Sea Psychrophilic Enzymes*

The deep sea is primarily a cold environment, and the majority of the water is present at 5 °C. Consequently, this biome harbours an abundance of cold-adapted psychrophiles, which have a restricted range of temperature for growth, and are extremophiles that are adapted to moderate or extreme cold and have been shown to achieve active metabolism at −25 °C and conduct DNA synthesis at −20 °C [69]. Psychrophiles are divided into the following two types according to their growth temperatures: eurypsychrophiles (formerly psychrotolerant microorganisms), which comprise the majority of isolates from the deep sea and have a broad temperature range and tolerate warmer environments, and stenopsychrophiles (formerly true psychrophiles), which cannot grow at temperatures above 20 °C [70]. Psychrophiles have developed several mechanisms that allow them to thrive in icy environments, including the production of cold-induced cold-shock proteins and RNA chaperones, enhanced tRNA flexibility, enhanced membrane fluidity for maintaining the semi-fluid state of the membranes, and the production of cold-active secondary metabolites, enzymes, pigments and antifreeze proteins [71,72]. The most common adaptive characteristic of psychrophilic enzymes is their high reaction rate at low temperatures, which is generally achieved by their flexible structures and low stabilities [73]. From a structural perspective, psychrophilic proteins have a higher content of α-helix than β-sheets, which is recognised as an essential feature for maintaining flexibility even at low temperatures [7]. Because cold-active enzymes maintain a high catalytic rate at low temperatures through the augmentation of the solvent connection and structural flexibility [73,74], they are capable of binding more tightly to the solvent, in a way similar to that of salt-adapted enzymes [75].

Enzymes that are adapted to low temperatures possess several features that are favourable for industrial applications [76], and have been used in industries as diverse as food processing, molecular biology and fine chemical synthesis [77,78]. Cold-active enzymes bring potential benefits to the food and feed industries, where it is crucial to avoid spoilage as this may result in a change in nutritional value and flavour of the original thermosensitive substrates and products [77,79]. Cold-adapted enzymes are also useful for molecular biology because of the need to use enzymes in sequential reactions and to inactivate enzymes once they have accomplished their functions. To this end, heat-labile enzymes have great potential, as heat inactivation can be performed at temperatures that do not cause the melting of double-stranded DNA (dsDNA), eliminating the need for additional chemical extraction steps [77]. The detergent, biofuel production and pulp and paper industries are also interested in cold-active hydrolases, such as proteases, lipases, amylases and cellulases, as these enzymes can provide economic benefits by reducing energy consumption and production costs [80,81].

Deep-sea psychrophiles are a promising source of industrially important cold-active enzymes (Table 2). Cold-active cellulose-degrading enzymes, such as glucosidases, are useful in the textile, beverage and biofuel industries. The first cold-active and alkali-stable β-glucosidase was isolated from the deep-sea bacterium *Martelella mediterranea* and showed favourable characteristics, being able to retain more than 50% of its maximum enzymatic activity at 4 °C and 80% of its maximum enzymatic activity at pH 11 for 11 h [82]. The deep-sea-sediment–dwelling bacterium *Exiguobacterium oxidotolerans* also produces a cold-active β-glycosidase, which maintains 61% of its maximum activity at 10 °C and in a pH range of 6.6–9.0 [83]. Several cold-adapted xylanases that have been isolated from the deep sea, such as from *Zunongwangia profunda* [84] and *Flammeovirga pacifica* [85], have potential uses in the food industry, such as as additives to wheat flour to improve dough handling and the quality of the baked products. Numerous cold-adapted amylases have also been isolated from deep-sea microorganisms over the past few years that have potential applications in the detergent, textile and food industries [86–88]; for example, Jiang et al. [89] reported a cold-adapted alpha-amylase from the deep-sea bacterium *Bacillus* sp. dsh19-1, which shows maximum activity at 20 °C. Cold-active lipases and esterases are important catalysts in the chemical, pharmaceutical, cosmetic, food, laundry detergent and environmental remediation industries and can be isolated from deep-sea microorganisms and metagenomic libraries derived from deep-sea samples [77]. For example, Chen reported a novel psychrophilic esterase Est11 from the deep-sea bacterium *Psychrobacter pacificensis*, which is highly active and stable at 10 °C and 5 M NaCl [90]. Furthermore, incubation with ethanol, isopropanol, propanediol, dimethyl sulphoxide (DMSO), acetonitrile and glycerol were shown to have remarkable positive effects on Est11 activity, indicating that this cold-active, halo-tolerant and organic solvent-resistant esterase may be useful in harsh industrial processes [90].

Table 2. Representative psychrophilic enzymes from deep-sea microorganisms.

Source	Habitat	Enzyme	Activities at Low Temperatures	References
Martelella mediterranea	deep-sea water	β-glucosidase	50% at 4 °C	[82]
Exiguobacterium oxidotolerans	deep-sea sediment	β-glycosidase	61% at 10 °C	[83]
Zunongwangia profunda	deep-sea sediment	xylanase	38% at 5 °C	[84]
Flammeovirga pacifica	deep-sea water	xylanase	50–70% at 10 °C	[85]
Luteimonas abyssi	deep-sea water	α-amylase	36% at 10 °C	[87]
Zunongwangia profunda	deep-sea sediment	α-amylase	39% at 10 °C	[88]
Pseudomonas strain	deep-sea sediment	α-amylase	50% at 5 °C	[91]
Wangia sp. C52	deep-sea sediment	α-amylase	50% at 25 °C	[92]
Bacillus sp. dsh19-1	deep-sea sediment	α-amylase	35.7% at 4 °C	[89]
Psychrobacter pacificensis	deep-sea water	esterase	70% at 10 °C	[90]
Metagenomic libraries	deep-sea sediment	esterase	100% at 10 °C	[25]
Metagenomic libraries	deep-sea sediment	esterase	38% at 15 °C	[26]
Metagenomic libraries	deep-sea sediment	lipase	most active below 30 °C	[93]
Pseudoaltermonas sp. SM9913	deep-sea sediment	serine protease	60% at 20 °C	[94]
Planococcus sp. M7	deep-sea sediment	protease	45% at 10 °C	[95]

3.3. Deep-Sea Halophilic Enzymes

Halophiles are capable of thriving in high salt concentrations, which can be found in DHABs or deep-sea hypersaline anoxic lakes. These extreme habitats have been discovered on the sea floor in different oceanic regions, such as the Red Sea, the eastern Mediterranean Sea and the Gulf of Mexico. In a DHAB, the dissolved evaporitic deposits are trapped in the sea floor sediments, forming very stable brine and a sharply stratified chemocline in the water column. The brines that are enclosed in these basins are characterised by hypersalinity (5–10 times the concentration of sea water), a high pressure (approximately 35 MPa), a lack of oxygen and highly reducing conditions, and an absence of light, making them one of the most extreme environments on the Earth, which has allowed these habitats to remain isolated for thousands of years [7,96]. Since the discovery of the first Mediterranean DHAB termed 'Tyro' in 1983, six more DHABs have been discovered termed 'l'Atalante', 'Bannock', 'Discovery', 'Medee', 'Thetis' and 'Urania' [97], all of which are sources of anaerobic halophilic microorganisms.

Halophilic microorganisms can be classified into the following three categories according to the optimal salt concentration for growth: (i) slight halophiles, which are capable of developing at 200–500 mM NaCl; (ii) moderate halophiles, which can develop at 500–2500 mM NaCl; and (iii) extreme halophiles, which can develop at 2500–5200 mM NaCl [98]. Certain halophiles are also thermostable and tolerant to a wide range of pHs, and halophiles have high metabolic diversity, comprising anoxic phototrophic, fermenter, aerobic heterotrophic, sulphate reducer, denitrifying and methanogenic organisms [99].

Halophiles have developed different adaptive strategies to survive the osmotic pressures that are induced by the high NaCl concentrations in the environments they inhabit. Some extremely halophilic bacteria use a type of 'salt-in' strategy to balance the osmotic pressure of the environment, whereby they accumulate inorganic ions (K^+, Na^+, Cl^-) in the cytoplasm [100]. However, moderate halophiles have distinct adaptations that allow them to biosynthesize and/or accumulate large amounts of specific organic osmolytes in the cytoplasm. These accumulated osmolytes act as osmoprotectants and help to maintain osmotic balance and low salt concentrations in the cytoplasm without interfering with the normal cellular metabolism [101]. Halophiles also produce enzymes that are active and stable in the presence of salts, with the enzymes employing different adaptation mechanisms and exhibiting very high stability at low water activity as well as in the presence of organic solvents and high salt concentrations [35,102]. Structural analyses have revealed that the major differences between non-halophilic and halophilic proteins occur on the surfaces of the molecules. Halophilic enzymes contain a greater percentage of certain amino acid residues, such as serine and threonine, a higher proportion of aspartic and glutamic acids, a lower percentage of lysine, and a higher occurrence of amino acids with low hydrophobic characters than non-halophilic enzymes, which allow a higher number of salt bridges to be created and cooperation with electrostatic interactions [103]. The stability of these enzymes relies on the negative charge of the acidic amino acids on the protein surface, the hydration of the protein surface due to the carboxylic groups that are present in aspartic and glutamic acids, and the occurrence of hydrophobic groups in the presence of high salt concentrations. In addition, the negative surface charges are believed to be important for the solvation of halophilic proteins and the prevention of denaturation, aggregation and precipitation [101,104]. Deep-sea halophilic enzymes provide great opportunities for the food, detergents, textile, bioremediation and biosynthetic industries [102], with their industrial potential lying in their activity and stability not only at high salt concentrations but also in the presence of organic solvents [105,106]. Moreover, several deep-sea halophilic enzymes are also active and stable at high or low temperatures [89,90]. These unique properties make deep-sea halophilic enzymes attractive wherever enzymatic conversion needs to occur under challenging physical and chemical conditions, such as at extreme salt concentrations and temperatures and in the presence of organic solvents.

Numerous halophilic enzymes isolated from the deep sea have been cloned and characterised to date (Table 3), with examples of industrially important halophilic enzymes including polysaccharide-hydrolysing enzymes, such as amylases and xylanases [10,102,107]. For instance, two cold-adapted and salt-tolerant alpha-amylases have been reported from the deep-sea bacteria *Bacillus* sp. dsh19-1 and *Zunongwangia profunda*, which are among the very few known alpha-amylases that can tolerate both cold and saline conditions [88,89]. The high activities and stabilities of these halophilic amylases in harsh conditions make them desirable for industrial applications, particularly for the treatment of waste water containing high salt concentrations and starch residues. In addition, a novel psychrophilic and halophilic β-1,3-xylanase (Xyl512) was recently characterised from the deep-sea bacterium *Flammeovirga pacifica* strain WPAGA1, and it was found that a high-saline concentration (1.5 M NaCl) could alter the optimum temperature and pH of Xyl512, as well as significantly improve its overall activity by two-fold compared with an absence of NaCl, which would meet the food industry's demands for low temperatures and high concentrations of salt [85]. Some deep-sea halophilic enzymes are lipolytic, such as esterases, which have particularly great potential in the production of biodiesel, polyunsaturated fatty acids and food [108,109]. Five esterase genes have been identified from a metagenome expression library derived from the DHAB Urania, some of which were highly active in high-salinity conditions and were able to function in polar solvents, making them suitable for use in the chemical, pharmaceutical and biofuel industries [110]. In addition, research regarding deep-sea extremophiles has identified and characterised other industrially important halophilic enzymes, such as proteases, mercuric reductase and the first reported DNA polymerase to exhibit halophilic and thermophilic features [111–113].

Table 3. Representative halophilic enzymes from deep-sea microorganisms.

Source	Habitat	Enzyme	Activities at High Saline Concentrations	References
Zunongwangia profunda	deep-sea sediment	α-amylase	93% activity at 4 M NaCl	[88]
Bacillus sp. dsh19-1	deep-sea sediment	α-amylase	60.5% activity at 5 M NaCl	[89]
Zunongwangia profunda	deep-sea sediment	xylanase	near 100% activity at 5 M NaCl	[84]
Flammeovirga pacifica	deep-sea water	xylanase	maximum at 1.5 M NaCl	[85]
Emericellopsis sp. TS11	deep-sea sponge	xylanase	maximum at 2 M NaCl	[114]
Metagenomic libraries	deep-sea brine	esterase	maximum at 3–4 M NaCl	[110]
Fosmid library	deep-sea sediment	esterase	maximum at 3.5 M NaCl	[27]
Psychrobacter pacificensis	deep-sea water	esterase	maximum at 5 M NaCl	[90]
Pseudoalteromonas spp.	deep-sea sediment	protease	maximum at 2 M NaCl	[111]
Metagenomic libraries	deep-sea brine	mercuric reductase	maximum at 4 M NaCl	[112]
candidate division MSBL1 archaeon SCGC-AAA261G05	deep-sea brine	DNA polymerase	maximum at 0.5 M NaCl	[113]

3.4. Deep-Sea Piezophilic Enzymes

The hydrostatic pressure can reach 70–110 MPa in the deepest parts of the oceans, making these environments highly challenging. These deep-sea habitats host a group of extremophiles known as piezophiles, which survive and thrive under conditions of extremely high hydrostatic pressure [115,116]. Piezophiles can be classified into the following two categories based on their pressure requirements for growth: 1) piezophilic microorganisms, which exhibit optimal growth at pressures above atmospheric pressure; and 2) piezotolerant microorganisms, which can grow at atmospheric pressure and high pressures but do not require high pressures for optimal growth [117]. High pressure plays a selective role on living organisms by affecting cellular structures and processes, such as cell motility and division. Consequently, the ability to live under extreme pressures requires substantial physiological adaptations that involve modifications to gene regulation and the cellular structure. The adaptative mechanisms of piezophiles have not yet been fully clarified but are known to involve a reduction in cell division, the production of compatible osmolytes and polyunsaturated fatty acids, a switch in the flexibility state, and the formation of multimeric and antioxidant proteins [118–121]. Lauro et al. have also described the occurrence of extended helices in the 16S ribosomal RNA (rRNA) genes for adaptation to high pressures [122].

So far, very little research has been conducted on deep-sea piezophilic enzymes [117,123], and many more experiments and computational studies on different enzymes from a variety of piezophiles are required to advance our understanding [120]. However, piezophilic proteins have shown high efficiency in several industrial processes [5], with particular applications for food production, where high pressures are employed for the processing and sterilisation of food materials [124]. For example, piezophilic α-amylase has been shown to produce trisaccharide instead of maltobiose and tetrasaccharide from maltooligosaccharide at high pressures with little energy, which is a useful reaction in the food processing industry [35,117]. In addition, a peptidase from *Pyrococcus horikoshii* demonstrates stability at high pressures and thus may be useful for food processing [35,125]. Deep-sea piezophiles often produce polyunsaturated fatty acids, such as omega-3 polyunsaturated fatty acids, to stabilise the cell membrane under high pressure. This increase in unsaturated fatty acids creates highly disordered phospholipid bilayers, which renders the membrane resistant against high pressure [116]. Thus, the lipid biochemistry of piezophilic microorganisms is a very interesting topic, and the enzymes that participate in these metabolic pathways under high pressures may have great potential for industrial applications [126]. Piezophilic endonucleases may also have potential in the biotechnology industry. For example, the 'star activity' that is exhibited by *Eco*RI and other restriction endonucleases under high-osmotic-pressure conditions, whereby they lose some specificity to their recognition sequences, can be reversed by piezophilic endonucleases operating under a hydrostatic pressure of 50–75 Mpa [117,127].

4. Conclusions and Prospects

Deep-sea extremophiles are emerging as an important source of novel industrially robust extremozymes. The biodiversity of deep-sea extremophiles and the evolutionary adaptations of their derived extremozymes to the harsh conditions that are found in deep-sea ecosystems has facilitated the selection of more robust biocatalysts, which have special properties that are not found in any other prokaryotes. These extremozymes will be beneficial for novel biocatalytic processes, allowing them to be more efficient, specific, accurate and environmentally friendly. Due to their special features and enormous potential in industrial applications, the number of studies on deep-sea extremophiles and their extremozymes has greatly increased over the last two decades. However, there are still only a few extremophiles available and only a minor fraction of the deep-sea extremophiles has been exploited for extremozymes to date. This limited exploitation of extremozymes is largely due to the special nutritional requirements and challenging growth conditions of deep-sea extremophiles, which make their isolation and maintenance difficult. Fortunately, however, the rapidly increasing number of extremophilic genomes and metagenomes that can now be easily obtained by next-generation sequencing technologies offers an ever-expanding resource for the identification of new extremozymes from non-cultivable deep-sea extremophiles. In addition, although enzyme engineering techniques have been established, the enzyme optimisation process is still a limiting factor for the development of new extremozyme-inspired industrial processes. Thus, the simultaneous development of protein engineering technologies will assist the further modification and improvement of biocatalytic features, which will increase the application of deep-sea extremophiles in industry. Moreover, important advances in our knowledge of the genetics, physiology, metabolism and enzymology of deep-sea extremophiles are expected, which will enable us to better understand the applications of their biocatalysts. Thus, the advancement of modern molecular techniques and deep-sea sampling approaches in the future will allow deep-sea extremozymes to have significant impacts on a wide range of industries.

Author Contributions: Writing-original draft preparation, M.J., R.Z.; writing—review and editing, M.J., Y.G., X.G., Y.H., R.Z.

Funding: This work was financially supported by the China Ocean Mineral Resources R&D Association (DY135-B-04), the Scientific Research Foundation of Third Institute of Oceanography, MNR (2019013), and the National Natural Science Foundation of China (41976084).

Conflicts of Interest: The authors declare that they have no competing interests.

References

1. Sogin, M.L.; Morrison, H.G.; Huber, J.A.; Welch, D.M.; Huse, S.M.; Neal, P.R.; Arrieta, J.M.; Herndl, G.J. Microbial diversity in the deep sea and the underexplored "rare biosphere". *Proc. Natl. Acad. Sci. USA* **2006**, *103*, 12115–12120. [CrossRef] [PubMed]
2. Horikoshi, K.; Bull, A.T. Prologue: Definition, categories, distribution, origin and evolution, pioneering studies, and emerging fields of extremophiles. In *Extremophiles Handbook*; Springer: Tokyo, Janpan, 2011; pp. 3–15.
3. Harrison, J.P.; Gheeraert, N.; Tsigelnitskiy, D.; Cockell, C.S. The limits for life under multiple extremes. *Trends Microbiol.* **2013**, *21*, 204–212. [CrossRef]
4. Cowan, D.A.; Ramond, J.-B.; Makhalanyane, T.P.; De Maayer, P. Metagenomics of extreme environments. *Curr. Opin. Microbiol.* **2015**, *25*, 97–102. [CrossRef] [PubMed]
5. Cavicchioli, R.; Amils, R.; Wagner, D.; McGenity, T. Life and applications of extremophiles. *Environ. Microbiol.* **2011**, *13*, 1903–1907. [CrossRef] [PubMed]
6. Nath, I.A.; Bharathi, P.L. Diversity in transcripts and translational pattern of stress proteins in marine extremophiles. *Extremophiles* **2011**, *15*, 129–153. [CrossRef]
7. Dalmaso, G.; Ferreira, D.; Vermelho, A. Marine extremophiles: A source of hydrolases for biotechnological applications. *Mar. Drugs* **2015**, *13*, 1925–1965. [CrossRef]
8. Zhang, C.; Kim, S.K. Research and application of marine microbial enzymes: Status and prospects. *Mar. Drugs* **2010**, *8*, 1920–1934. [CrossRef]

9. Samuel, P.; Raja, A.; Prabakaran, P. Investigation and application of marine derived microbial enzymes: Status and prospects. *Int. J. Ocean. Mar. Ecol. Syst.* **2012**, *1*, 1–10. [CrossRef]
10. Raddadi, N.; Cherif, A.; Daffonchio, D.; Neifar, M.; Fava, F. Biotechnological applications of extremophiles, extremozymes and extremolytes. *Appl. Microbiol. Biot.* **2015**, *99*, 7907–7913. [CrossRef]
11. Van Den Burg, B. Extremophiles as a source for novel enzymes. *Curr. Opin. Microbiol.* **2003**, *6*, 213–218. [CrossRef]
12. Irwin, J.A.; Baird, A.W. Extremophiles and their application to veterinary medicine. *Irish Vet. J.* **2004**, *57*, 348. [CrossRef] [PubMed]
13. Haki, G.; Rakshit, S. Developments in industrially important thermostable enzymes: A review. *Bioresour. Technol.* **2003**, *89*, 17–34. [CrossRef]
14. Gao, B.; Li, L.; Wu, H.; Zhu, D.; Jin, M.; Qu, W.; Zeng, R. A novel strategy for efficient agaro-oligosaccharide production based on the enzymatic degradation of crude agarose in *Flammeovirga pacifica* WPAGA1. *Front. Microbiol.* **2019**, *10*, 1231. [CrossRef] [PubMed]
15. Ferrer, M.; Golyshina, O.; Beloqui, A.; Golyshin, P.N. Mining enzymes from extreme environments. *Curr. Opin. Microbiol.* **2007**, *10*, 207–214. [CrossRef] [PubMed]
16. Amann, R.I.; Binder, B.J.; Olson, R.J.; Chisholm, S.W.; Devereux, R.; Stahl, D.A. Combination of 16S rRNA-targeted oligonucleotide probes with flow cytometry for analyzing mixed microbial populations. *Appl. Environ. Microbiol.* **1990**, *56*, 1919–1925.
17. Madhavan, A.; Sindhu, R.; Parameswaran, B.; Sukumaran, R.K.; Pandey, A. Metagenome analysis: A powerful tool for enzyme bioprospecting. *Appl. Biochem. Biotechnol.* **2017**, *183*, 636–651. [CrossRef]
18. López-López, O.; Cerdan, M.E.; Gonzalez Siso, M.I. New extremophilic lipases and esterases from metagenomics. *Curr. Protein Pept. Sci.* **2014**, *15*, 445–455. [CrossRef]
19. Popovic, A.; Tchigvintsev, A.; Tran, H.; Chernikova, T.N.; Golyshina, O.V.; Yakimov, M.M.; Golyshin, P.N.; Yakunin, A.F. Metagenomics as a tool for enzyme discovery: Hydrolytic enzymes from marine-related metagenomes. In *Prokaryotic Systems Biology*; Springer: Berlin/Heidelberg, Germany, 2015; pp. 1–20.
20. Lee, H.S.; Kwon, K.K.; Kang, S.G.; Cha, S.-S.; Kim, S.J.; Lee, J.H. Approaches for novel enzyme discovery from marine environments. *Curr. Opin. Biotechnol.* **2010**, *21*, 353–357. [CrossRef]
21. Escobar-Zepeda, A.; Vera-Ponce de León, A.; Sanchez-Flores, A. The road to metagenomics: From microbiology to DNA sequencing technologies and bioinformatics. *Front. Genet.* **2015**, *6*, 348. [CrossRef]
22. Ferrer, M.; Beloqui, A.; Timmis, K.N.; Golyshin, P.N. Metagenomics for mining new genetic resources of microbial communities. *J. Mol. Microbiol. Biotechnol.* **2009**, *16*, 109–123. [CrossRef]
23. Perner, M.; Ilmberger, N.; Köhler, H.U.; Chow, J.; Streit, W.R. Emerging fields in functional metagenomics and its industrial relevance: Overcoming limitations and redirecting the search for novel biocatalysts. In *Handbook of Molecular Microbial Ecology II: Metagenomics in Different Habitats*; Wiley-Blackwell: Hoboken, NJ, USA, 2011; pp. 481–498.
24. Leis, B.; Heinze, S.; Angelov, A.; Pham, V.T.T.; Thürmer, A.; Jebbar, M.; Golyshin, P.N.; Streit, W.R.; Daniel, R.; Liebl, W.J. Functional screening of hydrolytic activities reveals an extremely thermostable cellulase from a deep-sea archaeon. *Front. Bioeng. Biotechnol.* **2015**, *3*, 95. [CrossRef] [PubMed]
25. Jiang, X.; Xu, X.; Huo, Y.; Wu, Y.; Zhu, X.; Zhang, X.; Wu, M.J. Identification and characterization of novel esterases from a deep-sea sediment metagenome. *Arch. Microbiol.* **2012**, *194*, 207–214. [CrossRef] [PubMed]
26. Fu, C.; Hu, Y.; Xie, F.; Guo, H.; Ashforth, E.J.; Polyak, S.W.; Zhu, B.; Zhang, L.J. Molecular cloning and characterization of a new cold-active esterase from a deep-sea metagenomic library. *Appl. Microbiol. Biotechnol.* **2011**, *90*, 961–970. [CrossRef] [PubMed]
27. Zhang, Y.; Hao, J.; Zhang, Y.Q.; Chen, X.L.; Xie, B.B.; Shi, M.; Zhou, B.C.; Zhang, Y.Z.; Li, P. Identification and characterization of a novel salt-tolerant esterase from the deep-sea sediment of the South China Sea. *Front. Microbiol.* **2017**, *8*, 441. [CrossRef]
28. Vermelho, A.B.; Noronha, E.F.; Filho, E.X.F.; Ferrara, M.A.; Bon, E.P. Diversity and biotechnological applications of prokaryotic enzymes. In *The Prokaryotes: Applied Bacteriology and Biotechnology*; Springer: Berlin/Heidelberg, Germany, 2013; pp. 213–240.
29. Bornscheuer, U.; Huisman, G.; Kazlauskas, R.J.; Lutz, S.; Moore, J.; Robins, K. Engineering the third wave of biocatalysis. *Nature* **2012**, *485*, 185. [CrossRef]

30. Smith, M.E.; Schumacher, F.F.; Ryan, C.P.; Tedaldi, L.M.; Papaioannou, D.; Waksman, G.; Caddick, S.; Baker, J.R. Protein modification, bioconjugation, and disulfide bridging using bromomaleimides. *J. Am. Chem. Soc.* **2010**, *132*, 1960–1965. [CrossRef]
31. Denard, C.A.; Ren, H.; Zhao, H. Improving and repurposing biocatalysts via directed evolution. *Curr. Opin. Chem. Biol.* **2015**, *25*, 55–64. [CrossRef]
32. Tiwari, M.K.; Singh, R.; Singh, R.K.; Kim, I.W.; Lee, J.K. Computational approaches for rational design of proteins with novel functionalities. *Comput. Struct. Biotechnol. J.* **2012**, *2*, e201204002. [CrossRef]
33. Littlechild, J.A. Enzymes from extreme environments and their industrial applications. *Front. Bioeng. Biotechnol.* **2015**, *3*, 161. [CrossRef]
34. Bertoldo, C.; Antranikian, G. Starch-hydrolyzing enzymes from thermophilic archaea and bacteria. *Curr. Opin. Chem. Biol.* **2002**, *6*, 151–160. [CrossRef]
35. Dumorné, K.; Córdova, D.C.; Astorga-Eló, M.; Renganathan, P. Extremozymes: A potential source for industrial applications. *J. Microbiol. Biotechnol.* **2017**, *27*, 649–659. [CrossRef] [PubMed]
36. Canganella, F.; Wiegel, J. Anaerobic thermophiles. *Life* **2014**, *4*, 77–104. [CrossRef] [PubMed]
37. Takai, K.; Nakamura, K.; Toki, T.; Tsunogai, U.; Miyazaki, M.; Miyazaki, J.; Hirayama, H.; Nakagawa, S.; Nunoura, T.; Horikoshi, K. Cell proliferation at 122 C and isotopically heavy CH4 production by a hyperthermophilic methanogen under high-pressure cultivation. *Proc. Natl. Acad. Sci. USA* **2008**, *105*, 10949–10954. [CrossRef] [PubMed]
38. Colletier, J.-P.; Aleksandrov, A.; Coquelle, N.; Mraihi, S.; Mendoza-Barberá, E.; Field, M.; Madern, D. Sampling the conformational energy landscape of a hyperthermophilic protein by engineering key substitutions. *Mol. Biol. Evol.* **2012**, *29*, 1683–1694. [CrossRef]
39. Tehei, M.; Madern, D.; Franzetti, B.; Zaccai, G. Neutron scattering reveals the dynamic basis of protein adaptation to extreme temperature. *J. Biol. Chem.* **2005**, *280*, 40974–40979. [CrossRef]
40. Reed, C.J.; Lewis, H.; Trejo, E.; Winston, V.; Evilia, C. Protein adaptations in archaeal extremophiles. *Archaea* **2013**, *2013*. [CrossRef]
41. Mayer, F.; Küper, U.; Meyer, C.; Daxer, S.; Müller, V.; Rachel, R.; Huber, H. AMP-forming acetyl coenzyme A synthetase in the outermost membrane of the hyperthermophilic crenarchaeon Ignicoccus hospitalis. *J. Bacteriol.* **2012**, *194*, 1572–1581. [CrossRef]
42. Liszka, M.J.; Clark, M.E.; Schneider, E.; Clark, D.S. Nature versus nurture: Developing enzymes that function under extreme conditions. *Ann. Rev. Chem. Biomol.* **2012**, *3*, 77–102. [CrossRef]
43. Yeoman, C.J.; Han, Y.; Dodd, D.; Schroeder, C.M.; Mackie, R.I.; Cann, I.K. Thermostable enzymes as biocatalysts in the biofuel industry. In *Advances in Applied Aicrobiology*; Elsevier: Amsterdam, The Netherlands, 2010; Volume 70, pp. 1–55.
44. Jin, M.; Chen, C.; He, X.; Zeng, R. Characterization of an extreme alkaline-stable keratinase from the draft genome of feather-degrading *Bacillus* sp. JM7 from deep-sea. *Acta Oceanol. Sin.* **2019**, *38*, 87–95. [CrossRef]
45. Ghosh, M.; Grunden, A.M.; Dunn, D.M.; Weiss, R.; Adams, M.W. Characterization of native and recombinant forms of an unusual cobalt-dependent proline dipeptidase (prolidase) from the hyperthermophilic archaeon *Pyrococcus furiosus*. *J. Bacteriol.* **1998**, *180*, 4781–4789.
46. Zhu, Y.; Li, H.; Ni, H.; Xiao, A.; Li, L.; Cai, H. Molecular cloning and characterization of a thermostable lipase from deep-sea thermophile *Geobacillus* sp. EPT9. *World J. Microbiol. Biotechnol.* **2015**, *31*, 295–306. [CrossRef] [PubMed]
47. Tang, W.; Lan, D.; Zhao, Z.; Li, S.; Li, X.; Wang, Y. A thermostable monoacylglycerol lipase from marine *Geobacillus* sp. 12AMOR1: Biochemical characterization and mutagenesis Study. *Int. J. Mol. Sci.* **2019**, *20*, 780. [CrossRef] [PubMed]
48. Chen, X.L.; Hou, Y.P.; Jin, M.; Zeng, R.Y.; Lin, H.T. Expression and characterization of a novel thermostable and pH-stable β-agarase from deep-sea bacterium *Flammeovirga* sp. OC4. *J. Agric. Food Chem.* **2016**, *64*, 7251–7258. [CrossRef] [PubMed]
49. Hou, Y.; Chen, X.; Chan, Z.; Zeng, R. Expression and characterization of a thermostable and pH-stable β-agarase encoded by a new gene from *Flammeovirga pacifica* WPAGA1. *Process Biochem.* **2015**, *50*, 1068–1075. [CrossRef]
50. Ohta, Y.; Hatada, Y.; Nogi, Y.; Miyazaki, M.; Li, Z.; Akita, M.; Hidaka, Y.; Goda, S.; Ito, S.; Horikoshi, K.J. Enzymatic properties and nucleotide and amino acid sequences of a thermostable β-agarase from a novel species of deep-sea *Microbulbifer*. *Appl. Microbiol. Biotechnol.* **2004**, *64*, 505–514. [CrossRef]

51. Zhou, G.; Jin, M.; Cai, Y.; Zeng, R.J. Characterization of a thermostable and alkali-stable α-amylase from deep-sea bacterium *Flammeovirga pacifica*. *Int. J. Biol. Maromol.* **2015**, *80*, 676–682. [CrossRef]
52. Jiang, T.; Cai, M.; Huang, M.; He, H.; Lu, J.; Zhou, X.; Zhang, Y.J. Purification, characterization of a thermostable raw-starch hydrolyzing α-amylase from deep-sea thermophile *Geobacillus* sp. *Protein Expres. Purif.* **2015**, *114*, 15–22. [CrossRef]
53. Gao, C.; Jin, M.; Yi, Z.; Zeng, R.J. Characterization of a recombinant thermostable arylsulfatase from deep-sea bacterium *Flammeovirga pacifica*. *J. Microbiol. Biotechnol.* **2015**, *25*, 1894–1901. [CrossRef]
54. Li, X.; Li, D.; Park, K.H.J. An extremely thermostable amylopullulanase from Staphylothermus marinus displays both pullulan-and cyclodextrin-degrading activities. *Appl. Microbiol. Biotechnol.* **2013**, *97*, 5359–5369. [CrossRef]
55. Wu, S.; Liu, B.; Zhang, X.J. Characterization of a recombinant thermostable xylanase from deep-sea thermophilic *Geobacillus* sp. MT-1 in East Pacific. *Appl. Microbiol. Biotechnol.* **2006**, *72*, 1210–1216. [CrossRef]
56. Barzkar, N.; Homaei, A.; Hemmati, R.; Patel, S. Thermostable marine microbial proteases for industrial applications: Scopes and risks. *Extremophiles* **2018**, *22*, 335–346. [CrossRef] [PubMed]
57. Ward, D.E.; Shockley, K.R.; Chang, L.S.; Levy, R.D.; Michel, J.K.; Conners, S.B.; Kelly, R.M. Proteolysis in hyperthermophilic microorganisms. *Archaea* **2002**, *1*, 63–74. [CrossRef] [PubMed]
58. Aehle, W. *Enzymes in Industry: Production and Applications*; John Wiley & Sons: Hoboken, NJ, USA, 2007.
59. Bruins, M.E.; Janssen, A.E.; Boom, R.M. Thermozymes and their applications. *Appl. Biochem. Biotechnol.* **2001**, *90*, 155. [CrossRef]
60. Hasan, F.; Shah, A.A.; Hameed, A. Industrial applications of microbial lipases. *Enzyme Microb. Technol.* **2006**, *39*, 235–251. [CrossRef]
61. Jin, M.; Liu, H.; Hou, Y.; Chan, Z.; Di, W.; Li, L.; Zeng, R. Preparation, characterization and alcoholic liver injury protective effects of algal oligosaccharides from *Gracilaria lemaneiformis*. *Food Res. Int.* **2017**, *100*, 186–195. [CrossRef] [PubMed]
62. Kim, H.T.; Yun, E.J.; Wang, D.; Chung, J.H.; Choi, I.G.; Kim, K.H. High temperature and low acid pretreatment and agarase treatment of agarose for the production of sugar and ethanol from red seaweed biomass. *Bioresour. Technol.* **2013**, *136*, 582–587. [CrossRef]
63. Fu, X.T.; Kim, S.M.J. Agarase: Review of major sources, categories, purification method, enzyme characteristics and applications. *Mar. Drugs* **2010**, *8*, 200–218. [CrossRef]
64. Gao, B.; Jin, M.; Li, L.; Qu, W.; Zeng, R.J. Genome sequencing reveals the complex polysaccharide-degrading ability of novel deep-sea bacterium *Flammeovirga pacifica* WPAGA1. *Front. Microbiol.* **2017**, *8*, 600. [CrossRef]
65. Xu, H.; Fu, Y.; Yang, N.; Ding, Z.; Lai, Q.; Zeng, R.J. *Flammeovirga pacifica* sp. nov., isolated from deep-sea sediment. *Int. J. Syst. Evol. Micr.* **2012**, *62*, 937–941. [CrossRef]
66. Prakash, O.; Jaiswal, N.J. α-Amylase: An ideal representative of thermostable enzymes. *Appl. Biochem. Biotechnol.* **2010**, *160*, 2401–2414. [CrossRef]
67. Callen, W.; Richardson, T.; Frey, G.; Miller, C.; Kazaoka, M.; Mathur, E.; Short, J. Amylases and Methods for Use in Starch Processing. U.S. Patent No. 8,338,131, 25 December 2012.
68. Nedwin, G.E.; Sharma, V.; Shetty, J.K. Alpha-Amylase Blend for Starch Processing and Method of Use Thereof. U.S. Patent No. 8,545,907, 1 October 2013.
69. Mykytczuk, N.C.; Foote, S.J.; Omelon, C.R.; Southam, G.; Greer, C.W.; Whyte, L.G. Bacterial growth at −15°C; molecular insights from the permafrost bacterium *Planococcus halocryophilus* Or1. *ISME J.* **2013**, *7*, 1211. [CrossRef] [PubMed]
70. Cavicchioli, R. Cold-adapted archaea. *Nat. Rev. Microbiol.* **2006**, *4*, 331. [CrossRef] [PubMed]
71. Casanueva, A.; Tuffin, M.; Cary, C.; Cowan, D.A. Molecular adaptations to psychrophily: The impact of 'omic' technologies. *Trends Microbiol.* **2010**, *18*, 374–381. [CrossRef] [PubMed]
72. De Maayer, P.; Anderson, D.; Cary, C.; Cowan, D.A. Some like it cold: Understanding the survival strategies of psychrophiles. *EMBO Rep.* **2014**, *15*, 508–517. [CrossRef] [PubMed]
73. Siddiqui, K.S.; Cavicchioli, R. Cold-adapted enzymes. *Annu. Rev. Biochem.* **2006**, *75*, 403–433. [CrossRef] [PubMed]
74. Merlino, A.; Krauss, I.R.; Castellano, I.; De Vendittis, E.; Rossi, B.; Conte, M.; Vergara, A.; Sica, F. Structure and flexibility in cold-adapted iron superoxide dismutases: The case of the enzyme isolated from *Pseudoalteromonas haloplanktis*. *J. Struct. Biol.* **2010**, *172*, 343–352. [CrossRef]

75. Karan, R.; Capes, M.D.; DasSarma, S. Function and biotechnology of extremophilic enzymes in low water activity. *Aquat. Biosyst.* **2012**, *8*, 4. [CrossRef]
76. Sarmiento, F.; Peralta, R.; Blamey, J.M. Cold and hot extremozymes: Industrial relevance and current trends. *Front. Bioeng. Biotechnol.* **2015**, *3*, 148. [CrossRef]
77. Cavicchioli, R.; Charlton, T.; Ertan, H.; Omar, S.M.; Siddiqui, K.; Williams, T.J. Biotechnological uses of enzymes from psychrophiles. *Micr. Biotechnol.* **2011**, *4*, 449–460. [CrossRef]
78. Gomes, J.; Steiner, W.J. The biocatalytic potential of extremophiles and extremozymes. *Food Technol. Biotechnol.* **2004**, *42*, 223–225.
79. Luisa Tutino, M.; di Prisco, G.; Marino, G.; de Pascale, D.J. Cold-adapted esterases and lipases: From fundamentals to application. *Protein Pep. Lett.* **2009**, *16*, 1172–1180.
80. Santiago, M.; Ramírez-Sarmiento, C.A.; Zamora, R.A.; Parra, L.P. Discovery, molecular mechanisms, and industrial applications of cold-active enzymes. *Front. Microbiol.* **2016**, *7*, 1408. [CrossRef] [PubMed]
81. Barroca, M.; Santos, G.; Gerday, C.; Collins, T. Biotechnological aspects of cold-active enzymes. In *Psychrophiles: From Biodiversity to Biotechnology*; Springer: Berlin/Heidelberg, Germany, 2017; pp. 461–475.
82. Mao, X.; Hong, Y.; Shao, Z.; Zhao, Y.; Liu, Z.J. A novel cold-active and alkali-stable β-glucosidase gene isolated from the marine bacterium *Martelella mediterranea*. *Appl. Biochem. Biotechnol.* **2010**, *162*, 2136–2148. [CrossRef] [PubMed]
83. Chen, S.; Hong, Y.; Shao, Z.; Liu, Z.J. A cold-active β-glucosidase (Bgl1C) from a sea bacteria *Exiguobacterium oxidotolerans* A011. *Word J. Microbiol. Biotechnol.* **2010**, *26*, 1427–1435. [CrossRef]
84. Liu, X.; Huang, Z.; Zhang, X.; Shao, Z.; Liu, Z. Cloning, expression and characterization of a novel cold-active and halophilic xylanase from *Zunongwangia profunda*. *Extremophiles* **2014**, *18*, 441–450. [CrossRef]
85. Cai, Z.W.; Ge, H.H.; Yi, Z.W.; Zeng, R.Y.; Zhang, G.Y. Characterization of a novel psychrophilic and halophilic β-1, 3-xylanase from deep-sea bacterium, *Flammeovirga pacifica* strain WPAGA1. *Int. J. Biol. Macom.* **2018**, *118*, 2176–2184. [CrossRef]
86. Kuddus, M.; Roohi, A.J.; Ramteke, P.W.J.B. An overview of cold-active microbial α-amylase: Adaptation strategies and biotechnological potentials. *Biotechnology* **2011**, *10*, 246–258. [CrossRef]
87. Zhang, L.; Wang, Y.; Liang, J.; Song, Q.; Zhang, X.H. Degradation properties of various macromolecules of cultivable psychrophilic bacteria from the deep-sea water of the South Pacific Gyre. *Extremophiles* **2016**, *20*, 663–671. [CrossRef]
88. Qin, Y.; Huang, Z.; Liu, Z. A novel cold-active and salt-tolerant α-amylase from marine bacterium *Zunongwangia profunda*: Molecular cloning, heterologous expression and biochemical characterization. *Extremophiles* **2014**, *18*, 271–281. [CrossRef]
89. Dou, S.; Chi, N.; Zhou, X.; Zhang, Q.; Pang, F.; Xiu, Z. Molecular cloning, expression, and biochemical characterization of a novel cold-active α-amylase from *Bacillus* sp. dsh19-1. *Extremophiles* **2018**, *22*, 739–749. [CrossRef]
90. Wu, G.; Zhang, X.; Wei, L.; Wu, G.; Kumar, A.; Mao, T.; Liu, Z. A cold-adapted, solvent and salt tolerant esterase from marine bacterium *Psychrobacter pacificensis*. *Int. J. Biol. Macrom.* **2015**, *81*, 180–187. [CrossRef] [PubMed]
91. Zhang, J.; Zeng, R. Psychrotrophic amylolytic bacteria from deep sea sediment of Prydz Bay, Antarctic: Diversity and characterization of amylases. *World J. Microbiol. Biotechnol.* **2007**, *23*, 1551–1557. [CrossRef]
92. Liu, J.; Zhang, Z.; Liu, Z.; Zhu, H.; Dang, H.; Lu, J.; Cui, Z. Production of cold-adapted amylase by marine bacterium *Wangia* sp. C52: Optimization, modeling, and partial characterization. *Mar. Biotechnol.* **2011**, *13*, 837–844. [CrossRef] [PubMed]
93. Chan, Z.; Wang, R.; Fan, Y.; Zeng, R. Enhanced cold active lipase production by metagenomic library recombinant clone CALIP3 with a step-wise temperature and dissolved oxygen level control strategy. *Chin. J. Chem. Eng.* **2016**, *24*, 1263–1269. [CrossRef]
94. Chen, X.-L.; Zhang, Y.-Z.; Gao, P.-J.; Luan, X. Two different proteases produced by a deep-sea psychrotrophic bacterial strain, *Pseudoaltermonas* sp. SM9913. *Mar. Biol.* **2003**, *143*, 989–993. [CrossRef]
95. Chen, K.; Mo, Q.; Liu, H.; Yuan, F.; Chai, H.; Lu, F.; Zhang, H. Identification and characterization of a novel cold-tolerant extracellular protease from *Planococcus* sp. CGMCC 8088. *Extremophiles* **2018**, *22*, 473–484. [CrossRef]

96. Van der Wielen, P.W.; Bolhuis, H.; Borin, S.; Daffonchio, D.; Corselli, C.; Giuliano, L.; D'Auria, G.; de Lange, G.J.; Huebner, A.; Varnavas, S.P. The enigma of prokaryotic life in deep hypersaline anoxic basins. *Science* **2005**, *307*, 121–123. [CrossRef]
97. Yakimov, M.M.; La Cono, V.; Ferrer, M.; Golyshin, P.N.; Giuliano, L. Metagenomics of Deep Hypersaline Anoxic Basins. *Science* **2015**, 341–348. [CrossRef]
98. Pikuta, E.V.; Hoover, R.B.; Tang, J. Microbial extremophiles at the limits of life. *Crit. Rev. Microbiol.* **2007**, *33*, 183–209. [CrossRef]
99. Antunes, A.; Ngugi, D.K.; Stingl, U. Microbiology of the Red Sea (and other) deep-sea anoxic brine lakes. *Environ. Microbiol.* **2011**, *3*, 416–433. [CrossRef]
100. De Lourdes Moreno, M.; Pérez, D.; García, M.; Mellado, E. Halophilic bacteria as a source of novel hydrolytic enzymes. *Life* **2013**, *3*, 38–51. [CrossRef] [PubMed]
101. Ma, Y.; Galinski, E.A.; Grant, W.D.; Oren, A.; Ventosa, A. Halophiles 2010: Life in saline environments. *Am. Soc. Microbiol.* **2010**. [CrossRef] [PubMed]
102. Yin, J.; Chen, J.C.; Wu, Q.; Chen, G.Q. Halophiles, coming stars for industrial biotechnology. *Biotechnol. Adv.* **2015**, *33*, 1433–1442. [CrossRef]
103. Tadeo, X.; López-Méndez, B.; Trigueros, T.; Laín, A.; Castaño, D.; Millet, O. Structural basis for the aminoacid composition of proteins from halophilic archea. *PLoS Biol.* **2009**, *7*, e1000257. [CrossRef]
104. Tokunaga, H.; Arakawa, T.; Tokunaga, M. Engineering of halophilic enzymes: Two acidic amino acid residues at the carboxy-terminal region confer halophilic characteristics to *Halomonas* and *Pseudomonas* nucleoside diphosphate kinases. *Protein Sci.* **2008**, *17*, 1603–1610. [CrossRef] [PubMed]
105. Raddadi, N.; Cherif, A.; Daffonchio, D.; Fava, F. Halo-alkalitolerant and thermostable cellulases with improved tolerance to ionic liquids and organic solvents from *Paenibacillus tarimensis* isolated from the Chott El Fejej, Sahara desert, Tunisia. *Bioresour. Technol.* **2013**, *150*, 121–128. [CrossRef]
106. Datta, S.; Holmes, B.; Park, J.I.; Chen, Z.; Dibble, D.C.; Hadi, M.; Blanch, H.W.; Simmons, B.A.; Sapra, R. Ionic liquid tolerant hyperthermophilic cellulases for biomass pretreatment and hydrolysis. *Green Chem.* **2010**, *12*, 338–345. [CrossRef]
107. Elleuche, S.; Schroeder, C.; Sahm, K.; Antranikian, G. Extremozymes—Biocatalysts with unique properties from extremophilic microorganisms. *Cur. Opin. Biotechnol.* **2014**, *29*, 116–123. [CrossRef]
108. Litchfield, C.D. Potential for industrial products from the halophilic Archaea. *J. Int. Microbiol. Biot.* **2011**, *38*, 1635. [CrossRef]
109. Schreck, S.D.; Grunden, A.M. Biotechnological applications of halophilic lipases and thioesterases. *Appl. Microbiol. Biot.* **2014**, *98*, 1011–1021. [CrossRef]
110. Ferrer, M.; Golyshina, O.V.; Chernikova, T.N.; Khachane, A.N.; dos Santos, V.A.M.; Yakimov, M.M.; Timmis, K.N.; Golyshin, P.N. Microbial enzymes mined from the Urania deep-sea hypersaline anoxic basin. *Chem. Biol.* **2005**, *12*, 895–904. [CrossRef] [PubMed]
111. Xiong, H.; Song, L.; Xu, Y.; Tsoi, M.Y.; Dobretsov, S.; Qian, P.Y. Characterization of proteolytic bacteria from the Aleutian deep-sea and their proteases. *J. Ind. Microbiol. Biot.* **2007**, *34*, 63–71. [CrossRef] [PubMed]
112. Sayed, A.; Ghazy, M.A.; Ferreira, A.J.; Setubal, J.C.; Chambergo, F.S.; Ouf, A.; Adel, M.; Dawe, A.S.; Archer, J.A.; Bajic, V.B. A novel mercuric reductase from the unique deep brine environment of Atlantis II in the Red Sea. *J. Biol. Chem.* **2014**, *289*, 1675–1687. [CrossRef] [PubMed]
113. Takahashi, M.; Takahashi, E.; Joudeh, L.I.; Marini, M.; Das, G.; Elshenawy, M.M.; Akal, A.; Sakashita, K.; Alam, I.; Tehseen, M. Dynamic structure mediates halophilic adaptation of a DNA polymerase from the deep-sea brines of the Red Sea. *FASEB J.* **2018**, *32*, 3346–3360. [CrossRef]
114. Batista-García, R.A.; Sutton, T.; Jackson, S.A.; Tovar-Herrera, O.E.; Balcázar-López, E.; del Rayo Sanchez-Carbente, M.; Sánchez-Reyes, A.; Dobson, A.D.; Folch-Mallol, J.L. Characterization of lignocellulolytic activities from fungi isolated from the deep-sea sponge *Stelletta normani*. *PLoS ONE* **2017**, *12*, e0173750.
115. Kawamoto, J.; Sato, T.; Nakasone, K.; Kato, C.; Mihara, H.; Esaki, N.; Kurihara, T. Favourable effects of eicosapentaenoic acid on the late step of the cell division in a piezophilic bacterium, *Shewanella violacea* DSS12, at high-hydrostatic pressures. *Environ. Microbiol.* **2011**, *13*, 2293–2298. [CrossRef]
116. Zhang, Y.; Li, X.; Bartlett, D.H.; Xiao, X. Current developments in marine microbiology: High-pressure biotechnology and the genetic engineering of piezophiles. *Cur. Opin. Biot.* **2015**, *33*, 157–164. [CrossRef]
117. Abe, F.; Horikoshi, K. The biotechnological potential of piezophiles. *Trends Biot.* **2001**, *19*, 102–108. [CrossRef]

118. Daniel, I.; Oger, P.; Winter, R. Origins of life and biochemistry under high-pressure conditions. *Chem. Soc. Rev.* **2006**, *35*, 858–875. [CrossRef]
119. Nath, A.; Subbiah, K. Insights into the molecular basis of piezophilic adaptation: Extraction of piezophilic signatures. *J. Theor. Biol.* **2016**, *390*, 117–126. [CrossRef]
120. Ichiye, T. Enzymes from piezophiles. In *Seminars in Cell & Developmental Biology*; Elsevier: Amsterdam, The Netherlands, 2018; pp. 138–146.
121. Huang, Q.; Rodgers, J.M.; Hemley, R.J.; Ichiye, T. Extreme biophysics: Enzymes under pressure. *J. Comput. Chem.* **2017**, *38*, 1174–1182. [CrossRef] [PubMed]
122. Lauro, F.M.; Chastain, R.A.; Blankenship, L.E.; Yayanos, A.A.; Bartlett, D.H. The unique 16S rRNA genes of piezophiles reflect both phylogeny and adaptation. *Appl. Environ. Microbiol.* **2007**, *73*, 838–845. [CrossRef] [PubMed]
123. Mota, M.J.; Lopes, R.P.; Delgadillo, I.; Saraiva, J. Microorganisms under high pressure—Adaptation, growth and biotechnological potential. *Biot. Adv.* **2013**, *31*, 1426–1434. [CrossRef] [PubMed]
124. Balny, C.; Hayashi, R. *High Pressure Bioscience and Biotechnology*; Elsevier: Amsterdam, The Netherlands, 1996; Volume 13.
125. Rosenbaum, E.; Gabel, F.; Durá, M.A.; Finet, S.; Cléry-Barraud, C.; Masson, P.; Franzetti, B. Effects of hydrostatic pressure on the quaternary structure and enzymatic activity of a large peptidase complex from *Pyrococcus horikoshii. Arch. Biochem. Biophys.* **2012**, *517*, 104–110. [CrossRef] [PubMed]
126. Fang, J.; Kato, C.; Sato, T.; Chan, O.; McKay, D. Biosynthesis and dietary uptake of polyunsaturated fatty acids by piezophilic bacteria. *Comp. Biochem. Phys. B* **2004**, *137*, 455–461. [CrossRef] [PubMed]
127. Robinson, C.R.; Sligar, S.G. Hydrostatic and osmotic pressure as tools to study macromolecular recognition. In *Methods in Enzymology*; Elsevier: Amsterdam, The Netherlands, 1995; Volume 259, pp. 395–427.

marine drugs

MDPI

Article

Biochemical and Genomic Characterization of the Cypermethrin-Degrading and Biosurfactant-Producing Bacterial Strains Isolated from Marine Sediments of the Chilean Northern Patagonia

Patricia Aguila-Torres [1,*,†], Jonathan Maldonado [2,3,4,†], Alexis Gaete [2,3], Jaime Figueroa [5], Alex González [6], Richard Miranda [7], Roxana González-Stegmaier [5,8], Carolina Martin [1] and Mauricio González [2,3,*]

1 Laboratorio de Microbiología Molecular, Escuela de Tecnología Médica, Universidad Austral de Chile, Puerto Montt 5504335, Chile; carolina.martin@uach.cl
2 Laboratorio de Bioinformática y Expresión Génica, Instituto de Nutrición y Tecnología de los Alimentos, Universidad de Chile, Santiago 7810000, Chile; jomaldon@gmail.com (J.M.); alex.ignacio@live.com (A.G.)
3 Center for Genome Regulation, Santiago 7810000, Chile
4 Laboratorio de Biología de Sistemas de Plantas, Departamento Genética Molecular y Microbiología, Facultad de Ciencias Biológicas, Pontificia Universidad Católica de Chile, Santiago 8331150, Chile
5 Instituto de Bioquímica y Microbiología, Facultad de Ciencias, Universidad Austral de Chile, Valdivia 5090000, Chile; jefigueroa@uach.cl (J.F.); rgstegmaier@gmail.com (R.G.-S.)
6 Laboratorio de Microbiología Ambiental y extremófilos, Departamento de Ciencias Biológicas y Biodiversidad, Universidad de los Lagos, Osorno 5290000, Chile; alex.gonzalez@ulagos.cl
7 Escuela de Ingeniería Civil Industrial, Universidad Austral de Chile, Puerto Montt 5500000, Chile; rmiranda@spm.uach.cl
8 Laboratorio Medicina Traslacional, Instituto Clínico Oncológico, Fundación Arturo López Pérez, Santiago 8320000, Chile
* Correspondence: patricia.aguila@uach.cl (P.A.-T.); mgonzale@inta.uchile.cl (M.G.); Tel.: +56-65-2277118 (P.A.-T.); +56-2-29781440 (M.G.)
† These authors have contributed equally to this work.

Received: 15 April 2020; Accepted: 11 May 2020; Published: 13 May 2020

Abstract: Pesticides cause severe environmental damage to marine ecosystems. In the last ten years, cypermethrin has been extensively used as an antiparasitic pesticide in the salmon farming industry located in Northern Patagonia. The objective of this study was the biochemical and genomic characterization of cypermethrin-degrading and biosurfactant-producing bacterial strains isolated from cypermethrin-contaminated marine sediment samples collected in southern Chile (MS). Eleven strains were isolated by cypermethrin enrichment culture techniques and were identified by 16S rDNA gene sequencing analyses. The highest growth rate on cypermethrin was observed in four isolates (MS13, MS15a, MS16, and MS19) that also exhibited high levels of biosurfactant production. Genome sequence analyses of these isolates revealed the presence of genes encoding components of bacterial secondary metabolism, and the enzymes esterase, pyrethroid hydrolase, and laccase, which have been associated with different biodegradation pathways of cypermethrin. These novel cypermethrin-degrading and biosurfactant-producing bacterial isolates have a biotechnological potential for biodegradation of cypermethrin-contaminated marine sediments, and their genomes contribute to the understanding of microbial lifestyles in these extreme environments.

Keywords: cypermethrin; biosurfactants; biodegradation capacities; marine sediments

1. Introduction

Los Lagos region (S41°85′39″ W73°48′32″), located at the Chilean Northern Patagonia, has a high-density salmon farming industry with an extensive history of cypermethrin usage [1,2]. Cypermethrin [cyano-(3-phenoxyphenyl)methyl]-3-(2,2-dichloroethenyl)-2,2-dimethylcyclopro-pane-1-carboxylate is a synthetic pyrethroid pesticide used in agriculture and aquaculture [3], classified as a possible human carcinogen by the Environmental Protection Agency with moderate–acute toxicity according to World Health Organization [4,5]. This compound has an impact on marine ecosystems, affecting the biodiversity of fish and aquatic invertebrates [2,6]. Given its bioaccumulative effect and its further biomagnification in the food chain, the presence of this compound in sediment and soil water is of great concern [7]. As shown in a previous report [2], a high concentration of the pyrethroid cypermethrin, with values ranging from 18.0 to 1323.7 ng g^{-1}, was observed in marine sediments in the Northern Patagonia, the same region from which our bacterial isolates were obtained. These habitats are extreme environments with a wide range of temperatures, ranging from 4 to 20 °C, and salinity (range 32%–33%), and also a low nutrient availability, as is the case for nitrate (NO_3) and phosphate (PO_4).

Bioremediation has become an essential tool for removing these pollutants through biological methods, taking advantage of the degradative capabilities of microorganisms for cleaning contaminated environments [8,9]. The most recommended procedure is to use the local genetic resources, whose activity can be modified by modifying nutrients, water, air, and biosurfactants [9,10]. Natural degradation of cypermethrin is carried out by microorganisms that could produce the hydrolysis of the ester linkage, resulting in 3-phenoxybenzoic acid [11]. Diverse microorganisms isolated from soil have been reported to degrade cypermethrin, such as *Pseudomonas*, *Serratia*, *Streptomyces*, *Rhodobacter*, *Stenotrophomonas*, *Sphingomonas*, and *Bacillus* [12–17]. However, studies reporting cypermethrin-degrading bacterial strains obtained from marine environments are less frequent (i.e., *Cellulophaga lytica* DAU203) [18], especially from marine sediments.

Biosurfactant production increases the bioavailability of pollutants for microorganisms by increasing cell surface hydrophobicity [19]. This, in turn, improves the binding of organic compounds to the cell membrane, their adsorption, and ultimately, their biosorption [19,20]. Different microorganisms produce a diversity of biosurfactants [21]. However, there are only a few reported biosurfactant-producing microorganisms that have proven useful in cypermethrin biodegradation processes [4,22]. Therefore, the aims of this study were the identification and characterization of cypermethrin-degrading and biosurfactant-producing bacterial strains isolated from marine sediments in extreme environments, as is Chilean Northern Patagonia, and determining the presence of cypermethrin biodegradation pathway genes, integrating biochemical and genomics approaches.

2. Results

2.1. Isolation and Identification of Marine Bacterial Strains

Eleven cypermethrin-degrading and biosurfactant-producing bacteria were isolated from cypermethrin-polluted sediment sampled at Manao Bay, Ancud, Chiloé (Figure 1a). Strains were isolated after three subcultures by enrichment with cypermethrin, with concentrations ranging from 50 to 200 mg L^{-1} (Figure 1b). According to Gram-staining analyses, five isolates were Gram-negative and six were Gram-positive. Strains were cocci, bacilli, and rod-shaped (Table S1). All strains were catalase-positive, and five of them were motile. Four strains were capable of growth on 50 mg L^{-1} of cypermethrin as the sole carbon and energy source, while reaching the highest cell concentration measured by $OD_{600\ nm}$. These strains were selected for further analysis. The eleven marine bacterial strains (MS) obtained were compared using 16S rRNA gene identity; the results are summarized in Figure 1c. The phylogenic analysis showed that strains MS8, MS10, MS15a, and MS19 are closely related to *Pseudomonas*. MS1, MS11, MS12, MS13, MS14, and MS16 strains are closely related to *Rhodococcus*, and MS4 belongs to *Serratia* (Figure S2, Figure 1c).

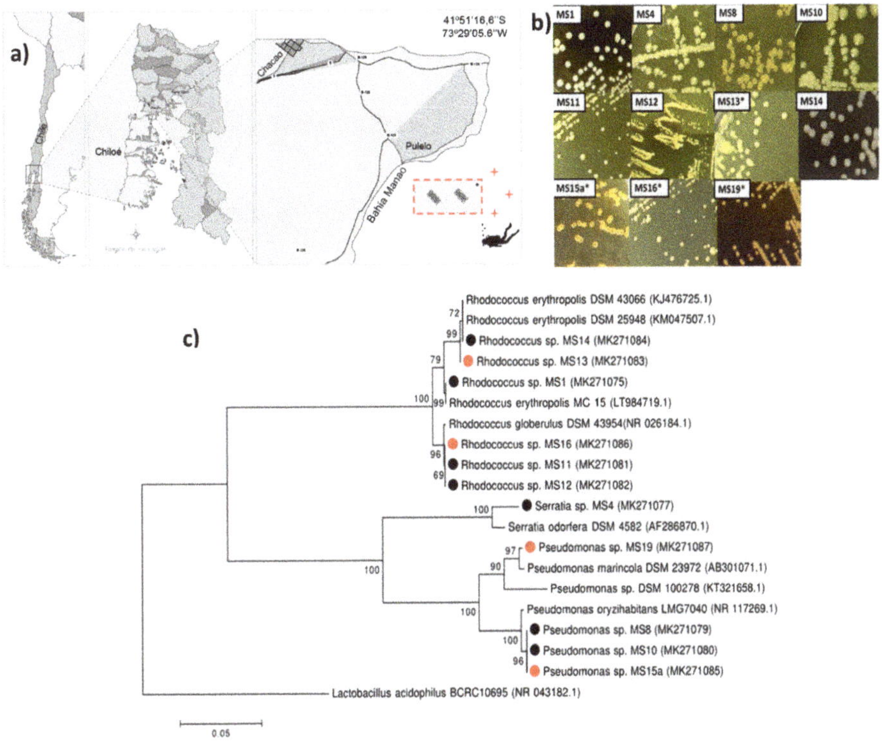

Figure 1. Map of sampling site, geographical position, colony morphologies, phylogeny, and biodiversity of cypermethrin-degrading and biosurfactant-producing bacterial strains isolated from the Chilean Northern Patagonia samples. (**a**) Map of the sampling sites in the Manao Bay: samples were collected from marine sediments at 25 m depth. The asterisk indicates salmon farming center. Crosses mark the three sampling sites. (**b**) Colony morphology, in TSA medium, of cypermethrin-degrading and biosurfactant-producing bacterial strains isolated by enrichment using cypermethrin as the sole carbon and energy source. (**c**) Phylogenetic tree of cypermethrin-degrading and biosurfactant-producing bacterial strains isolated from the Northern Patagonia; black circles indicate cypermethrin-degrading and biosurfactant-producing isolated bacterial strains. Red circles indicate strains selected for genomic analysis.

2.2. Surfactant-Producing Bacteria

The emulsion index (E_{24}) produced by each of the eleven bacterial strains was quantified in order to identify the bacterial strain with the highest capacity of biosurfactant production. All the strains grown in the ETMS medium were capable of emulsion production, which was observed after the addition of diesel petroleum. Strains MS13, MS15a, MS16, and MS19 showed the highest emulsion indexes (>60%) among all the bacterial strains in these conditions (Table S1).

2.3. SEM Studies

The morphologies of selected marine bacteria grown until the mid-exponential phase were studied by scanning electron microscopy (Figure 2). MS13, MS15a, MS16, and MS19 strains showed cell pleomorphism with a rod, bacilli, and coccoid shapes. Cells usually occurred in pairs. In strain MS16, anchor-like appendages forming bridges from one cell to the next were observed (Figure 2).

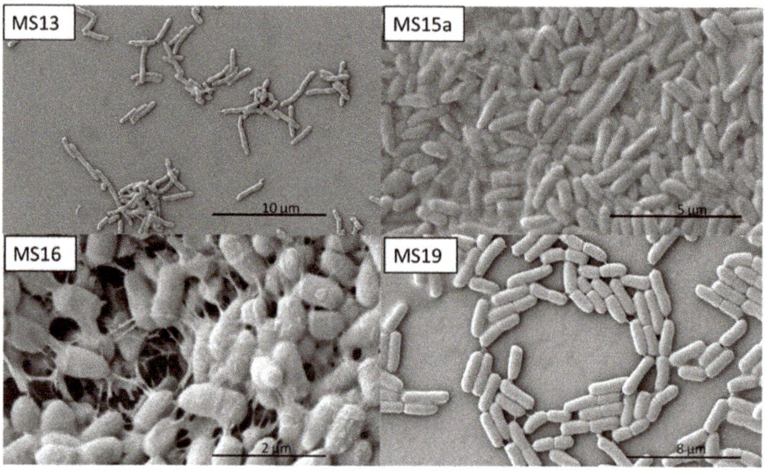

Figure 2. Scanning electron microscopy of cypermethrin-degrading and biosurfactant-producing bacterial strains. Cells tended to occur in pairs. The formation of inter-cellular bonds is highlighted in strain MS16.

2.4. Genome Characterization of Selected Strains

To further investigate the cypermethrin catabolic pathway in selected marine bacterial strains, the whole genome was sequenced. The assembled genomes of *Rhodococcus* sp. MS13 and *Rhodococcus* sp. MS16 consisted of 6,460,280 bp and 6,970,856 bp, and 23 and 37 scaffolds, respectively; the average G + C content was 62% for both strains (Table 1). The assembled genomes of *Pseudomonas* sp. MS15a and *Pseudomonas* sp. MS19 consisted of 5,249,999 bp and 4,496,051 bp, and 27 and 30 scaffolds, respectively; the average G + C content was 65% and 57%, respectively (Table 1). The four sequenced genomes represent high-quality assemblies with N50 indexes over 290Kb, BUSCO completeness indexes over 96%, single copy proportions of BUSCO markers over 94%, and near 0% fragmented markers (Table 1).

Table 1. Genome properties and features.

Property	*Rhodococcus* sp. MS13	*Rhodococcus* sp. MS16	*Pseudomonas* sp. MS15a	*Pseudomonas* sp. MS19
Genome size (bp)	6,460,280	6,970,856	5,249,999	4,496,051
N50 (bp)	557,702	745,857	371,249	290,555
G+C content	62%	62%	65%	57%
DNA scaffolds	23	37	27	30
Total genes	5964	6424	4849	4116
RNA genes	62	58	72	67
tRNA genes	54	52	59	56
Pseudogenes	58	158	65	39
Protein-coding genes	5844	6208	4712	4010
Complete BUSCOs	97%	96%	98%	100%

2.5. Identification of Secondary Metabolites and Detection of Genes Involved in Cypermethrin Catabolism in MS13, MS15, MS16, and MS19 Marine Bacterial Strains, and Comparison with Reference Strains

In order to establish catabolic and anabolic capabilities of the four sequenced strains, an analysis of the biosynthetic coding capacity (BGC) using antiSMASH was performed, and the *estA*, *pytH*, and *laccase* genes encoding the cypermethrin catabolic pathway were identified. BGC's analysis showed a differential pattern of bioactive compounds in all sequenced strains. Figure 3 describes the number of BGC detected in all studied strains compared with their respective reference strains using antiSMASH version 5.0. Of the four studied strains, *Rhodococcus* sp. MS13 had the highest number of gene clusters, with 17 BGC, followed by *Rhodococcus* sp. MS16, with 15 BGC. *Pseudomonas* sp. MS15a and MS19 had seven and five BGC, respectively. Compared with strains of the genus *Pseudomonas, Rhodococcus* showed a greater number of non-ribosomal peptide synthetases (NRPS). Regarding specific NRPS compounds, *Rhodococcus* sp. MS13 and *Rhodococcus* sp. MS16 presented siderophores, antifungals, and antibiotics, whereas *Pseudomonas* only had the first two. Figure 3 also describes the presence of genes involved in the cypermethrin degradation pathway and the biosurfactant compounds that MS13, MS15, MS16, and MS19 produce. Overall, laccases and carboxylesterases were detected in all analyzed genomes, but genes encoding esterases were identified only in *Pseudomonas* sp. strain (MS15a and MS19) genomes.

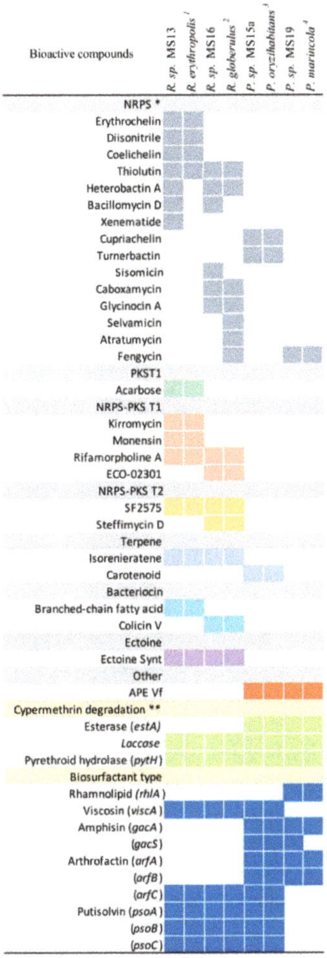

Figure 3. Biosynthetic gene clusters for secondary metabolites and cypermethrin degradation genes in isolated bacteria and reference strains. [1] Soil contaminated with fuel. [2] Rhizosphere of plants grown in soil contaminated with polychlorinated biphenyls (PCBs). [3] Groundwater of pea rhizoplane (*Pisum sativum* L.). [4] Deep-sea in the Fiji Sea. * Secondary metabolites identified through antiSMASH5.0 database and ** *in silico* analysis using a search by homology approach.

The proposed cypermethrin degradation pathway for MS13, MS16, MS15a, and MS19 isolates is described in Figure 4. Genomic analysis suggests that the cypermethrin degradation pathway could be carried out by esterase, carboxylesterase, and laccase.

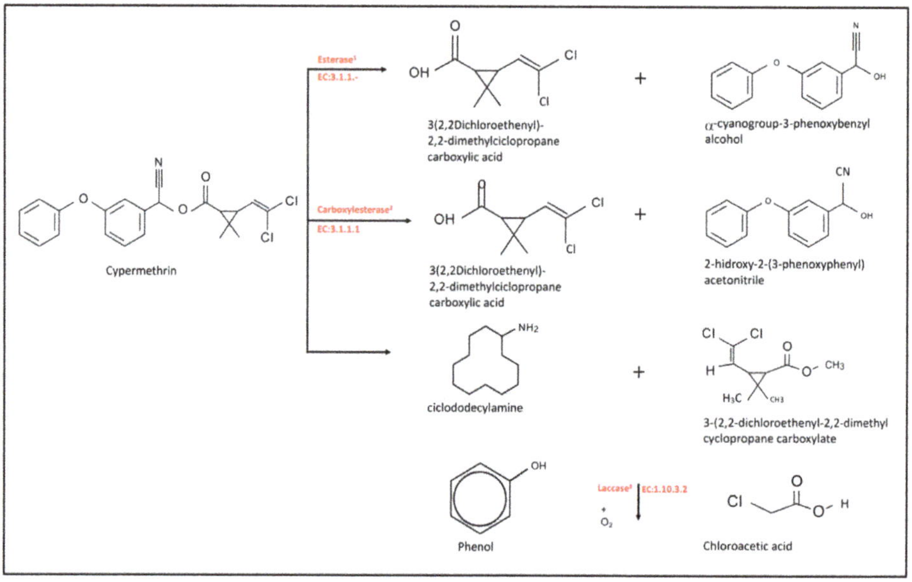

Figure 4. Proposed pathway of cypermethrin biodegradation based on the presence of esterase, laccase, and carboxylesterase-encoding genes in the genomes of MS13, MS16, MS15a, and MS19 isolates. Adapted from [1]Bhatt et al. [23], [2]Zhan et al. [24], and [3]Gangola et al. [17].

3. Discussion

Since 1997, *Caligus rogercresseyi* has been recorded as the most serious parasite in the salmon industry in Northern Patagonia, Chile [1]. Several products have been used to keep sea lice under control in Chile. Cypermethrin [2] is one of them. As a consequence of the extended exposure time to the drug, Northern Patagonia presents high concentrations of cypermethrin in marine sediments [2]. In this scenario, some microorganisms may have acquired the cypermethrin catabolic pathway as a mechanism to use this organic carbon source in an environment with low availability of carbon and hard environmental conditions.

In this study, cypermethrin-degrading and biosurfactant-producing bacterial strains isolated from marine sediment in Northern Patagonia were studied, along with their phenotypic, biochemical, and genomic properties, and their potential to bioremediate cypermethrin-polluted sediments. Based on 16S rRNA gene sequences analyses, bacterial isolates were related to the genera *Pseudomonas, Rhodococcus,* and *Serratia,* suggesting a lower abundance of bacterial genera associated with marine sediments in our sampling sites. Phylogenetic analyses indicate that these isolates are highly related to the reference strains *Rhodococcus erythropolis*, *Rhodococcus* sp., *Rhodococcus globerulus*, *Serratia odorifera*, *Pseudomonas oryzihabitans*, *Pseudomonas* sp., and *Pseudomonas marincola*. Isolates from the genus *Rhodococcus* were the most abundant. These results are consistent with those reported by Choi et al. [25], which indicated that *Actinobacteria* and *Gammaproteobacteria* were very prominent families in bacterial communities inhabiting the surfaces of such marine sediments [25].

Overall, clear morphological differences were observed between the eleven isolated strains; and all isolates were able to grow on cypermethrin as the sole carbon source and showed emulsion activity (biosurfactants). However, four of them (MS13, MS15a, MS16, and MS19) reached the maximum measurable growth on cypermethrin (measured by turbidity—optical density: OD_{600}). Emulsions were also achieved in the cell-free extracts of these strains, indicating that the emulsifying activities were extracellular. Therefore, strains MS13, MS15a, MS16, and MS19 were selected for further characterization towards their application for cypermethrin bioremediation.

Biosurfactants are amphipathic molecules with emulsifying and high surface activity; this turns them into attractive agents for bioremediation [26]. Strains MS13, MS15a, MS16, and MS19 were isolated from cypermethrin-contaminated sediment and showed high potential as biosurfactant-producing bacteria, reaching emulsion indexes of 77%, 60%, 79%, and 71% respectively. Techaoei et al. [27] reported biosurfactant-producing bacteria from soil samples that showed emulsifying activities ranging from 8% to 63% emulsification [27]. Borah and Yadav [28] reported that E24 tested with kerosene, crude oil, and engine oil reached lower values than the ones reported here; namely, 55%, 29%, and 20% emulsion indices, respectively [28]. Previously, it has been described that members of the *Rhodococcus* and *Pseudomonas* genera showed degrading activity of cypermethrin in polluted soils [10], along with *Serratia*, in in vitro assays [4], but to our knowledge, there are no studies on cypermethrin degradation in marine sediments. In this study we determined that, of all obtained isolates, four strains grew successfully in high cypermethrin concentrations, two *Rhodococcus* and two *Pseudomonas*.

Therefore, these bacteria are good candidates for biodegradation of cypermethrin-contaminated marine sediments. Electron microscopy showed that marine strains usually occur in pairs and form bridges via a net-like structure. It has been reported that genera *Rhodococcus* and *Pseudomonas* have nocardioform, that is, rod-shaped or coccoid elements [29,30].

The results of the assembled genome of *Rhodococcus* sp. MS13 and *Rhodococcus* sp. MS16 are comparable with a bacterial strain isolated from marine sediment in Comau fjord, North Patagonia, by Undabarrena [31]. The isolated marine bacterium was *Rhodococcus* sp. H-CA and its complete chromosome has 6.19 Mbp with a content of 62.45% G + C. However, the presence of a *Rhodococcus* sp. RHA1 (RHA1) strain has also been reported, which has the largest bacterial genome sequenced to date, comprising 9,702,737 bp (67% G + C) [29]. Regarding the assembled genomes of *Pseudomonas* sp. MS15a and *Pseudomonas* sp. MS19, our genome data was comparable with strain *Pseudomonas* sp. S.C.T. isolated from marine sediment, whose genome was sequenced and assembled with 4.79 Mbp and 62.5% G + C content [32].

Rhodococcus sp. MS13 and *Rhodococcus* sp. MS16 have great numbers of biosynthetic clusters compared to the other two isolated bacteria; they also have the largest genomes—6.5 and 6.9 Mb. Both strains have great numbers of biosynthetic gene clusters in their respective genomes. These data are similar to those obtained by Ceniceros et al. [33], and Undabarrena et al. [31], which explored the metabolic capacities of the genus *Rhodococcus* and sequence the genome of *Rhodococcus* sp. H-CA8f [31,33]. The strains with the fewest gene clusters are *Pseudomonas* sp. MS19, which has the smallest genome size, 4.5 Mb, together with *Pseudomonas* sp. MS15, with seven gene clusters. The most represented BGCs correspond to non-ribosomal peptide synthetases (NRPS). These results show the biosynthetic potentials of the studied strains.

In relation to NRPS, the strains studied presented siderophore, antifungal, and antibiotic bioactive compounds. Siderophores play an essential role in bacterial metabolism regarding iron uptake, since it has been described that there is a low concentration of iron in seawater (0.01–2 nM) [34,35]. It is interesting to note that *Rhodococcus* sp. MS13 contained more NRPS than *Rhodococcus erythropolis* PR4. One of them, glycinocin A, from *Rhodococcus* sp. MS16, generates lipopeptides, which can act like biosurfactants or antibiotics [34]; this strain showed the highest E24 index.

The cypermethrin degradation pathway depends on three enzymes: esterase, carboxylesterase, and laccase [36–38]. Laccase is an enzyme involved in the oxidation of aromatic compounds, which should play a role in cypermethrin biodegradation. Gangola et al. [17] described a novel cypermethrin degradation pathway in *B. subtilis* [17]: *pytH* gene encodes a pyrethroid-hydrolyzing carboxylesterase capable of degrading a variety of pyrethroids, including cypermethrin, suggesting that these strains could be good cypermethrin-degrading candidates [36], although chemical analyses are yet to be done; cypermethrin and its intermediate metabolites should be analyzed because sometimes toxic intermediates metabolites such as 3-phenoxybenzoic acid exist. This one metabolite is a toxic intermediate of cypermethrin degradation, a recalcitrant chemical [13].

Cypermethrin is first degraded by esterases into 3-(2,2-dichloroethenyl)-2,2-dimethylciclopropane carboxylic acid and α-cyanogroup-3-phenoxybenzyl alcohol; the latter is transformed into 3-PBA [23,36]; cypermethrin can also to be degraded by carboxylesterases through hydrolysis of the carboxyl ester bond, resulting in 3-(2,2-dichloroethenyl)-2,2-dimethylciclopropane carboxylic acid and 2-hydroxy-2-(3-phenoxyphenyl) acetonitrile [24,36]. The former is converted into CO_2 [36]. To selectmicroorganisms good for bioremediation is necessary so that the cypermethrin-degrading strain can transform pyrethroid into non-toxic intermediate metabolites. These bacteria first could be used for in situ treatment of bioaugmentation in an environmentally-sustainable strategy to reduce cypermethrin levels in cypermethrin-contaminated sediment. According to Chun et al. [37], the stimulation of PCB-dechlorinating and degrading microorganisms with electron-donors/-acceptors addition contributed to the degradation of PCBs in sediment.

There is an approach that made the biodegradation of β-cypermethrin and 3-PBA more efficient—using a coculture of *Bacillus licheniformis* B-1 and *Aspergillus oryzae* M-4 [38].

The enzyme laccase uses molecular oxygen and a phenolic substrate for degrading cypermethrin [17,24,39]. *Laccase* and *pytH* genes were present in all strains, but the *estA* gene was present only in *Pseudomonas* sp., MS15a and *Pseudomonas* sp. MS19 (*in silico*). Amplification of cypermethrin-degrading genes in the selected bacterial strains revealed that the *pytH* and *laccase* genes were present in all studied strains (data not shown). Kubicki et al. [40], have described some biosurfactants produced by marine microorganisms [40]. Our results suggest that both *Rhodococcus* sp. synthesize viscosin, arthrofactin, and putisolvin; *Pseudomonas* sp. M15a synthetizes viscosin, amphisin, and putisolvin; and *Pseudomonas* sp. MS19 synthesizes rhamnolipid, amphisin and arthrofactin; this indicates that our studied strains have a variety of surface-active metabolites.

In summary, these four cypermethrin-degrading and biosurfactant-producing bacterial strains isolated from marine sediments have great biotechnological potential for biodegradation of cypermethrin-contaminated marine sediments.

4. Materials and Methods

4.1. Sampling Site

Sediment samples were collected in April 2018 from cypermethrin-contaminated sediments ($n = 9$). These samples were obtained in triplicate from three sampling sites, near a salmon farm in the Manao Bay, Ancud, located in the district of Chiloé (S41°51′16.6″ W73°29′05.6″), at 25 meter depth (Figure 1a). Samples were transported and stored at 4 °C until analyses.

4.2. Culture Conditions

Bacteria were cultivated in Bushnell–Haas (BH) broth medium (composition per L: 1 g KH_2PO_4; 1 g K_2HPO_4; 1 g NH_4NO_3; 0.2 g $MgSO_4$; 0.02 g $CaCl_2$; and 0.05 g $FeCl_3$ at pH 7.0), containing 50 mg L^{-1}cypermethrin (Merck®) as the sole carbon source. Cypermethrin-degrading and biosurfactant-producing bacterial strains were grown in minimal ethanol salts medium (ETMS) (composition per L: 22.2 g $K_2HPO_4 \times 3H_2O$; 7.26 g KH_2PO_4; 0.2 g $MgSO_4 \times 7H_2O$; 0.4 g $(NH_4)_2SO_4$) and 25 mL of absolute ethanol (Merck®) [41]. Strains were also cultivated in Trypticase Soy Agar (TSA) (Difco®) and Trypticase Soy Broth (TSB) (Difco®). Cultures were grown at 28 °C in a gyratory shaker (model 3016A, Labtech) at 140 rpm. Cell growth was determined by optical density (O.D.) at 600 nm.

4.3. Isolation of Bacterial Strains from Cypermethrin-Contaminated Marine Sediments

Using enrichment culture techniques, several bacterial species were isolated (Figure 1b). To do this, a 5 g sample of marine sediment was added to a 250 mL Erlenmeyer flask containing 50 mL of sterilized

BH enrichment medium with an initial concentration of 50 mg L^{-1} of cypermethrin and incubated at 28 °C in a rotary shaker at 140 rpm for five days. After that, 5 mL of enrichment culture was inoculated into 50 mL of fresh BH medium containing 100 mg $L^{-1}$of cypermethrin. Later, the enrichment culture was incubated five days in fresh enrichment medium containing 200 mg L^{-1} of cypermethrin.

The final culture was serially diluted and spread on B.H. agar plates containing 50 mg L^{-1} cypermethrin for incubation at 28 °C for five days. To inhibit eukaryotic cell growth, 100 and 200 mg L^{-1} of cycloheximide (Sigma, St. Louis, MO, USA) were added to the first and second enrichments, respectively [11]. Plating was repeated until obtaining pure cultures and these were checked through Gram-staining using an Eclipse Ni-U (Nikon, Tokyo, Japan) optical microscope with 1000× magnification (Table S1). Isolates were stored in glycerol (15%) and kept at −80 °C until use. Strains (Table S2) were deposited in GenBank (MK271075, MK271077, MK271079, MK271080, MK271081, MK271082, MK271083, MK271084, MK271085, MK271086, and MK271087).

4.4. 16S rDNA Gene Sequencing

A colony of each isolated strain was obtained from the TSA medium, transferred to the TSB medium, and grown to OD_{600nm} = 0.6. Cells were harvested by centrifugation, and genomic DNA was extracted using the Wizard Genomic DNA Purification Kit (Promega, Madison, WI, USA), according to manufacturer's recommendations. Universal primers 27F (5′-AGA GTT TGA TCA TGG CTC AG-3′) and 1492R (5′-CGG TTA CCT TGT TAC GAC TT-3′) were used to amplify 16S rDNA [42]. Master Mix containing *Taq* DNA polymerase (Promega, Madison, WI, USA) was used for PCR-amplification. PCR thermal cycling conditions for the amplification of 16S rDNA genes were: initial denaturation for 4 min at 94 °C, followed by 30 cycles of 30 s at 94 °C denaturation temperature; 1 min at 58 °C as annealing temperature; 1 min at 72 °C as extension temperature; and a final extension of 7 min at 72 °C. PCR products were visualized through agarose gel electrophoresis. PCR products from 16S rRNA amplification were sequenced by Macrogen (Seoul, Korea), using the primer 800R (5′-TAC CAG GGT ATC TAA TCC-3′).

4.5. Determination of Emulsion Index (E_{24})

Emulsion activity was measured by mixing 2 mL of a cell-free supernatant obtained from cells grown in test tubes up to stationary phase (OD_{600nm} = 3.0) with 2 mL of petroleum diesel. The mixture was vortexed at high speed for 2 min. After vortexing, the tubes were left resting for 24 h and the emulsion layer was measured. The emulsion index (E_{24}) was calculated by dividing the height of the emulsion layer by the total height and multiplying that by 100 [43].

4.6. Scanning Electron Microscopy (SEM)

To study the bacterial morphologies of the isolated marine strains, cells were grown in TSB medium to stationary phase (OD_{600nm} = 3.0) and observed by scanning electron microscopy. For this, cells were prepared for SEM, washed with phosphate-buffered saline, and fixed with 2.5% glutaraldehyde at room temperature. Cells were gradually dehydrated in a series of ethanol dilutions and subsequently dried. Samples were then coated with a layer of palladium and examined under 15 kV accelerating voltage in an LEO-420 field emission scanning electron microscope (LEO electron microscopy, Carl Zeiss, S.M.T., Oberkochen, Germany).

4.7. Phylogenetic Analysis

Taxonomy was primarily assigned using sequences of 16S rDNA obtained by BLAST for comparison against the NCBI Non Redundant database. The sequences of strains under study and of type strains were aligned using Mega 6.0 program (Philadelphia, PA, USA) from a region of 600 bp approximately, and a phylogenetic tree was built. Phylogenetic distance between sequences was calculated with the neighbor-Joining algorithm and a bootstrap of 1000. Bootstrap values greater than 50% are shown in Figure 1c. *Lactobacillus acidophilus* 16S rDNA sequence was used as outgroup to root the tree.

4.8. Genome Sequencing and Sequence Information

Genome sequencing of MS13, MS15a, MS16, and MS19 bacterial strains was performed using Illumina Hiseq sequencing technology (Mr. DNA, Shallowater, TX, USA). Libraries were prepared using KAPA HyperPlus Kits (Kapa Biosystems, Wilmington, MA, USA) by following the manufacturer's user guide. The concentration of DNA was evaluated using the Qubit® dsDNA H.S. Assay Kit (Life Technologies, Madison, WI, USA) and the average library size was determined using the Agilent 2100 Bioanalyzer (Agilent Technologies, Santa Clara, CA, USA). Libraries were end-sequenced for 500 cycles. *De novo* assembly was carried out using C.L.C. Genomics Workbench version 11.0.1 under quality-filtered reads ($Q \geq 20$; no more than two ambiguities; final read length ≥500 bp), with length and similarity cutoffs of 60% and 90%, respectively, and minimum contig length of 5000 bp. Genomes were annotated using the NCBI Prokaryotic Genome Annotation Pipeline version 4.6, released in 2013 and approved on May 16th, 2019 [44]. Gene mining and genomic contexts were visualized using the RAST server [45]. Completeness of genome assemblies was evaluated with BUSCO software version 3.0.2 (Lausanne, Switzerland) and the bacteria subset version odb10 [46].

4.9. Identification of Secondary Metabolites, and Detection of Genes Involved in Cypermethrin Catabolism in MS13, MS15a, MS16, and MS19 Bacterial Marine Strains and a Subsequent Comparison with Reference Strains

Biosynthetic gene clusters (BGC) were determined through AntiSMASH bacterial version 5.0 [33] using the assembled genomes of selected isolated strains. The comparison was made with reference strains using NCBI information. Differences (discolored) or similarities (colored) of BGCs were established manually. To identify cypermethrin catabolic genes, specifically *est*, *pytH*, and *laccase* genes, *in silico* analyses were performed with a search by homology approach using BLAST and the following sequences as probes: AAB61674.1 (*est*), AEV51797.1 (*est*), AEY11370.1 (*pytZ*), RKM76030.1 (*laccase*), ERS87108.1 (*laccase*), ASO18034.1 (*pytH*), and KHF66595.1 (*pytH*). For genomic neighborhoods, five genes upstream and downstream to each *est*, *pytH*, and *laccase* gene were identified through the nucleotide and protein BLAST database (NCBI, Bethesda, MD, USA).

5. Conclusions

This study describes a taxonomic identification and biochemical characterization of cypermethrin-degrading and biosurfactant-producing bacterial strains isolated from a unique and extreme marine ecosystem in the Chilean Northern Patagonia. The availability of MS13, MS15a, MS16, and MS19 genome sequences offers new opportunities for systems metabolic engineering that could be useful for biodegradation of cypermethrin-polluted sediments by biosurfactants-producing microorganisms.

Supplementary Materials: The following information is available online at http://www.mdpi.com/1660-3397/18/5/252/s1. Table S1: Biochemical characteristics of cypermethrin-degrading and biosurfactant-producing bacterial strains isolated from the Chilean Northern Patagonia. Table S2: Identification of cypermethrin-degrading and biosurfactant-producing bacterial strains isolated from the Northern Chilean Patagonia by comparative sequence analyses.

Author Contributions: Conceptualization, P.A.-T., J.M., and M.G.; investigation, P.A.-T., J.M., and A.G. (Alexis Gaete); methodology, P.A.-T., J.M., and A.G. (Alexis Gaete); resources, P.A.-T., J.F., R.G.-S., A.G. (Alex González), R.M., C.M., and M.G.; visualization, P.A.-T., J.M., and A.G. (Alexis Gaete); writing—original draft, P.A.-T.; writing—review and editing, P.A.-T., J.M., A.G. (Alexis Gaete), A.G. (Alex González), R.M., R.G.-S., and M.G.; project administration, P.A.-T. All authors have read and agreed to the published version of the manuscript.

Funding: This study was funded by UACH Sede Puerto Montt project 2018-03 (54613903), 1000Genomes Chile, CONICYT/FONDECYT Postdoctorado 3170356 (R.G.S.). Project FONDAP-CRG 15090007 and INTA-U.Chile.

Conflicts of Interest: The authors declare no conflict of interest.

References

1. Bravo, S.; Silva, M.T.; Agustí, C.; Sambra, K.; Horsberg, T.E. The effect of chemotherapeutic drugs used to control sea lice on the hatching viability of egg strings from Caligus rogercresseyi. *Aquaculture* **2015**, *443*, 77–83. [CrossRef]
2. Tucca, F.; Moya, H.; Pozo, K.; Borghini, F.; Focardi, S.; Barra, R. Occurrence of antiparasitic pesticides in sediments near salmon farms in the Northern Chilean Patagonia. *Mar. Pollut. Bull.* **2017**, *115*, 465–468. [CrossRef] [PubMed]
3. Poley, J.D.; Braden, L.M.; Messmer, A.M.; Whyte, S.; Koop, B.F.; Fast, M.D. Cypermethrin exposure induces metabolic and stress-related gene expression in copepodid salmon lice (*Lepeophtheirus salmonis*). *Comp. Biochem. Physiol. Part D Genom. Proteom.* **2016**, *20*, 74–84. [CrossRef] [PubMed]
4. Zhang, C.; Jia, L.; Wang, S.; Qu, J.; Li, K.; Xu, L.; Shi, Y.; Yan, Y. Biodegradation of beta-cypermethrin by two *Serratia* spp. with different cell surface hydrophobicity. *Bioresour. Technol.* **2010**, *101*, 3423–3429. [CrossRef]
5. World Health Organization (WHO). *The WHO Recommended Classification of Pesticides by Hazardand Guidelines to Classification 2009*; World Health Organization: Geneva, Switzerland, 2009; Volume 61.
6. Ullah, S.; Zuberi, A.; Alagawany, M.; Farag, M.; Dadar, M.; Karthik, K.; Tiwari, R.; Dhama, K.; Iqbal, H.M. Cypermethrin induced toxicities in fish and adverse health outcomes: Its prevention and control measure adaptation. *J. Environ. Manag.* **2018**, *206*, 863–871. [CrossRef]
7. Sundaram, S.; Das, M.T.; Thakur, I.S. Biodegradation of cypermethrin by *Bacillus* sp. in soil microcosm and in-vitro toxicity evaluation on human cell line. *Int. Biodeterior. Biodegrad.* **2013**, *77*, 39–44. [CrossRef]
8. Navia, R.; Seeger, M. (Eds.) *Biorremediación de Suelos Contaminados con Compuestos Orgánicos Persistentes (COPs)*; Ediciones Universidad de La Frontera: Temuco, Chile, 2006; 225p; ISBN 956-236-170-5.
9. Fuentes, S.; Méndez, V.; Aguila, P.; Seeger, M. Bioremediation of petroleum hydrocarbons: Catabolic genes, microbial communities, and applications. *Appl. Microbiol. Biotechnol.* **2014**, *98*, 4781–4794. [CrossRef]
10. Saavedra, J.M.; Acevedo, F.; González, M.; Seeger, M. Mineralization of PCBs by the genetically modified strain *Cupriavidus necator* JMS34 and its application for bioremediation of PCBs in soil. *Appl. Microbiol. Biotechnol.* **2010**, *87*, 1543–1554. [CrossRef]
11. Akbar, S.; Sultan, S.; Kertesz, M. Determination of Cypermethrin Degradation Potential of Soil Bacteria Along with Plant Growth-Promoting Characteristics. *Curr. Microbiol.* **2014**, *70*, 75–84. [CrossRef]
12. Boricha, H.; Fulekar, M. *Pseudomonas plecoglossicida* as a novel organism for the bioremediation of cypermethrin. *Biol. Med.* **2009**, *1*, 1–10.
13. Chen, S.; Luo, J.; Hu, M.; Lai, K.; Geng, P.; Huang, H. Enhancement of cypermethrin degradation by a coculture of *Bacillus cereus* ZH-3 and *Streptomyces aureus* HP-S-01. *Bioresour. Technol.* **2012**, *110*, 97–104. [CrossRef] [PubMed]
14. Yin, L.; Zhao, L.; Liu, Y.; Zhang, D.; Zhang, S.; Xiao, K. Isolation and Characterization of Cypermethrin Degrading Bacteria Screened from Contaminated Soil. In *Biodegradation of Hazardous and Special Products*; Chamy, R., Ed.; IntechOpen: Valparaíso, Chile, 2013; ISBN 978-953-51-1155-9. [CrossRef]
15. Gür, Ö.; Ozdal, M.; Algur, O.F. Biodegradation of the synthetic pyrethroid insecticide α-cypermethrin by Stenotrophomonas maltophilia OG2. *Turk. J. Boil.* **2014**, *38*, 684–689. [CrossRef]
16. Liu, F.; Chi, Y.; Wu, S.; Jia, D.; Yao, K. Simultaneous Degradation of Cypermethrin and Its Metabolite, 3-Phenoxybenzoic Acid, by the Cooperation of *Bacillus licheniformis* B-1 and *Sphingomonas* sp. SC-1. *J. Agric. Food Chem.* **2014**, *62*, 8256–8262. [CrossRef] [PubMed]
17. Gangola, S.; Sharma, A.; Bhatt, P.; Khati, P.; Chaudhary, P. Presence of esterase and laccase in *Bacillus subtilis* facilitates biodegradation and detoxification of cypermethrin. *Sci. Rep.* **2018**, *8*, 12755. [CrossRef] [PubMed]
18. Lee, J.H.; Lee, Y.-S.; You, A.-Y.; Choi, Y.-L. Biological degradation of cypermethrin by marine bacteria, *Cellulophaga lytica* DAU203. *J. Life Sci.* **2018**, *28*, 483–487.
19. Pacwa-Płociniczak, M.; Płaza, G.A.; Piotrowska-Seget, Z.; Cameotra, S.S. Environmental Applications of Biosurfactants: Recent Advances. *Int. J. Mol. Sci.* **2011**, *12*, 633–654. [CrossRef]
20. Krasowska, A.; Sigler, K. How microorganisms use hydrophobicity and what does this mean for human needs? *Front. Microbiol.* **2014**, *4*, 112. [CrossRef]
21. Tripathi, L.; Irorere, V.; Marchant, R.; Banat, I.M. Marine derived biosurfactants: A vast potential future resource. *Biotechnol. Lett.* **2018**, *40*, 1441–1457. [CrossRef]

22. Zhang, S.; Yin, L.; Liu, Y.; Zhang, D.; Luo, X.; Cheng, J.; Cheng, F.; Dai, J. Cometabolic biotransformation of fenpropathrin by Clostridium species strain ZP3. *Biodegradation* **2010**, *22*, 869–875. [CrossRef]
23. Bhatt, P.; Huang, Y.; Zhan, H.; Chen, S. Insight into Microbial Applications for the Biodegradation of Pyrethroid Insecticides. *Front. Microbiol.* **2019**, *10*, 1778. [CrossRef]
24. Zhan, H.; Huang, Y.; Lin, Z.; Bhatt, P.; Chen, S. New insights into the microbial degradation and catalytic mechanism of synthetic pyrethroids. *Environ. Res.* **2020**, *182*, 109138. [CrossRef] [PubMed]
25. Choi, H.; Koh, H.-W.; Kim, H.; Chae, J.-C.; Park, S.-J. Microbial Community Composition in the Marine Sediments of Jeju Island: Next-Generation Sequencing Surveys. *J. Microbiol. Biotechnol.* **2016**, *26*, 883–890. [CrossRef] [PubMed]
26. Floris, R.; Rizzo, C.; Giudice, A.L. Biosurfactants from Marine Microorganisms. *Bacteriology* **2018**, 1–16. [CrossRef]
27. Techaoei, S.; Leelapornpisid, P.; Santiarwarn, D.; Lumyong, S. Preliminary screening of biosurfactant producing microorganisms isolated from hot spring and garages in northern Thailand. *KMITL Sci. Tech. J.* **2007**, *7*, S1.
28. Borah, D.; Yadav, R. Bioremediation of petroleum based contaminants with biosurfactant produced by a newly isolated petroleum oil degrading bacterial strain. *Egypt. J. Pet.* **2017**, *26*, 181–188. [CrossRef]
29. Elsayed, Y.; Refaat, J.; Abdelmohsen, U.R.; Fouad, M.A. The Genus *Rhodococcus* as a source of novel bioactive substances: A review. *J. Pharmacogn. Phytochem.* **2017**, *6*, 83–92.
30. Romanenko, L.A.; Tanaka, N.; Svetashev, V.I.; Mikhailov, V.V. *Pseudomonas glareae* sp. nov., a marine sediment-derived bacterium with antagonistic activity. *Arch. Microbiol.* **2015**, *197*, 693–699. [CrossRef] [PubMed]
31. Undabarrena, A.; Salvà-Serra, F.; Jaén-Luchoro, D.; Castro-Nallar, E.; Mendez, K.; Valencia, R.; Ugalde, J.; Moore, E.; Seeger, M.; Cámara, B. Complete genome sequence of the marine *Rhodococcus* sp. H-CA8f isolated from Comau fjord in Northern Patagonia, Chile. *Mar. Genom.* **2018**, *40*, 13–17. [CrossRef]
32. Harada, M.; Ito, K.; Nakajima, N.; Yamamura, S.; Tomita, M.; Suzuki, H.; Amachi, S. Genomic Analysis of *Pseudomonas* sp. Strain SCT, an Iodate-Reducing Bacterium Isolated from Marine Sediment, Reveals a Possible Use for Bioremediation. *Genes Genomes Genet.* **2019**, *9*, 1321–1329. [CrossRef]
33. Ceniceros, A.; Dijkhuizen, L.; Petrusma, M.; Medema, M.H. Genome-based exploration of the specialized metabolic capacities of the genus *Rhodococcus*. *BMC Genom.* **2017**, *18*, 593. [CrossRef]
34. Blin, K.; Shaw, S.; Steinke, K.; Villebro, R.; Ziemert, N.; Lee, S.Y.; Medema, M.H.; Weber, T. antiSMASH 5.0: Updates to the secondary metabolite genome mining pipeline. *Nucleic Acids Res.* **2019**, *47*, W81–W87. [CrossRef] [PubMed]
35. Chen, J.; Guo, Y.; Lu, Y.; Wang, B.; Sun, J.; Zhang, H.; Wang, H. Chemistry and Biology of Siderophores from Marine Microbes. *Mar. Drugs* **2019**, *17*, 562. [CrossRef] [PubMed]
36. Wang, B.-Z.; Guo, P.; Hang, B.-J.; Li, L.; He, J.; Li, S.-P. Cloning of a Novel Pyrethroid-Hydrolyzing Carboxylesterase Gene from *Sphingobium* sp. Strain JZ-1 and Characterization of the Gene Product. *Appl. Environ. Microbiol.* **2009**, *75*, 5496–5500. [CrossRef] [PubMed]
37. Chun, C.; Paine, R.; Sowers, K.; May, H. Electrical stimulation of microbial PCB degradation in sediment. *Water Res.* **2013**, *47*, 141–152. [CrossRef] [PubMed]
38. Zhao, J.; Chi, Y.; Xu, Y.; Jia, D.; Yao, K. Co-metabolic degradation of β-cypermethrin and 3-phenoxybenzoic acid by coculture of *Bacillus liqueniformis* B-1 and *Aspergillus oryzae* M-4. *PLoS ONE* **2016**, *29*, 11.
39. Shraddha; Shekher, R.; Sehgal, S.; Kamthania, M.; Kumar, A. Laccase: Microbial Sources, Production, Purification, and Potential Biotechnological Applications. *Enzym. Res.* **2011**, *2011*, 1–11. [CrossRef]
40. Kubicki, S.; Bollinger, A.; Katzke, N.; Jaeger, K.-E.; Loeschcke, A.; Thies, S. Marine Biosurfactants: Biosynthesis, Structural Diversity and Biotechnological Applications. *Mar. Drugs* **2019**, *17*, 408. [CrossRef]
41. Shabtai, Y.; Gutnick, D.L. Tolerance of *Acinetobacter calcoaceticus* RAG-1 to the cationic surfactant cetyltrimethylammonium bromide: Role of the bioemulsifier emulsan. *Appl. Environ. Microbiol.* **1985**, *49*, 192–197. [CrossRef]
42. Maza, F.; Maldonado, J.; Vásquez-Dean, J.; Mandakovic, D.; Gaete, A.; Cambiazo, V.; González, M. Soil Bacterial Communities from the Chilean Andean Highlands: Taxonomic Composition and Culturability. *Front. Bioeng. Biotechnol.* **2019**, *7*, 10. [CrossRef]
43. Bento, F.M.; Camargo, F.A.D.O.; Okeke, B.C.; Frankenberger, W.T. Diversity of biosurfactant producing microorganisms isolated from soils contaminated with diesel oil. *Microbiol. Res.* **2005**, *160*, 249–255. [CrossRef]

44. Tatusova, T.; DiCuccio, M.; Badretdin, A.; Chetvernin, V.; Nawrocki, E.P.; Zaslavsky, L.; Lomsadze, A.; Pruitt, K.D.; Borodovsky, M.; Ostell, J. NCBI prokaryotic genome annotation pipeline. *Nucleic Acids Res.* **2016**, *44*, 6614–6624. [CrossRef] [PubMed]
45. Aziz, R.K.; Bartels, D.; Best, A.A.; DeJongh, M.; Disz, T.; Edwards, R.A.; Formsma, K.; Gerdes, S.Y.; Glass, E.; Kubal, M.; et al. The RAST Server: Rapid Annotations using Subsystems Technology. *BMC Genom.* **2008**, *9*, 75. [CrossRef] [PubMed]
46. Seppey, M.; Manni, M.; Zdobnov, E.M. BUSCO: Assessing Genome Assembly and Annotation Completeness. In *Methods in Molecular Biology*; Springer Science and Business Media LLC: Lausanne, Switzerland, 2019; Volume 1962, pp. 227–245.

marine drugs

MDPI

Review

Deep-Sea Fungi Could Be the New Arsenal for Bioactive Molecules

Muhammad Zain ul Arifeen, Yu-Nan Ma, Ya-Rong Xue and Chang-Hong Liu *

State Key Laboratory of Pharmaceutical Biotechnology, School of Life Sciences, Nanjing University, Nanjing 210023, China; m.z.arifeen@gmail.com (M.Z.u.A.); mayunan994727@163.com (Y.-N.M.); xueyr@nju.edu.cn (Y.-R.X.)

* Correspondence: chliu@nju.edu.cn; Tel./Fax: +86-25-8968-5469

Received: 28 November 2019; Accepted: 17 December 2019; Published: 20 December 2019

Abstract: Growing microbial resistance to existing drugs and the search for new natural products of pharmaceutical importance have forced researchers to investigate unexplored environments, such as extreme ecosystems. The deep-sea (>1000 m below water surface) has a variety of extreme environments, such as deep-sea sediments, hydrothermal vents, and deep-sea cold region, which are considered to be new arsenals of natural products. Organisms living in the extreme environments of the deep-sea encounter harsh conditions, such as high salinity, extreme pH, absence of sun light, low temperature and oxygen, high hydrostatic pressure, and low availability of growth nutrients. The production of secondary metabolites is one of the strategies these organisms use to survive in such harsh conditions. Fungi growing in such extreme environments produce unique secondary metabolites for defense and communication, some of which also have clinical significance. Despite being the producer of many important bioactive molecules, deep-sea fungi have not been explored thoroughly. Here, we made a brief review of the structure, biological activity, and distribution of secondary metabolites produced by deep-sea fungi in the last five years.

Keywords: deep-sea; extreme; ecosystem; fungi; bioactive compounds; secondary metabolites

---

1. Deep-Sea Fungi: A Novel Source of Bioactive Molecules

Antibiotics and antifungal drugs are the most commonly used drugs in the world, but their role in treating human diseases has been greatly reduced due to the development of pathogen resistance against these drugs. Scientists are now looking for new, untapped and renewable resources for the isolation of novel compounds to with clinical importance. Despite the fact that the ocean provides habitats to a huge number of microbes, both fungi and bacteria for thousands of years, the microbes of these extreme ecosystems and their potential for new drug discovery have not yet been fully realized due to methodological and technical limitations. Fungi are the most diverse and abundant eukaryotic organisms on the planet, and their presence in all possible extreme ecosystems make them an ideal source for investigations of new drug development. Scientists are interested in the extraction of novel and unique natural products, having clinical importance, from different organisms living in the extreme environments. In addition to terrestrial extreme environments, the ocean could also be considered a good reservoir of bioactive metabolites [1–4]. Fungi living in the deep-sea environments are known to produce novel bioactive compounds. Although, it is not fully understood why the fungi living in the extreme environments produce unique and novel products, it is assumed that fungal genome has evolved to make necessary adjustments in order to sustain life in such harsh conditions and might be involved in chemical defense and communication [5].

The ocean is considered to be one of the most diverse ecosystems. Compared to terrestrial and coastal ecosystems, the deep-sea (water depths below 1000 m) has a variety of extreme environments, such as temperatures ranging from 0 to 400 °C, lack of light and oxygen, high hydrostatic pressure up to 400 atm, and limited supply of nutrient substrates, making these habitats extremely difficult for life [6,7]. In order to inhabit such extreme ecosystems, organisms should have the potential to adjust to these conditions with different mechanism, such as regulating temperature, pH, and solute concentration, as well as the production of biomolecules to control DNA, protein, and lipid damage. This may be why microorganisms growing in these environments produce special metabolites.

Previously, drug investigators mainly considered bacteria, especially actinomycetes, as an important source of antifungal and antibacterial drugs. Cephalosporin C was the first compound derived from the marine fungus *Cephalosporium* sp. in 1949. After that, a number of important drugs— for instance, polyketide griseofulvin, terpenoid fusidic acid, cephalosporins, etc.—have been isolated from the marine fungi. Despite being the source of such important products, deep-sea fungi have not received full attention [8]. With the increasing demand for new drugs, scientists are now looking for new and unexplored resources for bioactive compounds, and the deep-sea consists of some extreme ecosystems that are worth exploring for new metabolites. Studies about isolating new bioactive molecules from marine environments are growing at an increasing rate, and hundreds of new compounds are reported every year; for instance, in 2017, a total of 448 new compounds were reported [9].

In this review, we present an overview of all those new and important bioactive metabolites isolated from deep-sea fungi during the last five years. We include only those molecules which were extracted from the deep-sea fungi associated with some kind of extreme environments, irrespective of its isolation from terrestrial counterparts, while all those compounds were excluded which were isolated from marine fungi and were not associated with extreme environments. This review will benefit all those who are interested in extreme-marine-environment fungi and their bioactive molecules. For more detailed information about other important secondary metabolites extracted from marine fungi, one should refer to our previous review papers [10–12].

2. Bioactive Compounds from Deep-Sea Fungi

According to the literature survey, we found 151 novel bioactive compounds isolated from marine fungi extracted from different extreme environments in the last five years. The majority of these compounds were isolated from two fungal genera i.e., *Penicillium* (63, 41.2% of the total compounds) and *Aspergillus* (43, 28.1% of the total compounds). Table 1 lists the detail of these compounds, which fall into different categories according to their structure.

2.1. Polyketide Compounds

Twenty-four polyketide compounds (**1–24**; Figure 1) with important biological activities were isolated from fungi extracted from different deep-sea environments. Among them, compounds **1** and **2** were isolated from *Penicillium* spp., which showed antibiotic activity (MIC of 32 μg/mL against *Bacillus subtilis*) and nuclear factor NF-kB inhibition activity, respectively [13,14]. Compounds **3–11** were from *Aspergillus* sp. 16-02-1, which exhibited cytotoxicity (with a 10%–80% inhibition rate at 100 μg/mL against various cancer cell lines i.e., K562, HL-60, HeLa, and BGC-823) [15]. Similarly, compounds **12–24** were isolated from the species belonging to *Ascomycetes*, *Engyodontium*, and *Lindgomycetaceae*, out of which compounds **12–13** and **23–24** showed strong antibiotic activities against *Bacillus subtilis*, *Acinetobacter baumannii*, *Escherichia coli*, *Staphylococcus aureus*, *Enterococcus faecalis*, *Staphylococcus epidermidis*, and *Propionibacterium acnes*, while compounds **14–22** exhibited strong cytotoxic activity (IC_{50} 4.9 μM) against U937 cells (Table 1) [16–18].

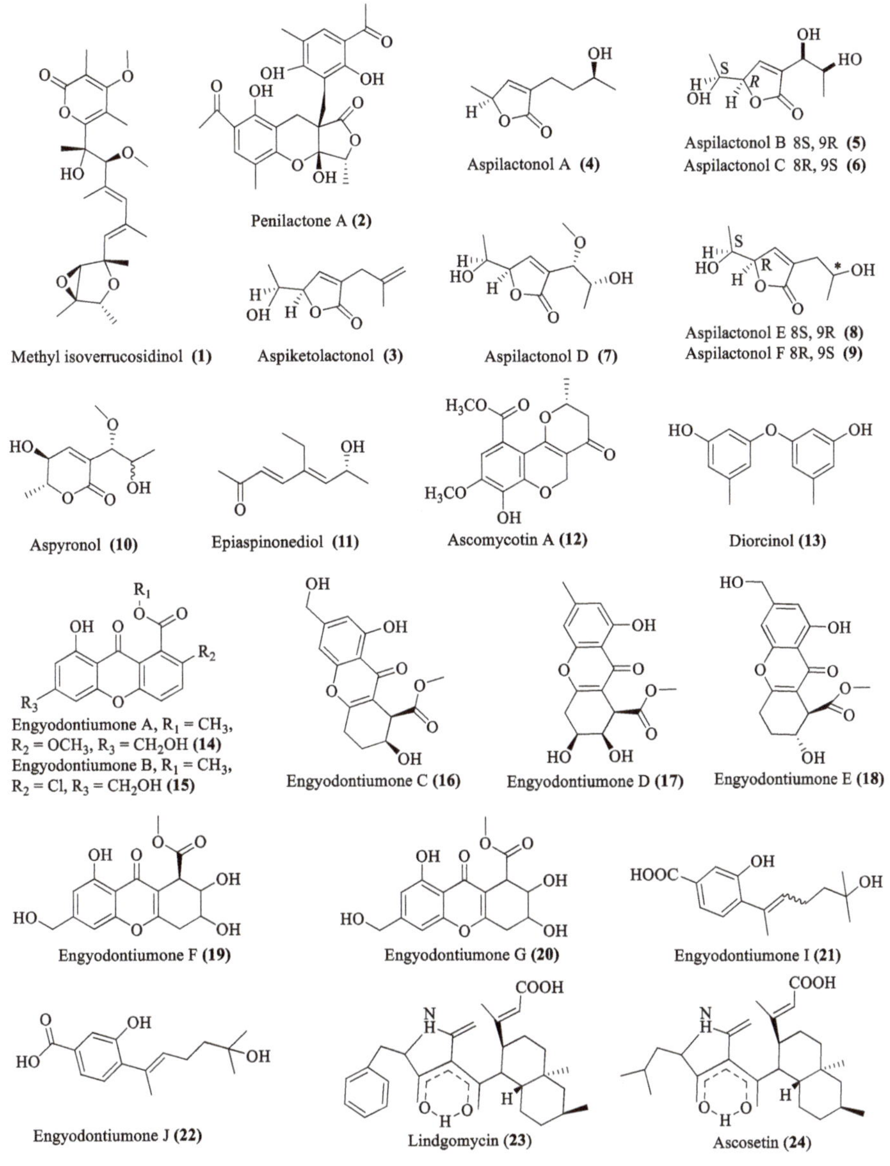

Figure 1. Structures of polyketide secondary metabolites obtained from deep-sea fungi.

2.2. Nitrogen-Containing Compounds

Twenty-four novel alkaloid-bioactive compounds (**25–48**; Figure 2) have been reported from deep-sea fungi since 2013, out of which compounds **25–40** were isolated from *Penicillium* spp., and showed cytotoxic activities against BV2 cell (IC_{50} of 27–45 μg/mL), brine shrimp (IC_{50} of 14.1 to 38.5 μg/mL), SMMC-7721 (IC_{50} of 54.2 μM), BEL-7402 ((IC_{50} of 17.5 μM), and BEL-7402 (IC_{50} of 19.8 μM) [19–21]. Compounds **41–46** were identified from *Aspergillus* spp., in which compounds **41** and **45–46** displayed antibiotic activity (MIC of 30 to 40 μg/mL) against BCG, *Candida albicans*, *Bacillus subtilis*, *Staphylococcus aureus*, *Pseudomonas aeruginosa*, *Bacillus cereus*, *Klebsiella pneumoniae*, and *Escherichia coli*, while compounds **47** and **48** were extracted from other genera and showed antimicrobial activity (MIC between 16 and 64 μg/mL against *Escherichia coli*, *Aeromonas hydrophila*, *Micrococcus luteus*, *Staphylococcus aureus*, *Vibrio anguillarum*, *Vibrio harveyi*, and *Vibrio parahaemolyticus*) and cytotoxic activity against human cervical carcinoma HeLa, respectively [22–26].

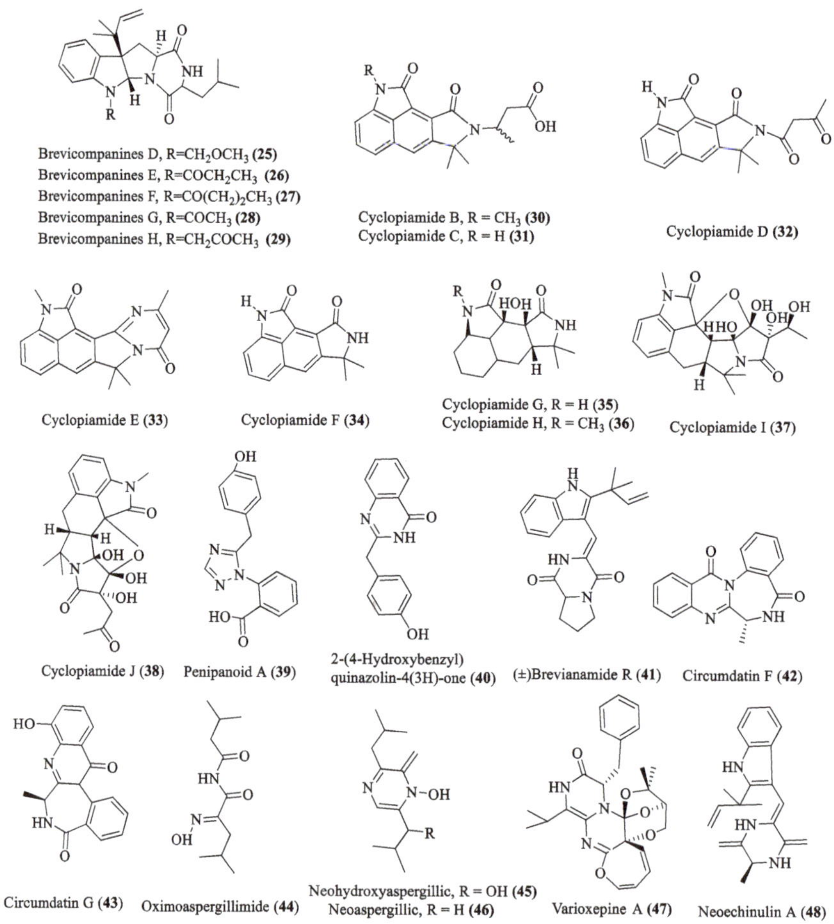

Figure 2. Bioactive alkaloid compounds isolated from deep-sea fungi.

2.3. Polypeptides

Twenty-two polypeptides with novel structures (**49–70**; Figure 3) were reported from fungi inhabiting different marine environments during 2013–2019. Compounds **49** and **50** were isolated from *Penicillium canescens* and displayed antibiotic activity against *Bacillus amyloliquefaciens* and *Pseudomonas aeruginosa* at 100 μM, while compounds **51–55** were extracted from *Aspergillus* spp., in which **51–54** showed cytotoxic activity (IC_{50} of 15–25 μg/mL) against HepG2, SMMC-7721, Bel-7402, and human glioma U87 cell lines, while compound **55** showed inhibitory effects (IC_{50} value of 5.11 μmol/L) against *Mycobacterium tuberculosis* protein tyrosine phosphatase B (MptpB) [27–30]. However, compounds **56–64**, which were obtained from *Simplicillium obclavatum*, and **65–70**, obtained from *Trichoderma asperellum*, displayed cytotoxicity (IC_{50} of 39.4–100 μM) against human leukemia HL-60 and K562 cell lines and antibiotic activity (IC_{50} of 39.4–100 μM) against Gram-positive bacteria (e.g., *Bacillus amyloliquefaciens*, *Staphylococcus aureus*) and Gram-negative bacteria (e.g., *Pseudomonas aeruginosa* and *Escherichia coli*), respectively [28,31].

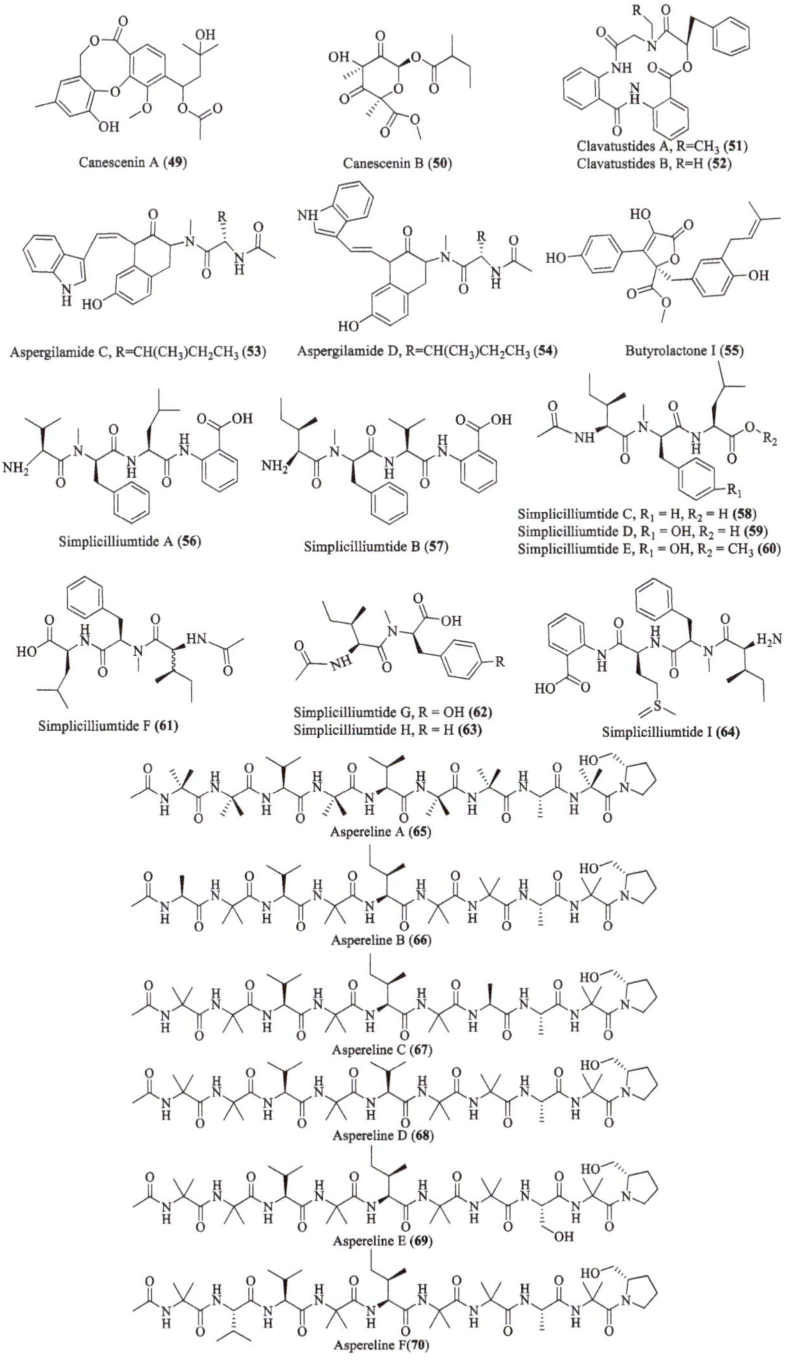

Figure 3. Bioactive polypeptides isolated from deep-sea fungi.

2.4. Ester and Phenolic Derivatives

Six new ester derivatives (**71–76**; Figure 4) were extracted from *Aspergillus ungui* NKH-007 and showed inhibition of sterol O-acyltransferase (SOAT) enzymes in Chinese hamster ovary (CHO) cells and are thus considered to be good candidates for an anti-atherosclerotic agent [32]. Five new phenolic compounds (**77–81**; Figure 4) isolated from *Penicillium* sp. and *Aspergillus versicolor* showed potent activity against *Staphylococcus aureus* and *Bacillus subtilis*, with MIC values of 2–8 μg/mL [33,34]. However, compounds **78–81** expressed antiviral activity toward HSV-1, with EC_{50} values of 3.12–6.25 μM [34].

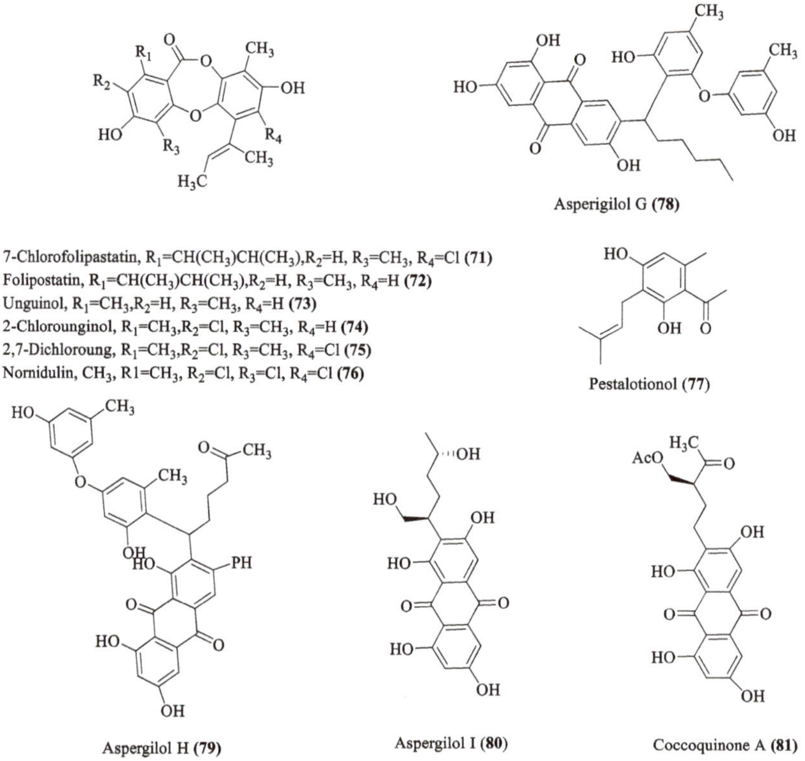

Figure 4. Ester and phenolic derivatives obtained from deep-sea fungi.

2.5. Piperazine Derivatives

Fourteen new piperazine derivatives (**82–95**; Figure 5) reported from marine fungi during the last five years. These derivatives were isolated from genera of *Penicillium*, *Aspergillus*, and *Dichotomomyces* collected from deep-sea sediments. Compounds **82–84** showed strong cytotoxicity with IC_{50} of 1.7 and 2 μM against K562 and mouse lymphoma cell line, respectively; similarly, compounds **91–95** also showed strong cytotoxic activity [35–37]. Compounds **85–89** showed antibacterial activity against *Staphylococcus aureus* with the MIC values of 6.25–12.5 μg/mL [21]. The new compound **90** also showed stronger inhibition activity against α-glucosidase with IC_{50} value of 138 μM [37].

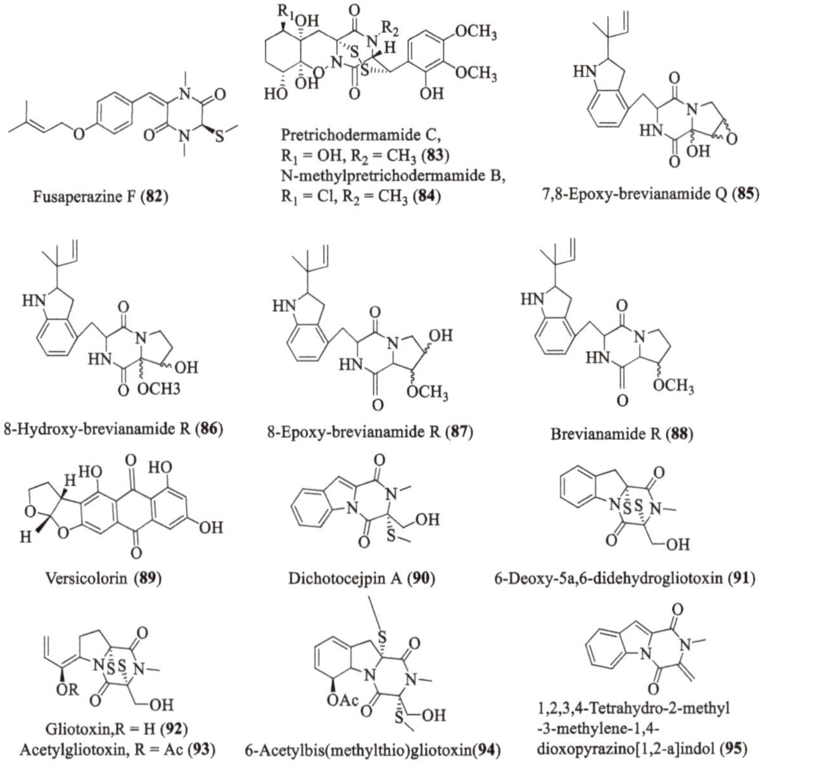

Figure 5. Piperazine derivatives isolated from deep-sea fungi.

2.6. Terpenoid Compounds

Thirty-six new and important bioactive terpenoids (**96–131**; Figure 6) have been isolated from marine fungi extracted from the deep-sea sediments since 2013. Compounds **96–113** were isolated from *Penicillium* spp., while compounds **114–131** were extracted from *Aspergillus* spp. Breviones (**96–99**), isolated from the deepest sediment-derived fungus *Penicillium* sp. (5115 m depth), displayed diverse activities, such as cytotoxicity against HeLa, MCF-7, and A549 cells with IC_{50} values of 7.44 to 32.5 μM, respectively, and growth inhibition of HIV-1 with EC_{50} value of 14.7 μM against C8166 cells [22,38]. Compounds **100–110** showed antibiotic and inhibition activities against silkworm, while 20-nor-isopimarane diterpenoids, including aspewentins (**114–118**), asperethers (**121–125**), asperoloids (**119–120**), and compounds **130** and **131**, showed cytotoxic activities [33,39–45]. However, the spirocyclic diterpenes (**111–113**) exhibited strong anti-allergic effect with 18% inhibition at 20 μg/mL [46]. Interestingly, four new compounds (**126–129**) were extracted from hydrothermal vent-derived *Aspergillus sydowii*, through activation of a new pathway for secondary metabolite production by the addition of a 5-azacytidine (a DNA methyltransferase inhibitor). These compounds showed anti-inflammatory and antidiabetic activities and are thus the first secondary metabolites isolated from fungi which have both antidiabetic and anti-inflammatory activities [47].

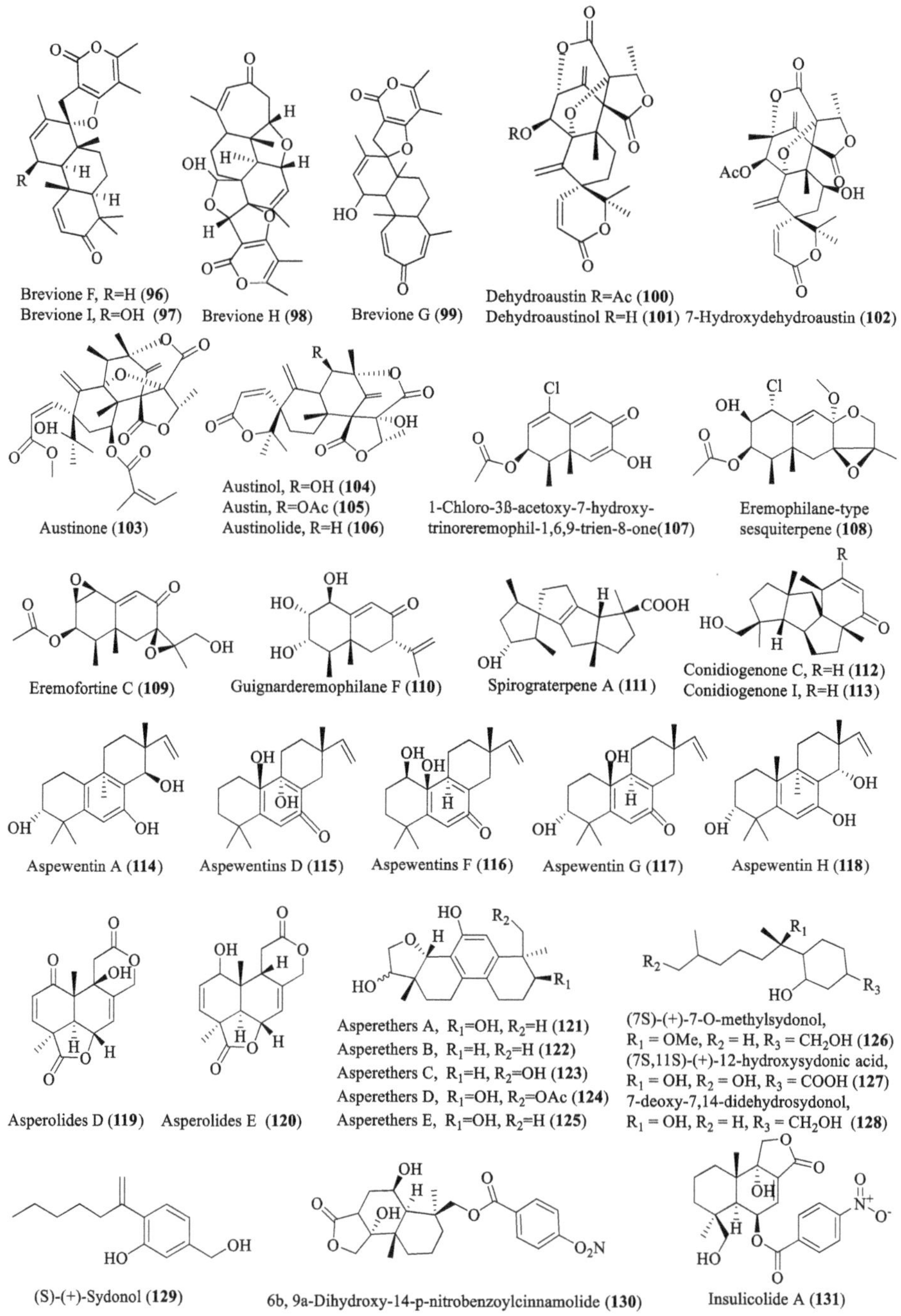

Figure 6. Structures of terpenoid secondary metabolites obtained from deep-sea fungi.

2.7. Other Unrelated Compounds

Twenty secondary metabolites with different structures were isolated from deep-sea fungi, mainly from *Penicillium* spp. and *Aspergillus* spp. (**132–151**; Figure 7). Penipacids A–F (**134–139**), polyoxygenated sterol (**132**), dicitrinone B (**133**) and butanolide A (**140**), which were isolated from deep-sea sediments-derived *Penicillium* spp., showed cytotoxic activities against RKO, MCF-7, PTP1B and A375 cancer cell lines with IC_{50} values of 8.4–28.4 μM [38,42,48,49]. Similarly, four isocoumarins, penicillisocoumarin A–D (**147–150**), and an isocoumarins aspergillumarin B (**151**) were also isolated from *Penicillium* which showed weak antibacterial activities [33]. Four antibiotic cyclopenin derivatives compounds (**141–144**) and a series of antitumor wentilactones (**145,146**) were isolated from *Aspergillus* spp. [50,51].

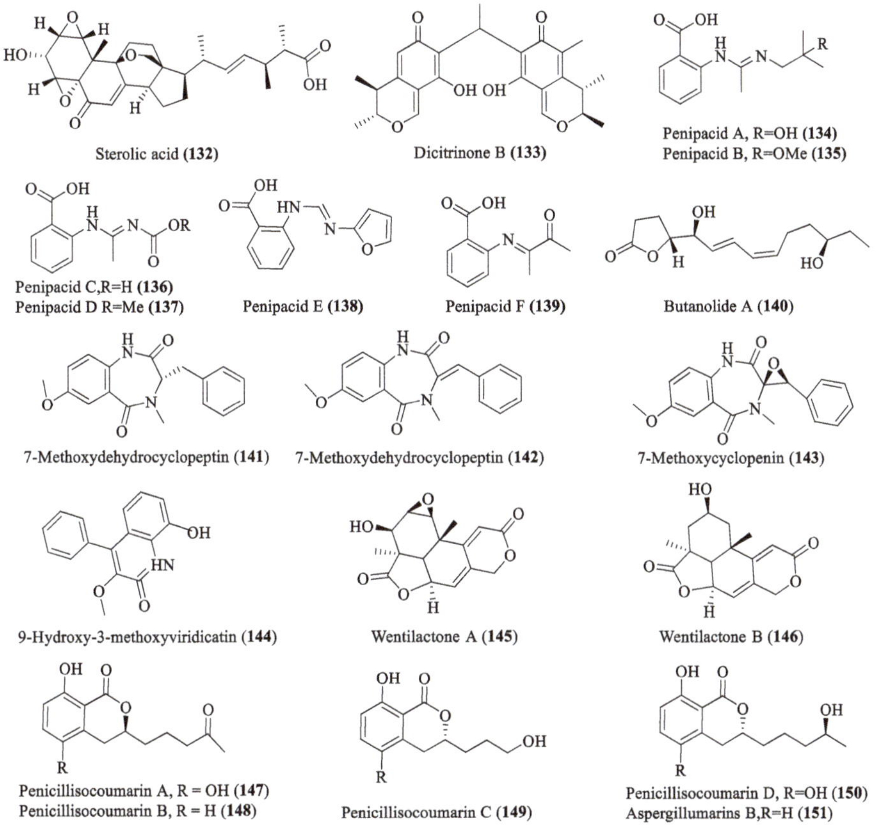

Figure 7. Bioactive metabolites derived from deep-sea fungi.

Table 1. Secondary metabolites extracted from deep-sea fungi during 2013–2019.

Metabolites	Fungal Species	Source	Location	Depth (m) *	Bioactivity	Ref.
		Polyketide				
Methyl-isoverrucosidinol **(1)**	*Penicillium* sp. Y-50-10	Sulfur-rich Sediment	hydrothermal vent, Taiwan	_	Antibiotic	[13]
Penilactone A **(2)**	*Penicillium crustosum* PRB-2	Sediment	Prydz Bay, Antarctica	526	NF-kB inhibition	[14]
Aspiketolactonol **(3)** Aspilactonols A–F **(4-9)** Aspyronol **(10)** Epiaspinonediol **(11)**	*Aspergillus* sp. 16-02-1	Hydrothermal vent water	Lau Basin, Southwest Pacific Ocean,	2255	Cytotoxic	[15]
Ascomycotin A **(12)** Diorcinol **(13)**	*Ascomycota* sp. Ind19F07	Sediment	Indian Ocean	3614	Antibiotic	[16]
Engyodontiumones A–J **(14-22)**	*Engyodontium album* DFFSCS021	Sediment	South China Sea	3739	Cytotoxic	[18]
Lindgomycin **(23)** Ascosetin **(24)**	*Lindgomycetaceae* strains KF970 and LF327	Sediment	Greenland Sea, Baltic Sea	3650	Antibiotic	[17]
		Nitrogen-containing compounds				
Brevicompanines D–H **(25-29)**	*Penicillium* sp. F1	Sediment	_	5080	LPS-induced inflammation	[22]
Cyclopiamide B–J **(30-38)**	*Penicillium commune* DFFSCS026	Sediment	South China Sea	3563	Cytotoxic	[24]
Penipanoid A **(39)** Quinazolinone **(40)**	*Penicillium paneum* SD-44	Sediment	South China Sea	201	Cytotoxic	[23]
(±) Brevianamide R **(41)**	*Aspergillus* versicolor MF180151	Sediment	Bohai Sea, China	_	Antibacterial	[21]
Circumdatin F and G **(42-43)**	*Aspergillus westerdijkiae* SCSIO 05233	Sediment	South China Sea	4593	Cytotoxic	[20]
Oximoaspergillimide **(44)** Neohydroxyaspergillic **(45)** Neoaspergillic **(46)**	*Aspergillus* sp. (CF07002)	Water	Pacific Ocean off the coast of Panama		Cytotoxic Antibiotic	[19]
Varioxepine A **(47)**	*Paecilomyces variotii* EN-291	Deep sea water	_	_	Antibiotic	[26]
Neoechinulin A **(48)**	*Microsporum* sp. (MFS-YL)	Red alga	Guryongpo, Korea	_	Cytotoxic	[25]
		Polypeptide				
Canescenin A and B **(49-50)**	*Penicillium canescens* SCSIO z053	Water	East China Sea	2013	Antibacterial	[27]
Clavatustide A and B **(51-52)**	*Aspergillus clavatus* C2WU	Hydrothermal vent crab	Taiwan Kueishantao	_	Cytotoxic	[29]
Aspergillamides C and D **(53-54)** Butyrolactone I **(55)**	*Aspergillus terreus* SCSIO 41008	Sponge	Guangdong, China	_	Cytotoxic Antibiotic	[30]
Simplicilliumtides A–I **(56-64)**	*Simplicillium obclavatum* EIODSF 020	Sediment	East Indian Ocean	4571	Cytotoxic	[31]
Asperelines A–F **(65-70)**	*Trichoderma asperellum*	Sediment	Antarctic Penguin Island	_	Antibiotic	[28]

Table 1. *Cont.*

Metabolites	Fungal Species	Source	Location	Depth (m) *	Bioactivity	Ref.
			Esters			
7-chlorofolipastatin **(71)** Folipostatin B **(72)** Unguinol **(73)** 2-chlorounginol **(74)** 2,7-dichlorounguinol **(75)** Nornidulin **(76)**	*Aspergillus ungui* NKH-007	Sediment	Suruga Bay, Japan	–	Anti-atherosclerotic Cytotoxic Antibiotic	[32]
			Phenolic			
Pestalotionol **(77)**	*Penicillium* sp. Y-5-2	Hydrothermal vent water	Kueishantao off Taiwan	–	Antibiotic	[33]
Aspergilol G–I **(78-80)** Coccoquinone A **(81)**	*Aspergillus versicolor* SCSIO 41502	Sediment	South China Sea	2326	Anti-HSV-1 Antioxidant Antifouling	[34]
			Piperazine			
Fusaperazine F **(82)**	*Penicillium crustosum* HDN153086	Sediment	Prydz Bay, Antarctica	–	Cytotoxic	[35]
N-methyl-pretrichodermamide B **(83)** Pretrichodermamide C **(84)**	*Penicillium* sp. (WN-11-1-3-1-2)	Hypersaline sediment	Wadi El-Natrun, Egypt	–	Cytotoxic	[36]
(±) 7,8-epoxy-brevianamide Q **(85)** (±) 8-hydroxy-brevianamide R **(86)** (±) 8-epihydroxy-brevianamide R **(87)** Brevianamide R **(88)** Versicolorin B **(89)**	*Aspergillus versicolor* MF180151	Sediment	Bohai Sea, China	–	Antibiotic	[21]
Dichotocejpins A **(90)** 6-deoxy-5a,6-didehydrogliotoxin **(91)** Gliotoxin **(92)** Acetylgliotoxin **(93)** 6-acetylbis(methylthio)-gliotoxin **(94)** 1,2,3,4-tetrahydro-2-methyl-3-methylene-1,4-dioxopyrazino [1,2-a] indole **(95)**	*Dichotomomyces cejpii* FS110	Sediment	South China Sea	3941	α-Glucosidase inhibition Cytotoxic	[37]
			Terpenoid			
Brevione F–I **(96-99)**	*Penicillium* sp. (MCCC 3A00005)	Sediment	Pacific Ocean	5115	Cytotoxic HIV-1 inhibition	[22,38]
Dehydroaustin **(100)** Dehydroaustinol **(101)** 7-hydroxydehydroaustin **(102)** Austinone **(103)** Austinol **(104)** Austin **(105)** Austinolide **(106)**	*Penicillium* sp. Y-5-2	Hydrothermal vent water	Kueishantao off Taiwan	8	Antibacterial Anti-insectal	[33]

Table 1. *Cont.*

Metabolites	Fungal Species	Source	Location	Depth (m) *	Bioactivity	Ref.
1-chloro-3β-acetoxy-7-hydroxytrinoreremophil-1,6,9-trien-8-one **(107)** Eremophilane-type sesquiterpenes **(108)** Eremofortine C **(109)**	*Penicillium* sp. PR19N-1	Sediment	Prydz Bay, Antarctica	526	Cytotoxic	[40,41]
Guignarderemophilane F **(110)**	*Penicillium* sp. S-1-18	Sediment	Antarctic	1393	Antibacterial	[42]
Spirograterpene A **(111)** Conidiogenone C and I **(112-113)**	*Penicillium granulatum* MCCC 3A00475	Water	Prydz Bay of Antarctica	2284	Antiallergic	[46]
Aspewentin A and D–H **(114-118)** Asperethers A–E **(121-125)** Asperolides D and E **(119-120)**	*Aspergillus wentii* SD-310	Sediment	South China Sea	2038	Antimicrobial Cytotoxic Anti-inflammatory	[39,43,44]
(7S)-(+)7-O-methylsydonol **(126)** (7S,11S)-(+)-12-hydroxysydonic acid **(127)** 7-deoxy-7,14-didehydrosydonol **(128)** (S)-(+)-sydonol **(129)**	*Aspergillus sydowii*	Sediment	Hsinchu, Taiwan	–	Anti-inflammatory	[47]
6b,9a-dihydroxy-14-p-nitrobenzoylcinnamolide **(130)** Insulicolide A **(131)**	*Aspergillus ochraceus* Jcma1F17	Marine alga *Coelarthrum* sp.	South China Sea	–	Antiviral Cytotoxic	[45]
			Other compounds			
Sterolic acid **(132)**	*Penicillium* sp. MCCC 3A00005	Sediment	East Pacific Ocean	5115	Cytotoxic	[38]
Dicitrinone B **(133)**	*Penicillium citrinum*	Sediment	Langqi Island, Fujian, China	–	Antitumor	[49]
Penipacids A–F **(134-139)**	*Penicillium paneum* SD-44	Sediment	South China Sea	–	Cytotoxic	[48]
Butanolide A **(140)**	*Penicillium* sp. S-1-18	Sediment	Antarctic seabed	1393	Cytotoxic	[42]
7-Methoxycyclopeptin **(141)** 7-Methoxy dehydro cyclopeptin **(142)** 7-Methoxy cyclopenin **(143)** 9-Hydroxy-3-methoxyviridicatin **(144)**	*Aspergillus versicolor* XZ-4	Hydrothermal vent crab	Kueishantao, Taiwan		Antibiotic	[50]
Wentilactone A and B **(145-146)**	*Aspergillus dimorphicus* SD317	Sediment	South China Sea	2038	Antitumor	[51]
Penicillisocoumarin A–D **(147-150)** Aspergillumarins B **(151)**	*Penicillium* sp. Y-5-2	Hydrothermal vent water	Kueishantao off Taiwan	8	Antibacterial	[33]

* Depth represents water depth below the surface.

3. Conclusions and Perspective

The results of current studies indicate that the deep-sea extreme environmental fungi are one of the rich and unexploited sources of important medicinal lead compounds. Most of the fungi (e.g., *Penicillium* spp. and *Aspergillus* spp.) living in the extreme environments of the deep-sea have the potential to synthesize new bioactive compounds. However, the research on deep-sea fungi and their metabolites is very limited due to the difficulty of sampling and the limitation of culture technology. Thanks to the advances in genome technology and the implementation of the deep-sea drilling program, novel compounds with great biological activities are expected from these fungi in the near future. From the literature review, we can say these fungi from the extreme environments have the potential to produce clinically important natural products. The compounds we discussed in this review show strong bioactivities and might have the potential to be a future anticancer drug. Among them, terpenoid derivatives were the most important and abundant compound category which were mainly isolated from deep-sea derived *Penicillium* spp. and *Aspergillus* spp. This class of compounds showed strongest antibiotic and cytotoxic activities as compared to other classes of compounds and has the potential to be a future candidate for anticancer drugs, especially brevione, which was isolated from the deepest part of the sea and showed the strongest cytotoxic activity.

Author Contributions: Writing—original draft preparation, M.Z.u.A.; writing—review and editing, Y.-N.M., Y.-R.X. and C.-H.L. All authors have read and agreed to the published version of the manuscript.

Funding: This work was financially supported by the National Natural Science Foundation of China (General Program: 41773083, 41973073; Major Program: 91951121).

Conflicts of Interest: The authors declare that they have no competing interests.

References

1. König, G.M.; Kehraus, S.; Seibert, S.F.; Abdel-Lateff, A.; Müller, D. Natural products from marine organisms and their associated microbes. *Chem. Bio. Chem.* **2006**, *7*, 229–238. [CrossRef] [PubMed]
2. Chen, G.; Wang, H.-F.; Pei, Y.-H. Secondary metabolites from marine-derived microorganisms. *J. Asian Nat. Prod. Res.* **2014**, *16*, 105–122. [CrossRef] [PubMed]
3. Agrawal, S.; Adholeya, A.; Deshmukh, S.K. The pharmacological potential of non-ribosomal peptides from marine sponge and tunicates. *Front. Pharmacol.* **2016**, *7*, 333. [CrossRef] [PubMed]
4. Deshmukh, S.K.; Prakash, V.; Ranjan, N. Recent advances in the discovery of bioactive metabolites from *Pestalotiopsis*. *Phytochem. Rev.* **2017**, *16*, 883–920. [CrossRef]
5. Deshmukh, S.K.; Prakash, V.; Ranjan, N. Marine fungi: A source of potential anticancer compounds. *Front. Microbiol.* **2018**, *8*, 2536. [CrossRef]
6. Danovaro, R.; Corinaldesi, C.; Dell'Anno, A.; Snelgrove, P.V. The deep-sea under global change. *Curr. Biol.* **2017**, *27*, R461–R465. [CrossRef]
7. Barone, G.; Varrella, S.; Tangherlini, M.; Rastelli, E.; Dell'Anno, A.; Danovaro, R.; Corinaldesi, C. Marine fungi: Biotechnological perspectives from deep-hypersaline anoxic basins. *Diversity* **2019**, *11*, 113. [CrossRef]
8. Hamilton-Miller, J. Development of the semi-synthetic *penicillins* and *cephalosporins*. *Int. J. Antimicrob.* **2008**, *31*, 189–192. [CrossRef]
9. Carroll, A.R.; Copp, B.R.; Davis, R.A.; Keyzers, R.A.; Prinsep, M.R. Marine natural products. *Nat. Prod. Rep.* **2019**, *36*, 122–173. [CrossRef]
10. Wang, Y.-T.; Xue, Y.-R.; Liu, C.-H. A brief review of bioactive metabolites derived from deep-sea fungi. *Mar. Drugs* **2015**, *13*, 4594–4616. [CrossRef]
11. Arifeen, M.Z.U.; Liu, C.-H. Novel enzymes isolated from marine-derived fungi and its potential applications. *United J. Biochem. Biotechnol.* **2018**, *1*, 1–11.
12. Arifeen, M.Z.U.; Xue, Y.-R.; Liu, C.-H. Deep-sea fungi: Diversity, enzymes, and bioactive metabolites. In *Fungi in Extreme Environments: Ecological Role and Biotechnological Significance*; Springer: Berlin, Germany, 2019; pp. 331–347.

13. Pan, C.; Shi, Y.; Auckloo, B.; Chen, X.; Chen, C.-T.; Tao, X.; Wu, B. An unusual conformational isomer of verrucosidin backbone from a hydrothermal vent fungus, *Penicillium* sp. Y-50-10. *Mar. Drugs* **2016**, *14*, 156. [CrossRef]
14. Wu, G.; Ma, H.; Zhu, T.; Li, J.; Gu, Q.; Li, D. Penilactones A and B, two novel polyketides from Antarctic deep-sea derived fungus *Penicillium crustosum* PRB-2. *Tetrahedron* **2012**, *68*, 9745–9749. [CrossRef]
15. Chen, X.-W.; Li, C.-W.; Cui, C.-B.; Hua, W.; Zhu, T.-J.; Gu, Q.-Q. Nine new and five known polyketides derived from a deep sea-sourced *Aspergillus* sp. 16-02-1. *Mar. Drugs* **2014**, *12*, 3116–3137. [CrossRef]
16. Tian, Y.-Q.; Lin, X.-P.; Liu, J.; Kaliyaperumal, K.; Ai, W.; Ju, Z.-R.; Yang, B.; Wang, J.; Yang, X.-W.; Liu, Y. Ascomycotin A, a new citromycetin analogue produced by *Ascomycota* sp. Ind19F07 isolated from deep sea sediment. *Nat. Prod. Res.* **2015**, *29*, 820–826. [CrossRef]
17. Wu, B.; Wiese, J.; Labes, A.; Kramer, A.; Schmaljohann, R.; Imhoff, J. Lindgomycin, an unusual antibiotic polyketide from a marine fungus of the *Lindgomycetaceae*. *Mar. Drugs* **2015**, *13*, 4617–4632. [CrossRef]
18. Yao, Q.; Wang, J.; Zhang, X.; Nong, X.; Xu, X.; Qi, S. Cytotoxic polyketides from the deep-sea-derived fungus *Engyodontium album* DFFSCS021. *Mar. Drugs* **2014**, *12*, 5902–5915. [CrossRef]
19. Cardoso-Martínez, F.; de la Rosa, J.M.; Díaz-Marrero, A.R.; Darias, J.; D'Croz, L.; Cerella, C.; Diederich, M.; Cueto, M. Oximoaspergillimide, a fungal derivative from a marine isolate of *Aspergillus* sp. *Eur. J. Org. Chem.* **2015**, *2015*, 2256–2261. [CrossRef]
20. Fredimoses, M.; Zhou, X.; Ai, W.; Tian, X.; Yang, B.; Lin, X.; Xian, J.-Y.; Liu, Y. Westerdijkin A, a new hydroxyphenylacetic acid derivative from deep sea fungus *Aspergillus westerdijkiae* SCSIO 05233. *Nat. Prod. Res.* **2015**, *29*, 158–162. [CrossRef]
21. Hu, J.; Li, Z.; Gao, J.; He, H.; Dai, H.; Xia, X.; Liu, C.; Zhang, L.; Song, F. New diketopiperazines from a marine-derived fungus strain *Aspergillus versicolor* MF180151. *Mar. Drugs* **2019**, *17*, 262. [CrossRef]
22. Zhang, X.; Li, S.-J.; Li, J.-J.; Liang, Z.-Z.; Zhao, C.-Q. Novel natural products from extremophilic fungi. *Mar. Drugs* **2018**, *16*, 194. [CrossRef] [PubMed]
23. Li, C.-S.; An, C.-Y.; Li, X.-M.; Gao, S.-S.; Cui, C.-M.; Sun, H.-F.; Wang, B.-G. Triazole and dihydroimidazole alkaloids from the marine sediment-derived fungus *Penicillium paneum* SD-44. *J. Nat. Prod.* **2011**, *74*, 1331–1334. [CrossRef] [PubMed]
24. Xu, X.; Zhang, X.; Nong, X.; Wei, X.; Qi, S. Oxindole alkaloids from the fungus *Penicillium commune* DFFSCS026 isolated from deep-sea-derived sediments. *Tetrahedron* **2015**, *71*, 610–615. [CrossRef]
25. Wijesekara, I.; Li, Y.-X.; Vo, T.-S.; Van Ta, Q.; Ngo, D.-H.; Kim, S.-K. Induction of apoptosis in human cervical carcinoma HeLa cells by neoechinulin A from marine-derived fungus *Microsporum* sp. *Process Biochem.* **2013**, *48*, 68–72. [CrossRef]
26. Zhang, P.; Mandi, A.; Li, X.-M.; Du, F.-Y.; Wang, J.-N.; Li, X.; Kurtan, T.; Wang, B.-G. Varioxepine A, a 3 H-oxepine-containing alkaloid with a new oxa-cage from the marine algal-derived endophytic fungus *Paecilomyces variotii*. *Org. Lett.* **2014**, *16*, 4834–4837. [CrossRef]
27. Dasanayaka, S.; Nong, X.-H.; Liang, X.; Liang, J.-Q.; Amin, M.; Qi, S.-H. New dibenzodioxocinone and pyran-3, 5-dione derivatives from the deep-sea-derived fungus *Penicillium canescens* SCSIO z053. *J. Asian Nat. Prod. Res.* **2019**, 1–8. [CrossRef]
28. Ren, J.; Xue, C.; Tian, L.; Xu, M.; Chen, J.; Deng, Z.; Proksch, P.; Lin, W. Asperelines A– F, peptaibols from the marine-derived fungus *Trichoderma asperellum*. *J. Nat. Prod.* **2009**, *72*, 1036–1044. [CrossRef]
29. Jiang, W.; Ye, P.; Chen, C.-T.; Wang, K.; Liu, P.; He, S.; Wu, X.; Gan, L.; Ye, Y.; Wu, B. Two novel hepatocellular carcinoma cycle inhibitory cyclodepsipeptides from a hydrothermal vent crab-associated fungus *Aspergillus clavatus* C2WU. *Mar. Drugs* **2013**, *11*, 4761–4772. [CrossRef]
30. Luo, X.W.; Yun, L.; Liu, Y.J.; Zhou, X.F.; Liu, Y.H. Peptides and polyketides isolated from the marine sponge-derived fungus *Aspergillus terreus* SCSIO 41008. *Chin. J. Nat. Med.* **2019**, *17*, 149–154. [CrossRef]
31. Liang, X.; Zhang, X.-Y.; Nong, X.-H.; Wang, J.; Huang, Z.-H.; Qi, S.-H. Eight linear peptides from the deep-sea-derived fungus *Simplicillium obclavatum* EIODSF 020. *Tetrahedron* **2016**, *72*, 3092–3097. [CrossRef]
32. Uchida, R.; Nakajyo, K.; Kobayashi, K.; Ohshiro, T.; Terahara, T.; Imada, C.; Tomoda, H. 7-Chlorofolipastatin, an inhibitor of sterol O-acyltransferase, produced by marine-derived *Aspergillus ungui* NKH-007. *J. Antibiot.* **2016**, *69*, 647. [CrossRef] [PubMed]
33. Pan, C.; Shi, Y.; Auckloo, B.N.; ul Hassan, S.S.; Akhter, N.; Wang, K.; Ye, Y.; Chen, C.-T.A.; Tao, X.; Wu, B. Isolation and antibiotic screening of fungi from a hydrothermal vent site and characterization of secondary metabolites from a *Penicillium* isolate. *Mar. Biotechnol.* **2017**, *19*, 469–479. [CrossRef] [PubMed]

34. Huang, Z.; Nong, X.; Ren, Z.; Wang, J.; Zhang, X.; Qi, S. Anti-HSV-1, antioxidant and antifouling phenolic compounds from the deep-sea-derived fungus *Aspergillus versicolor* SCSIO 41502. *Bioorg. Med. Chem. Lett.* **2017**, *27*, 787–791. [CrossRef] [PubMed]
35. Liu, C.-C.; Zhang, Z.-Z.; Feng, Y.-Y.; Gu, Q.-Q.; Li, D.-H.; Zhu, T.-J. Secondary metabolites from Antarctic marine-derived fungus *Penicillium crustosum* HDN153086. *Nat. Prod. Res.* **2019**, *33*, 414–419. [CrossRef] [PubMed]
36. Orfali, R.S.; Aly, A.H.; Ebrahim, W.; Abdel-Aziz, M.S.; Müller, W.E.; Lin, W.; Daletos, G.; Proksch, P. Pretrichodermamide C and N-methylpretrichodermamide B, two new cytotoxic epidithiodiketopiperazines from hyper saline lake derived *Penicillium* sp. *Phytochem. Lett.* **2015**, *11*, 168–172. [CrossRef]
37. Fan, Z.; Sun, Z.-H.; Liu, Z.; Chen, Y.-C.; Liu, H.-X.; Li, H.-H.; Zhang, W.-M. Dichotocejpins A–C: New diketopiperazines from a deep-sea-derived fungus *Dichotomomyces cejpii* FS110. *Mar. Drugs* **2016**, *14*, 164. [CrossRef]
38. Li, Y.; Ye, D.; Shao, Z.; Cui, C.; Che, Y. A sterol and spiroditerpenoids from a *Penicillium* sp. isolated from a deep sea sediment sample. *Mar. Drugs* **2012**, *10*, 497–508. [CrossRef]
39. Li, X.-D.; Li, X.-M.; Li, X.; Xu, G.-M.; Liu, Y.; Wang, B.-G. Aspewentins D–H, 20-nor-isopimarane derivatives from the deep sea sediment-derived fungus *Aspergillus wentii* SD-310. *J. Nat. Prod.* **2016**, *79*, 1347–1353. [CrossRef]
40. Wu, G.; Lin, A.; Gu, Q.; Zhu, T.; Li, D. Four new chloro-eremophilane sesquiterpenes from an Antarctic deep-sea derived fungus, *Penicillium* sp. PR19N-1. *Mar. Drugs* **2013**, *11*, 1399–1408. [CrossRef]
41. Lin, A.; Wu, G.; Gu, Q.; Zhu, T.; Li, D. New eremophilane-type sesquiterpenes from an antarctic deep-sea derived fungus, *Penicillium* sp. PR19 N-1. *Arch. Pharm. Res.* **2014**, *37*, 839–844. [CrossRef]
42. Zhou, Y.; Li, Y.-H.; Yu, H.-B.; Liu, X.-Y.; Lu, X.-L.; Jiao, B.-H. Furanone derivative and sesquiterpene from antarctic marine-derived fungus *Penicillium* sp. S-1-18. *J. Asian Nat. Prod. Res.* **2018**, *20*, 1108–1115. [CrossRef] [PubMed]
43. Li, X.-D.; Li, X.; Li, X.-M.; Xu, G.-M.; Zhang, P.; Meng, L.-H.; Wang, B.-G. Tetranorlabdane diterpenoids from the deep sea sediment-derived fungus *Aspergillus wentii* SD-310. *Planta Med.* **2016**, *82*, 877–881. [CrossRef] [PubMed]
44. Li, X.; Li, X.-M.; Li, X.-D.; Xu, G.-M.; Liu, Y.; Wang, B.-G. 20-Nor-isopimarane cycloethers from the deep-sea sediment-derived fungus *Aspergillus wentii* SD-310. *RSC Adv.* **2016**, *6*, 75981–75987. [CrossRef]
45. Fang, W.; Lin, X.; Zhou, X.; Wan, J.; Lu, X.; Yang, B.; Ai, W.; Lin, J.; Zhang, T.; Tu, Z. Cytotoxic and antiviral nitrobenzoyl sesquiterpenoids from the marine-derived fungus *Aspergillus ochraceus* Jcma1F17. *MedChemComm* **2014**, *5*, 701–705. [CrossRef]
46. Niu, S.; Fan, Z.-W.; Xie, C.-L.; Liu, Q.; Luo, Z.-H.; Liu, G.; Yang, X.-W. Spirograterpene A, a tetracyclic spiro-diterpene with a fused 5/5/5/5 ring system from the deep-sea-derived fungus *Penicillium granulatum* MCCC 3A00475. *J. Nat. Prod.* **2017**, *80*, 2174–2177. [CrossRef]
47. Chung, Y.-M.; Wei, C.-K.; Chuang, D.-W.; El-Shazly, M.; Hsieh, C.-T.; Asai, T.; Oshima, Y.; Hsieh, T.-J.; Hwang, T.-L.; Wu, Y.-C. An epigenetic modifier enhances the production of anti-diabetic and anti-inflammatory sesquiterpenoids from *Aspergillus sydowii*. *Bioorg. Med. Chem.* **2013**, *21*, 3866–3872. [CrossRef]
48. Li, C.-S.; Li, X.-M.; Gao, S.-S.; Lu, Y.-H.; Wang, B.-G. Cytotoxic anthranilic acid derivatives from deep sea sediment-derived fungus *Penicillium paneum* SD-44. *Mar. Drugs* **2013**, *11*, 3068–3076. [CrossRef]
49. Chen, L.; Gong, M.-W.; Peng, Z.-F.; Zhou, T.; Ying, M.-G.; Zheng, Q.-H.; Liu, Q.-Y.; Zhang, Q.-Q. The marine fungal metabolite, dicitrinone B, induces A375 cell apoptosis through the ROS-related caspase pathway. *Mar. Drugs* **2014**, *12*, 1939–1958. [CrossRef]
50. Pan, C.; Shi, Y.; Chen, X.; Chen, C.-T.A.; Tao, X.; Wu, B. New compounds from a hydrothermal vent crab-associated fungus *Aspergillus versicolor* XZ-4. *Org. Biomol. Chem.* **2017**, *15*, 1155–1163. [CrossRef]
51. Xu, R.; Xu, G.-M.; Li, X.-M.; Li, C.-S.; Wang, B.-G. Characterization of a newly isolated marine fungus *Aspergillus dimorphicus* for optimized production of the anti-tumor agent wentilactones. *Mar. Drugs* **2015**, *13*, 7040–7054. [CrossRef]

marine drugs

MDPI

Review

Halophiles and Their Biomolecules: Recent Advances and Future Applications in Biomedicine

Paulina Corral [1,2], Mohammad A. Amoozegar [3] and Antonio Ventosa [2,*]

1 Department of Biology, University of Naples Federico II, 80126 Naples, Italy; pcv@us.es
2 Department of Microbiology and Parasitology, Faculty of Pharmacy, University of Sevilla, 41012 Sevilla, Spain
3 Department of Microbiology, School of Biology, College of Science, University of Tehran, Tehran 14155-6955, Iran; amoozegar@ut.ac.ir
* Correspondence: ventosa@us.es; Tel.: +34-954556765

Received: 30 November 2019; Accepted: 28 December 2019; Published: 30 December 2019

Abstract: The organisms thriving under extreme conditions better than any other organism living on Earth, fascinate by their hostile growing parameters, physiological features, and their production of valuable bioactive metabolites. This is the case of microorganisms (bacteria, archaea, and fungi) that grow optimally at high salinities and are able to produce biomolecules of pharmaceutical interest for therapeutic applications. As along as the microbiota is being approached by massive sequencing, novel insights are revealing the environmental conditions on which the compounds are produced in the microbial community without more stress than sharing the same substratum with their peers, the salt. In this review are reported the molecules described and produced by halophilic microorganisms with a spectrum of action in vitro: antimicrobial and anticancer. The action mechanisms of these molecules, the urgent need to introduce alternative lead compounds and the current aspects on the exploitation and its limitations are discussed.

Keywords: halophilic bacteria; archaea and fungi; biomolecules; biomedicine; antimicrobial compounds; anticancer compounds

1. Halophilic Microorganisms

Halophiles are organisms represented by archaea, bacteria, and eukarya for which the main characteristic is their salinity requirement, halophilic "salt-loving". Halophilic microorganisms constitute the natural microbial communities of hypersaline ecosystems, which are widely distributed around the world [1]. They require sodium ions for their growth and metabolism. Thus, based on the NaCl optimal requirement for growth the halophiles are classified in three different categories: slight (1–3%); moderate (3–15%); and extreme (15–30%) [2,3]. In contrast to halotolerant organisms, obligate halophiles require NaCl concentrations higher than 3% NaCl or above of seawater, with about 3.5% NaCl [4]. The tolerance parameters and salt requirements are dependent on temperature, pH, and growth medium. In this way, the halophiles are adapted and limited by specific environmental factors. Those microorganisms able to survive and optimally thrive under a wide spectrum of extreme environmental factors are designed polyextremophiles [5,6]. In fact, a halophilic microorganism can also be alkaliphile, designated as haloalkaliphile, growing optimally or very well at pH values above 9.0, but cannot grow at the near neutral pH value of 6.5 [7].

The general features of halophilic microorganisms are the low nutritional requirements and resistance to high concentrations of salt with the capacity to balance the osmotic pressure of the environment [8]. Their mechanisms of haloadaptation are based on the intracellular storage of KCl over 37% (5 M) (salt-in strategy) or the accumulation of compatible solutes (salt-out strategy) to keep the balance of sodium into the cytoplasm and counteract the osmotic pressure of the external environment given by the high salinity [9].

They are physiologically diverse; mostly aerobic and as well anaerobic, heterotrophic, phototrophic, and chemoautotrophic [10,11]. Ecologically, the halophilic microorganisms inhabit different ecosystems characterized by a salinity higher than seawater, i.e., 3.5% NaCl, these niches go from hypersaline soils, springs, salt lakes, sabkhas, and other naturally-occurring coastal saline habitats, marshes, marine abyssal sediments to endophytes [12]. Other known habitats are the result of human intervention like salted foods, brines, oil fields, saltern ponds and tanneries [13]. The high salinity reduces the number of organisms where just halophilic or halotolerant ones can survive in such hypersaline ecosystem, with archaea typically dominating the higher salinity environments. The predominant natural habitats better studied are the hypersaline lakes of oceanic (thalassohaline) or non-oceanic (athalassohaline) origin and solar salterns [14–16]. The better known hypersaline environments are the Great Salt Lake and the Dead Sea, with pH values around 7, and soda lakes with highly alkaline values of pH 9–11, among them are the Lake Magadi in Kenya, the Wadi Natrun lakes in Egypt, Mono Lake, Big Soda Lake, Soap Lake in Western USA, and Kulunda Steppe soda lakes in Russia [17]. Many new species of bacteria and archaea have been reported from various hypersaline regions located in different countries, mainly China, Spain, USA, Austria, Australia, Egypt, Korea, Japan, Iran, Thailand, Indonesia, Russia, Argentina, Kenya, Mexico, France, Poland, Philippines, Taiwan, Romania, and India [10,18,19]. The vast majority of halophilic bacteria and archaea produce carotenoid pigments, present in high amount in their membranes. The dense community of halophiles and the algae *Dunaliella*, also producer of carotenoids, are the responsible of the typical pink, red, and purple coloration of the hypersaline environments [20].

2. Biotechnological Importance/Interest of Haloarchaea and Halophilic Bacteria

The exploitation of extremophiles is having special importance in the development of new molecules with potential applications in biomedicine. Current efforts are focused primarily to cover the urgent health needs, especially those that represent the main global threats, cancer and antibiotic resistance. The great metabolic versatility of halophilic microorganisms, their low nutritional requirements and their genetic machineries of adaptation to harsh conditions, like nutrient starvation, desiccation, high sun radiation, and high ionic strength, make them promising candidates and a hope for drug discovery [21]. Continuous advances in "omics" and bioinformatic tools are revealing uncountable encoding genes for the production of several active compound in response to the extreme conditions [22,23]. The concomitant application of cutting-edge technologies is helping to deciphering the molecular, physiological, and metabolic mechanisms for the production of new bioactive compounds [24].

Halophilic microorganisms are recognized producers of carotenoid pigments, retinal proteins, hydrolytic enzymes, and compatible solutes as macromolecules stabilizers, biopolymers, and biofertilizers [19,25]. Halophilic bacteria and extremely halophilic aerobic archaea, also known as haloarchaea, play a significant role in the industry with a large number of applications like fermented food products, cosmetics, preservatives, manufacturing of bioplastics, photoelectric devices, artificial retinas, holograms, biosensors, etc. [26–31].

In this review, we focus on the biomolecules described as antimicrobial or anticancer compounds produced by halophilic bacteria, archaea, or fungi and discuss current and future perspectives in this field.

3. Antimicrobial Compounds

The current situation of antibiotic resistance propagation poses a global threat to public health. Over the past decades, antibiotics have saved millions of lives, but their misuse has led to the emergence of multi-drug resistant bacteria (MDR), reducing or nullifying their effectiveness. Recently, the continuous increase in antibiotic resistance is reaching critical levels, which implies an increase in morbidity in the healthy population and an imminent risk for hospitalized patients [32,33]. In fact, the main cause of death of inpatients are attributable to complications due to MDR infections [34]. Preventing the return to the pre-antibiotic era is one of the main challenges for science. The urgent need to introduce new effective antimicrobial therapies is leading to the exploitation of all possible natural and sustainable resources, including extreme environments as a promising resource for new antibiotic discovery.

The first antimicrobial compounds from halophilic microorganisms were reported in 1982 by Rodriguez-Valera et al. Halocin was the term coined for substances secreted by several members of the genus *Halobacterium* capable of causing death and lysis of the surrounding microbiota. Halocins are the proteins and antimicrobial peptides (AMPs) produced by haloarchaea [35,36]. Despite the ecological and environmental role of several halocins, their action against human pathogens has been less studied.

In the fight against time, the clinical significance of halophilic microorganisms is minorly reported and the antimicrobial action against the most important risk group of human pathogens ESKAPE: *Enterococcus faecium, Staphylococcus aureus, Klebsiella pneumoniae, Acinetobacter baumannii,* and *Pseudomonas aeruginosa,* still remains as a potential.

According to the data inferred, the antagonistic action identified and the production of bioactive compounds by halophilic microorganisms are derived from bacteria, archaea, and fungi. In the chronology of AMPS discovery, several authors have gone beyond the primary screenings deciphering the chemical structure of the molecules in bacteria (Table 1), while the vast majority of inhibitory studies are solely limited to the activity (Table 2).

3.1. Bacteria

Members of the phylum *Actinobacteria* are mainly responsible for the inhibitory activity against human pathogens with clinical significance. As in non-extreme environments, in saline and hypersaline environments heterotrophic bacteria are also present in soils, being *Actinobacteria* frequently isolated from solar salterns, mangroves, and seafloor sediments [37,38]. The most frequent producers of metabolites reported come from species of the genus *Nocardiopsis* and *Streptomyces,* hence constituting the main producers of bioactive compounds. In fact, members of the genus *Streptomyces* are widely recognized as fruitful producers of natural compounds [39]. The chemical elucidation of molecules known from halophilic members of *Nocardiopsis* are: (i) pyrrolo (1,2-A (pyrazine-1,4-dione, hexahydro-3-[2-methylpropyl]-) and Actinomycin C2, two compounds produced by the haloalkaliphilic strain *Nocardiopsis* sp. AJ1, isolated from saline soil of Kovalam solar salterns in India [40]; (ii) Angucyclines and Angucyclinones are produced by *Nocardiopsis* sp. HR-4, isolated from a salt lake soil in Algerian Sahara, the new natural compound was established as 7-deoxy-8-O-methyltetrangomycin, which is also effective against Methicillin-Resistant *Staphylococcus aureus* (MRSA) ATCC 43300 [41]; (iii) Borrelidin C and D are produced by *Nocardiopsis* sp. HYJ128, isolated from topsoil saltern in Jeungdo, Jeollanamdo, Republic of Korea, exhibited antimicrobial action against *Salmonella enterica* ATCC 14028 [42]; (iv) Quinoline alkaloid (4-oxo-1,4-dihydroquinoline-3-carboxamide) was identified as a new natural product from *Nocardiopsis terrae* YIM 90022 isolated from saline soils in China. The antibacterial activity of the quinolone was reported in *S. aureus, B. subtilis* and *E. coli*; the quinolone has also antifungal activity against the pathogenic fungi, as it was observed against *Pyricularia oryzae*. Another five known compounds were also produced by *N. terrae* YIM 90022 [43]; (v) new p-terphenyls: p-terphenyl 1 and a novel p-terphenyl derivative bearing a benzothiazole moiety are produced by halophilic actinomycete *Nocardiopsis gilva* YIM 90087, isolated from a hypersaline soil Xinjiang, China. Furthermore, of the antimicrobial activity against clinical strains, these compounds exhibit antifungal activity against species of *Fusarium, Trichophyton, Aspergillus, Candida,* and *Pyricularia*. Known molecules like p-terphenyl 2, novobiocin, cyclodipeptides, and aromatic acids are also produced by *N. gilva* YIM 90087, which is considered as a new source for novobiocin [44].

Regarding the metabolites produced by members of the genus *Streptomyces*, only a low number of strains has been isolated from hypersaline environments; however, members of this genus are frequently isolated from marine deep or coastal sediments where the salinity is higher than that of seawater. Among the molecules identified are: (i) 1-hydroxy-1-norresistomycin, this quinone-related antibiotic was extracted from *Streptomyces chibaensis* AUBN1/7, isolated from marine sediment samples of the Bay of Bengal, India. This compound exhibited antibacterial activities against Gram-positive and Gram-negative bacteria, besides of a potent in vitro cytotoxic activity against cell lines HMO2 (gastric adenocarcinoma) and HePG2 (hepatic carcinoma) [45]; (ii) Himalomycin A and Himalomycin B, two new anthracycline antibiotics produced by *Streptomyces* sp. strain B692, isolated from sandy sediment of a coastal site of Mauritius (Indian Ocean). In addition, known metabolites like rabelomycin, fridamycin D, N benzylacetamide, and N-(2′-phenylethyl) acetamide were also produced by *Streptomyces* sp. strain B692 [46]; (iii) 7-demethoxy rapamycin was produced by a moderately halophilic strain *Streptomyces hygroscopicus* BDUS 49, isolated from seashore of Bigeum Island, South West coast of South Korea; the molecule displayed a broad spectrum antimicrobial activity against Gram-positive and Gram-negative bacteria. Antifungal and cytotoxic action was also identified on this strain [47]; (iv) Streptomonomicin (STM) is an antibiotic lasso peptide from *Streptomonospora alba* YIM 90003, isolated from a soil sample in Xinjiang province, China. STM is active against several Gram-positive bacteria, in particular species of *Bacillus, Listeria, Enterococcus, Mycobacterium* and *Staphylococcus*. Despite that STM has an inhibitory action against a wide panel of Gram-positive pathogens, the activity against fungi and Gram-negative bacteria was not evidenced [48].

In addition to the mentioned genera of *Actinobacteria* (*Nocardiopsis* and *Streptomyces*), recognized as the more prolific producers of natural substances, other halophilic species belonging to different genera have also been described as producers of molecules like: (i) cyclic antimicrobial lipopeptides: Gramicidin S and four cyclic dipeptides (CDPs), named cyclo(L-4-OH-Pro-L-Leu), cyclo(L-Tyr-L-Pro), cyclo(L-Phe-L-Pro), and cyclo(L-Leu-L-Pro), were extracted from *Paludifilum halophilum* strain SMBg3, which constitute a new genus of the family *Thermoactinomycetaceae*, isolated from superficial sediment collected from Sfax marine solar saltern in Tunisia. These CDPs possess an inhibitory effect against the plant pathogen *Agrobacterium tumefaciens* and the human pathogens *Staphylococcus aureus, Salmonella enterica, Escherichia coli,* and *Pseudomonas aeruginosa* [49]; (ii) A semi synthetic derivative N-(4-aminocyclooctyl)-3,5-dinitrobenzamide, obtained from the precursor of the novel natural product cyclooctane-1,4-diamine and a known compound 3-([1H-indol-6-yl] methyl) hexahydropyrrolo [1,2-a] pyrazine-1,4-dione were obtained from *Pseudonocardia endophytica* VUK-10, isolated from sediment of Nizampatnam mangrove ecosystem in Bay of Bengal, India. The new compound, semi synthetic derivative N-(4-aminocyclooctyl)-3,5-dinitrobenzamide showed a strong antimicrobial and antifungal activity against *Streptococcus mutans, Pseudomonas aeruginosa, Candida albicans,* and *Aspergillus niger*. Significant anticancer activities at nanomolar concentrations were also observed in carcinoma cell lines MDA-MB-231 (breast), HeLa (cervical), OAW-42 (ovarian), and MCF-7 (breast) reported as resistant to cancer drugs [50]. In minor grade, other halophilic bacteria not belonging to the phylum *Actinobacteria* produce antimicrobial compounds, as for example halophilic strains of the genus *Vibrio*, like *Vibrio* sp. A1SM3-36-8, isolated from Colombian solar salterns, which produces 13-cis-docosenamide with special antimicrobial action against Methicillin-resistant *Staphylococcus aureus* (MRSA) and cytotoxic activity against cervical adenocarcinoma (SiHa) and lung carcinoma (A-549) [51]. Within this genus, *Vibrio parahaemolyticus* strain B2 is recognized by producing Vibrindole A, and was also effective against *Staphylococcus aureus* [52].

Finally, *Bacillus* sp. BS3 [53] and *Halomonas salifodinae* MPM-TC [54] showed antimicrobial action against *Pseudomonas aeruginosa*. Both strains were isolated from solar salterns in Thamaraikulam, Tamil Nadu, India. In the case of *Halomonas salifodinae* MPM-TC, besides of the inhibition of bacterial growth also exhibits an antiviral action against the White Spot Syndrome Virus (WSSV) in the white shrimp *Fenneropenaeus indicus*. The effect suppressor of the virus and the boosting of immune system of the shrimps make of the extracted compound a feasible alternative to commercially banned antibiotics and excellent candidate to develop new antiviral drugs against shrimp viruses such as WSSV.

A genome-mining study conducted on 2699 genomes across the three domains of life demonstrated the widespread distribution of non-ribosomal peptide synthetase (NRPSs) and modular polyketide synthase (PKSs) biosynthetic pathways. Among 31 phyla of bacteria inferred, *Actinobacteria* is the most representative exhibiting the presence of 1225 gene clusters between NRPS, PKS and hybrids from a total of the 271 genomes studied. It was observed that *Salinispora arenicola* CNS-205 and *Salinispora tropica* CNB-440 harbor PKS and NRPS gene clusters, respectively. The halophilic bacterium *Halomonas elongata* DSM 2581 also contains NPRS [55].

Table 1. Chronological report of halophilic bacteria and their molecules with antimicrobial activity in vitro against human pathogens.

Isolation Source	Genus	Antimicrobial Activity	Molecule	Formula	Reference
Saline soil of Kovalam solar salterns India	*Nocardiopsis* sp. AJ1	*E. coli*, *S. aureus*, *P. aeruginosa*, *V. parahaemolyticus*, *A. hydrophila*	Pyrrolo (1,2-A (pyrazine-1,4-dione, hexahydro-3-(2-methylpropyl)-)	$C_{11}H_{18}N_2O_2$	[40]
			Actinomycin C2	$C_{63}H_{88}N_{12}O_{16}$	
Sfax solar saltern, Tunisia	*Paludifilum halophilum* SMBg3	*E. coli* BW25113, *S. henoxaz* ATCC43972, *P. aeruginosa* ATCC 49189 Gram-positive *M. luteus* LB 14110, *S. aureus* ATCC6538, and *L. ivanovii* BUG 496)	Cyclic lipopeptide:		[49]
			Gramicidin S	$C_{60}H_{92}N_{12}O_{10}$	
			Cyclic dipeptides (CDPs):		
			Cyclo(L-4-OH-Pro-L-Leu)	$C_{11}H_{18}N_2O_3$	
			Cyclo(L-Tyr-L-Pro)	$C_{14}H_{16}N_2O_3$	
			Cyclo(L-Phe-L-Pro)	$C_{14}H_{16}N_2O_2$	
			Cyclo(L-Leu-L-Pro)	$C_{11}H_{18}N_2O_2$	
Brine and sediments from Manaure solar saltern. La Guajira, Colombia	*Vibrio* sp. A1SM3–36-8	Methicillin-resistant *S. aureus* (MRSA) ATCC BAA-44, *B. subtilis* ATCC 21556	13-*cis*-docosenamide	$C_{22}H_{43}NO$	[51]
Salt lake soil, Algerian Sahara. Algeria	*Nocardiopsis* sp. HR-4	*S. aureus* ATCC 25923, Methicillin-Resistant *S. aureus* (MRSA) ATCC 43300, *M. luteus* ATCC 4698, *E. faecalis* ATCC 29212	Angucyclines and angucyclinones:		[41]
			Compound **1**: (−)-8-*O*-methyltetrangomycin	$C_{20}H_{16}O_5$	
			Compound **2**: (−)-7-deoxy-8-*O* methyltetrangomycin	$C_{20}H_{18}O_5$	
Topsoil saltern in Jeungdo, Jeollanam-do, Republic of Korea	*Nocardiopsis* sp. HYJ128	*Salmonella enterica* ATCC 14028	Borrelidin C	$C_{28}H_{43}NO_7$	[42]
			Borrelidin D	$C_{28}H_{43}NO_7$	
Sediments of mangrove Nizampatnam, Bay of Bengal, Andhra Pradesh, India	*Pseudonocardia endophytica* VUK-10	*B. cereus* (MTCC 430), *S. mutans* (MTCC 497), *S. aureus* (MTCC 3160), *S. epidermis* (MTCC 120), *B. subtilis* (ATCC 6633), *B. megaterium* (NCIM 2187), *E. coli* (ATCC 35218), *P. aeruginosa* (ATCC 9027), *P. vulgaris* (MTCC 7299), *S. marcescens* (MTCC 118), *X. campestris* (MTCC 2286), *X. malvacearum* (NCIM 2954) and *S. typhi* (ATCC 14028)	*N*-(4-aminocyclooctyl)-3,5-dinitrobenzamide	$C_{15}H_{20}N_4O_5$	[50]
			3-((1H-indol-6-yl) methyl) hexahydropyrrolo [1,2-a] pyrazine-1,4-dione	$C_{16}H_{17}N_3O_2$	

Table 1. *Cont.*

Isolation Source	Genus	Antimicrobial Activity	Molecule	Formula	Reference
Soil sample, Xinjiang Province, China	*Streptomonospora alba* YIM 90003	*B. anthracis*, *B. halodurans*, *B. cereus* ATCC 4342, ATCC 13472, *B. subtilis*, *L. monocytogenes*, *E. faecalis*, *S. aureus* and *M. smegmatis*	Streptomonomicin (STM)	$C_{107}H_{160}N_{22}O_{30}$	[48]
Great Barrier Reef (GBR) sponges, Queensland, Australia	*Salinisporaarenicola*	*M. avium*, *M. leprae*, *M. lepromatosis*, *M. tuberculosis*	Rifamycin B	$C_{39}H_{49}NO_{14}$	[56]
			Rifamycin S	$C_{37}H_{45}NO_{12}$	
			Rifamycin W	$C_{35}H_{45}NO_{11}$	
Saline soil, Qaidam Basin, north-west China	*Nocardiopsis terrae* YIM 90022	*S. aureus*, *E. coli* and *B. subtilis*	Quinoloid alkaloid 4-oxo-1,4-dihydroquinoline-3-carboxamide	$C_{10}H_7N_2O_2$	[43]
			p-hydroxybenzoic acid	$C_7H_6O_3$	
			N-acetyl-anthranilic acid	C_9H_9NO	
			Indole-3-carboxylic acid	$C_9H_7NO_2$	
			Cyclo (Trp-Gly)	$C_{13}H_{13}N_3O_2$	
			Cyclo (Leu-Ala)	$C_9H_{16}N_2O_2$	
Condenser water, solar salt works in Thamaraikulam, Kanyakumari district, Tamil Nadu, India	*Bacillus* sp. BS3	*E. coli*, *S. aureus*, *P. aeruginosa* and *S. typhi*	Lipopeptide biosurfactants		[53]
			13-Docosenamide, (Z)	$CH_3(CH_2)_7CH{=}CH(CH_2)_{11}CONH_2$	
			Mannosamine	$C_6H_{13}NO_5.HCl$	
			9-Octadecenamide, (Z)	$C_{18}H_{35}NO$	
			2-Octanol, 2-methyl-6-methylene	$C_{12}H_{22}O_2$	
			Cylohex-1,4,5-triol-3-one-1-carbo	$C_5H_8FN_3$	
			2-Butanamine, 2-methyl-	$C_5H_{13}N$	
			1,2-Ethanediamine, *N,N,N′,N′*-tetramethyl-	$C_6H_{16}N_2$	
Hypersaline soil, Xinjiang, China	*Nocardiopsis gilva* YIM 90087	*B. subtilis*, *S. aureus*	*p*-Terphenyl: 6′-Hydroxy-4,2′,3′,4′′-tetramethoxy-p-terphenyl	$C_{22}H_{22}O_5$	[44]
			p-Terphenyl derivative: 4,7-bis(4-methoxyphenyl)-6-hydroxy-5-methoxybenzo[d]thiazole	$C_{22}H_{19}NO_4S$	

Table 1. *Cont.*

Isolation Source	Genus	Antimicrobial Activity	Molecule	Formula	Reference
Solar salt condenser, Thamaraikulam solar saltern, Kanyakumari district, Tamil Nadu, India	*Halomonas salifodinae* MPM-TC	*V. harveyi*, *V. parahaemolyticus*, *P. aeruginosa* and *A. hydrophila*	Perfluorotributylamine	$C_{12}F_{27}N$	[54]
			Cyclopentane, 1-butyl-2-ethyl-	$C_{11}H_{22}$	
			1,1′-Biphenyl]-3-amine	$C_{12}H_{11}N$	
			Pyridine, 4-(phenylmethyl)-	$C_{12}H_{11}N$	
			Hexadecane, 2-methyl-	$C_{17}H_{36}$	
			Nonadecane	$C_{19}H_{40}$	
			Phytol	$C_{20}H_{40}O$	
Seashore soil, Bigeum Island, South West coast of South Korea	*Streptomyces hygroscopicus* BDUS 49	*B. subtilis*, *S. aureus*, *E. coli*, *S. typhi*	7-Demethoxy rapamycin	$C_{50}H_{75}NO_{12}$	[47]
Marine sediment of Mission Bay, San Diego, South California	*Marinispora* sp. NPS12745	*S. aureus* ATCC 29213-MSSA, *S. aureus* ATCC 43300-MRSA, *S. epidermidis* ATCC 700578, *S. epidermidis* ATCC 700582, *S. pneumoniae* ATCC 49619-Penicillin sensitive, *S. pneumoniae* ATCC 51915-Penicillin resistant, *E. faecalis* ATCC 29212-Vancomycin sensitive, *E. faecium* ATCC 700221-Vancomycin resistant, *Haemophilus influenzae* ATCC 49247, *Haemophilus influenzae* ATCC 49766 *E. coli* permeable mutant	Chlorinated bisindole pirroles:		[57]
			Lynamicin A	$C_{22}H_{16}N_3O_2Cl_2$	
			Lynamicin B	$C_{22}H_{14}N_3O_2Cl_3Na$	
			Lynamicin C	$C_{20}H_{12}N_3Cl_4$	
			Lynamicin D	$C_{24}H_{18}N_3O_4Cl_2$	
			Lynamicin E	$C_{24}H_{19}N_3O_4Cl$	
Platinum Coast on the Mediterranean Sea, north of Egypt	*Streptomyces* sp. Merv8102	*E. coli* ATCC 10536, *P. aeruginosa* ATCC 10145), *B. subtilis* ATCC 6051, *S. aureus* ATCC 6538 and *M. luteus* ATCC 9341	Essramycin Triazolopyrimidine [1,2,4] Triazolo[1,5-a]pyrimidin-7(4H)-one, 5-methyl-2-(2-oxo-2-phenylethyl)-	$C_{14}H_{12}N_4O_2$	[58]
Marine sediment, La Jolla, California	*Streptomyces* sp. CNQ-418	Methicillin-resistant *S. aureus* (MRSA)	Marinopyrroles A	$C_{22}H_{12}Cl_4N_2O_4$	[59]
			Marinopyrroles B	$C_{22}H_{11}BrCl_4N_2O_4$	

Table 1. *Cont.*

Isolation Source	Genus	Antimicrobial Activity	Molecule	Formula	Reference
Sediment of Bay of Bengal, India	*Streptomyces chibaensis* sp. AUBN1/7	*B. subtilis* ATCC 6633, *B. pumilus* ATCC 19164, *S. aureus* ATCC 29213, *E. coli* ATCC 25922, *P. aeruginosa* ATCC 27853 *P. vulgaris* ATCC 6897	1-Hydroxy-1-norresistomycin	$C_{21}H_{14}O_7$	[45]
Sediment of the Lagoon de Terminos at the Gulf of Mexico	*Streptomyces* B8005*Streptomyces* B4842	*E. coli*, *S. aureus*, *S. viridochromogenes*	Resistomycin 1-Hydroxy-1-norresistomycin	$C_{21}H_{14}O_7$	[60]
			Resistoflavin Resistoflavin methyl ether	$C_{23}H_{18}O_7$	
Marine sediment from Scripps Canyon. La Jolla, California, Pacific Coast, United States	*Streptomyces nodosus* NPS007994	Drug-sensitive and drug-resistant Gram-positive reaction bacteria	Lajollamycin Nitro-tetraene Spiro-β-lactone-γ-lactam	$C_{36}H_{53}N_3O_{10}$	[61]
Sediment of Jiaozhou Bay, China	*Actinomadura* sp. M048	*S. aureus*, *B. subtilis*, and *S. viridochromogenes*	Chandrananimycin A Acetamide, *N*-(9-hydroxy-3-oxo-3H-phenoxazin-2-yl)-	$C_{14}H_{10}N_2O_4$	[62]
			Chandrananimycin B Acetamide, 2-hydroxy-*N*-(3-oxo-3H-phenoxazin-2-yl)-	$C_{14}H_{10}N_2O_4$	
			Chandrananimycin C 1-Methoxy-3-methyl-1,2,3,4-tetrahydro-5H-pyrido[3,2-a]phenoxazin-5-one	$C_{17}H_{16}N_2O_3$	
Sandy sediment, coastal site of Mauritius, Indian Ocean	*Streptomyces* sp. B6921	*S. aureus*, *E. coli*, *B. subtilis*, and *S. viridochromogenes*	Fridamycin D	$C_{31}H_{32}O_{12}$	[46]
			Himalomycin A	$C_{43}H_{52}O_{16}$	
			Himalomycin B	$C_{43}H_{56}O_{16}$	
Mucus secreted by the box-fish *Ostracion cubicus*, Israel	*Vibrio parahaemolyticus* B2	*S. aureus*, *S. albus* and *B. subtilis*	Vibrindole A	$C_{18}H_{16}N_2$	[52]

Table 2. Chronological report of bacteria with antimicrobial activity in vitro against human pathogens which molecules have not been chemically identified.

Isolation Source	Genus	Antimicrobial Activity	Reference
Khewra Salt Range, Punjab, Pakistan	*Aquisalibacillus elongatus* MB592, *Salinicoccus sesuvii* MB597, and *Halomonas aquamarina* MB598	*B. subtilis*, *B. pumilus*, *E. faecalis*, *B. cereus*, *K. pneumoniae*, *Alcaligenes faecalis*, *P. geniculata*, *E. faecium*	[63]
Hypersaline soils (solonchaks, solonetz and takyr) from Kostanay, Auliekol and Mendykara. Almaty region, Balkhash, Kazakhstan	*Actinomycetes* spp.	*S. aureus* MRSA, *E. coli* (pMG223)	[64]
Marine water, Gujarat, Western India	*Kocuria* sp. strain rsk4	Antibiotic-resistant *S. aureus*	[65]
Crystallizer pond sediments of Ribandar saltern, Goa, India	*Streptomyces radiopugnans*	*S. typhimurium*, *P. vulgaris*, *E. coli*	[66]
	Streptomyces sporocinereus	*S. typhimurium*, *P. vulgaris*, *E. coli*	
	Kocuria palustris	*S. aureus*	
	Micromonospora sp.	*V. cholerae*	
	Nocardiopsis sp.	*S. citreus*	
Coastal Solar Saltern, India	*Nonomuraea* sp. JAJ18	Methicillin-Resistant *S. aureus* (MRSA), *B. subtilis* MTCC 441, *K. pneumonia* MTCC 109, *S. typhi* MTCC 733, and *P. vulgaris* MTCC 426	[67]
Sediment of estuarine coastal brackish, Chilika Lake, Khurdha Odisha, India	*Streptomyces chilikensis* RC 1830	*E. coli*, *S. aureus*, *B. cereus* and *S. typhi*	[67]
Mangrove sediment of Visakhapatnam, Andhra Pradesh, India	*Streptomyces* sp.	*S. aureus*, *B. subtilis*, *B. cereus*, *E. coli*, *P. aeruginosa*, *P. vulgaris*	[68]
Mangrove sediment, Nizampatnam, Andhra Pradesh, India	*Pseudonocardia* VUK-10	*S. aureus*, *S. mutans*, *B. subtilis*, *E. coli*, *E. faecalis*, *P. aeruginosa*	[69]

Table 2. *Cont.*

Isolation Source	Genus	Antimicrobial Activity	Reference
Salt pans Batim and Ribandar, Goa, India	*Bacillus* spp. *Virgibacillus* spp.	*A. baumanii*, *A. hydrophila*, *Citrobacter diversus*, *Citrobacter freundii*, *E. coli* ATCC 25922, *K. pneumoniae*, *Morganella morganii*, *P. mirabilis*, *P.* ATCC 27855, *P.* spp., *S. paratyphi* A, *S. typhi*, *S. typhimurium*, *S. boydii*, *S. flexneri*, *V. cholerae*, Methicillin Resistant *S. aureus* (MRSA), Methicillin Sensitive *S. aureus* (MSSA), *S. aureus* ATCC 25923, *S. citreus*	[70]
Salt pans, Kodiakarai, Tamil Nadu, India	*Streptoverticillium album*	*S. aureus*, *K. pneumoniae* and *E. coli*	[71]
Nonrhizospheric soil, Saharan regions, south of Algeria	*Actinopolyspora* spp. *A. halophila*, *A. mortivallis*, *A. erythraea*, *A. xinjiangensis*, *A. alba.Nocardiopsis* spp. *N. litoralis*, *N. xinjiangensis* *N. valliformis* and *N. exhalans* *Saccharomonospora* spp. *S. paurometabolica*, *S. halophila* *Streptomonospora* spp. *S. alba*, *S. amylolytica*, *S. flavalba* *Saccharopolyspora* sp.	*B. subtilis*, *S. aureus*, *M. luteus*, *K. pneumoniae*, *L. monocytogenes*	[72]

Table 2. *Cont.*

Isolation Source	Genus	Antimicrobial Activity	Reference
Crystallizer pond, Madurai, India	*Nocardiopsis* sp. JAJ16	*S. aureus*, *B. subtilis*, *S. typhi*, Methicillin-resistant *S. aureus* (MRSA), *K. pneumoniae*, *Enterobacter* sp. and *P. aeruginosa*	[73]
Bay of Bengal coast of Puducherry and Marakkanam, India	*Streptomyces* sp. VITSVK9	*B. subtilis*, *Escherchia coli*, *K. pneumoniae*, *S. aureus* and *S.* species	[74]
Marine sediment of Marakkanam, Bay of Bengal Coast, Tamil Nadu. India	*Saccharopolyspora salina* VITSDK4	*S. aureus* ATCC 25923, *B. subtilis* ATCC 6633, *E. coli* ATCC 25922, *K. pneumoniae* ATCC 10273	[75]
Marakkanam coast of Tamil Nadu, India	*Streptomyces* sp. VITSDK1	*S. aureus* ATCC 25923, *B. subtilis* ATCC 6633, *E. coli* ATCC 25922, *K. pneumoniae* ATCC 10273	[76]
Salt Lake Hami in Xinjiang, China	*Actinomyces* sp.	*B. subtilis*	[77]
Salt lakes of Bay of Bengal, India	*Actinomyces* sp. *Streptomyces* sp.	*P. aeruginosa*, *B. subtilis*, *S. epidermidis*, *E. coli*	[78]
Water samples Asen fjord in the Trondheim fjord and Steinvikholmen, Norway	*Streptomyces* sp.	Gram-negative and Gram-positive bacteria	[79]
Salt Lake Bardawil, Egypt	*Streptomyces viridiviolaceus*	*E. coli*, *Edwardsiella tarda*, *Corynebacterium michiganese* B-33, *P. solanacearum* B-3212 and *Staphilococcus* spp.	[77]

Table 2. *Cont.*

Isolation Source	Genus	Antimicrobial Activity	Reference
Soil from salt pan regions of Cuddalore and Parangipettai (Porto-Novo). Tamil Nadu, India	*Streptomyces* sp., *Saccharomonospora* sp.	*E. coli*, *K. pneumoniae*, *P. aeruginosa*, *V. cholerae*, *S. typhi*, *S. aureus*, and *S. dysenteriae*	[80]
Bismarck and Solomon Sea off the coast of Papua New Guinea	*Micromonospora nigra* DSM 43818, *Micromonospora rhodorangea*, *Micromonospora halophytica* DSM 43171	Multidrug-resistant (MDR) Gram-positive pathogens, vancomycin-resistant enterococci (VRE), and methicillin-resistant *S. aureus* (MRSA)	[81]
Marine sediment, Alibag coast, Maharashtra, India	*Actinopolyspora* spp. AH1, *A.halophila*, *A. mortivallis*, *A. iraqiensis*	*S. aureus*, *S. epidermidis*, *B. subtilis*	[82]

Noted: American Type Culture Collection (ATCC); Deutsche Sammlung von Mikroorganismen und Zellkulturen (DSMZ); Multidrug-resistant (MDR); Microbial Type Culture Collection and Gene Bank (MTCC). Microorganisms: *Acinetobacter (A.): A. baumanii. Aeromonas (A.): A. hydrophila. Alcaligenes (A.): A. faecalis. Bacillus (B.): B. cereus, B. halodurans, B. megaterium, B. pumilus, B. subtilis. Burkholderia (B.): B. metallica. Candida (C.): C. albicans. Citrobacter (C.): C. diversus, C. freundii. Corynebacterium (C.): C. michiganese. Edwardsiella (E.): E. tarda. Enterobacter (E.): E. aerogenes. Enterococcus (E.): E. faecalis, E. faecium*, Vancomycin resistant *Enterococcus faecium (VREF)*, Vancomycin sensitive *Enterococcus faecalis (VSEF)*, Vancomycin resistant enterococci (*VRE*). *Escherichia (E.): E. coli. Haemophilus (H.): H. influenzae. Klebsiella (K.): K. pneumonia. Listeria (L.): L. ivanovii, L. monocytogenes. Micrococcus (M.): M. luteus. Morganella (M.): M. morganii. Mycobacterium (M.): M. avium, M. leprae, M. lepromatosis, M. smegmatis, M. tuberculosis. Proteus (P.): P. mirabilis, P. vulgaris. Pseudomonas (P.): P. aeruginosa, P. geniculata, P. solanacearum. Salmonella (S.): S. henoxaz, S. paratyphi, S. typhi, S. typhimurium. Serratia (S.): S. marcescens. Shigella (S.): S. boydii, S. dysenteriae, S. flexneri. Staphylococcus (S.): S. aureus, S. citreus, S. epidermidis*, Antibiotic-resistant *Staphylococcus aureus (ARSA)*, Methicillin Sensitive *Staphylococcus aureus (MSSA)*, Methicillin-resistant *Staphylococcus aureus (MRSA). Streptococcus (S.): S. mutans, S. pneumoniae*, Penicillin resistant *Streptococcus pneumoniae (PRSP)*, Penicillin sensitive *Streptococcus pneumoniae (SPPS). Streptomyces (S.): S. viridochromogenes. Vibrio (V.): V. cholerae, V. harveyi, V. parahaemolyticus. Xanthomonas (X.): X. campestris, X. malvacearum.*

The biotechnological potential of halophilic bacteria, especially for antimicrobial exploitation, still remains in progress, in spite that the occurrence of new several groups of microorganisms is high, the rate of discovery of new biomolecules is low compared with non-halophilic bacteria. Despite periodic descriptions of new species and attempts to culture hidden microbiota, there are no significant studies focused on the discovery of new bioactive metabolites produced by microorganisms from hypersaline ecosystems. The genome-guided studies are currently the best support to take novel strategies in drug discovery. All the antimicrobial compounds described herein derived from halophilic bacteria in which the molecule has been elucidated are summarized in Table 1 and the strains capable of inhibiting pathogens in primary tests whose molecules are unknown are shown in Table 2.

3.2. *Archaea*

Since the discovery of halocins and their action against the surrounding microbiota in their habitats [35] no new or known antimicrobial compounds derived from archaea capable of inhibiting human pathogens have been reported in the literature to date. At an ecological level, the role of archaeocins in microbial communities is the interspecies competition, the antimicrobial activity of halocins suggests that its function is to dominate a given niche occupied by microorganisms having similar adaptations and nutritional requirements [83–85]. Members of *Halorubrum* and *Haloferax* have been identified as the preponderant halocin-producing genera, the cross-domanin antimicrobial action was observed against bacterial members of the genera *Halomonas*, *Rhodovibrio*, *Salisaeta*, or *Pontibacillus*, all isolated from hypersaline samples [86].

To understand the current situation, it is necessary that a comprehensive analysis of the possible reasons why haloarchaea are under-explored at the biotechnological level and why the antimicrobial exploitation is scarce in comparison with other microorganisms prevenient of non-halophilic environments. The first limitation found is the cultivation time of haloarchaea, observed at around 5 to 30 days to yield colonies or cellular density in broth cultures [12]. Once the cultivation is reached, the upcoming drawback is the evaluation of the inhibitory capacity of haloarchaea against a panel of human pathogens. The main obstacle to overcome is when the primary screening (isolate vs. pathogen) is performed due to the high salinity requirements of haloarchaea to grow, greater than 20% of NaCl until saturation, while in halophilic bacteria the screening can be adapted at lower range of salinity, under 15% of NaCl.

Tests such a direct spot-inoculation of the supernatant, diffusion discs, and cross-streak require the adaptation of an appropriate protocol. Finding the same and suitable conditions to test both microorganisms drive to set-up alternative technical procedures, like dual-media and crude extracts for testing those strains growing above the seawater salinity, ca. 3.5 % [87]. Another possible reason is that the study of extremophilic microbiota has been approached at an ecological level and the vast biotechnological exploitation of these extremophiles is more recognized on their enzymes and compatible solutes. The low metabolic requirements, the hypersaline conditions where they thrive, or the low competition for nutrients with their peers determine their behavior, i.e., the production of halocins, which action is limited to the closest members inhabiting in the same environment [88,89]. This could explain that the production of antimicrobials against the non-halophilic community of microorganisms seems to be unnecessary.

Constituted as a powerful tool, "omics" approaches as metagenomics and genomics effectively support ecological and bioprospecting studies deciphering new insights into halophilic microorganisms [90–92]. Extremely rare is the interdomain horizontal gene transfer (IHGT) across bacteria, archaea, and fungi of homologous DNA. However, a genomic-guided study revealed for the first time a potent antibacterial gene encoding a glycosyl hydrolase 25 muramidases (GH25-muramidase) identified in archaea after co-cultivation with a bacterial competitor [93]. In the genome-mining study conducted by Wang et al. (2014), an atlas of nonribosomal peptide synthetase (NRPSs) and modular polyketide synthase (PKSs) gene clusters was built based on 2699 genomes of bacteria, archaea, and fungi. In this study, were included 25 members of *Halobacteria: Haloarcula hispanica* ATCC 33960,

Halalkalicoccus jeotgali B3, *Haloarcula marismortui* ATCC 43049, *Halobacterium* sp. NRC-1, *Halobacterium salinarum* R1, *Haloferax mediterranei* ATCC 33500, *Haloferax volcanii* DS2, *Halogeometricum borinquense* DSM 11551, *Halomicrobium mukohataei* DSM 12286, *Halopiger xanaduensis* SH-6, *Haloquadratum walsbyi* C23, *Haloquadratum walsbyi* DSM 16790, *Halorhabdus tiamatea* SARL4B, *Halorhabdus utahensis* DSM 12940, *Halorubrum lacusprofundi* ATCC 49239, *Haloterrigena turkmenica* DSM 5511, *Halovivax ruber* XH-70, *Natrialba magadii* ATCC 43099, *Natrinema* sp. J7-2, *Natrinema pellirubrum* DSM 15624, *Natronobacterium gregoryi* SP2, *Natronococcus occultus* SP4, *Natronomonas moolapensis* 8.8.11, *Natronomonas pharaonis* DSM 2160, *Salinarchaeum* sp. Harcht-Bsk1. Of a total of 3339 cataloged gene clusters, no PKS, NPKS or hybrid in *Halobacteria* were reported. Within the studied archaea, only two and one NRPS were identified in *Methanobacteria* and *Methanomicrobia*, respectively [55]. Despite these results and considering that the class *Halobacteria* is wide represented with seven families, these results do not exclude the biosynthetic capacity of nonribosomal peptide and polyketide, and nor discourage the biotechnological interest of haloarchaea for future natural product discovery.

3.3. Fungi

Along the years of research on natural products, fungi represent the basis of antimicrobial discovery. Halotolerant and halophilic fungal communities that inhabit the natural hypersaline environments are not strictly salt requiring, as they can grow and adjust to the whole salinity range, from freshwater to almost saturated NaCl solutions [94,95]. Despite this versatility, the vast majority of antimicrobial molecules from halophilic fungi have been produced under low or moderate salinity conditions since the primary screenings against SKAPE microorganisms are easier without NaCl. The mycobiota of hypersaline environments is dominated by members of *Aspergillus*, *Penicillium*, and other genera, such as *Alternaria*, *Cladosporium*, *Fusarium*, *Debaryomyces*, *Scopulariopsis*, *Chaetomium*, *Wallemia*, and *Hortaea*, which are well represented in ecological and biodiversity studies [96,97]. The species *Gymnoascus halophilus*, *Aspergillus penicillioides*, *Hortaea werneckii*, *Phaeotheca triangularis*, *Aureobasidium pullulans*, *Trimmatostroma salinum*, and some species of the genus *Wallemia*, like *W. ichthyophaga*, are recognized as obligately halophilic, or require high levels of salt above that of seawater [98,99]. However, antimicrobial compounds have not been reported from these species.

The halophilic species of the genus *Aspergillus* are the most prolific and several strains of *Aspergillus* sp. have been isolated from Arctic sub-sea sediments from the Barents Sea (Table 3). In particular, strain 8Na identified as *A. protuberus*, a polyextremophilic fungus able to grow in a wide range of pH, temperature and salinity (up to 25% (*w/v*)) showed an antimicrobial efficacy against human pathogens. The strongest power inhibitory action was observed against *Staphylococcus aureus*. The molecule responsible of the activity was identified as Bisvertinolone, a compound member of the family Sorbicillinoid [87]. *Aspergillus flocculosus* PT05-1 and *Aspergillus terreus* PT06-2, both isolated from sediment of Putian sea saltern of Fujian, China, showed antimicrobial activity against *Enterobacter aerogenes*, *Pseudomonas aeruginosa*, and *Candida albicans*. Strain PT05-1 produces 11 metabolites among which two are new ergosteroids and pyrrole derivative compounds [100], and strain PT06-2 produces the novel compounds: Terrelactone A and Terremides A and B [101]. Other strains of the genus *Aspergillus*, like *A. terreus* Tsp22 [101–103], *A. flavus*, *A. gracilis*, and *A. penicillioids* [102] have antibacterial and antioxidant activities in crude extracts but the molecule has not been identified. In the atlas of Wang et al. (2014), 360 fungi were genome-mined cataloguing a total of 307 gene clusters from 30 strains of the phylum *Ascomycota*. Within this group, strains of the genus *Aspergillus*: *A. nidulans* FGSC A4, *A. fumigatus*, *A. niger* CBS 513 88, and *A. oryzae* RIB40 harbor NRPSs, PKSs and hybrids gene clusters [55]. These results confirm that the genus *Aspergillus* is among the most prolific producers of antimicrobial metabolites. In spite of the prosperous production of compounds from fungi, the active molecules derived from extremely halophilic fungi are still scarce (Table 3). It is highly probable that through genome-driven studies in halophilic fungi, NRPSs and PKSs are substantially present as their peers providing new insights into the fungal biosynthetic pathways.

Table 3. Halophilic fungi showing antimicrobial activity.

Isolation Source	Species	Antimicrobial Activity	Molecule	Formula	Reference
Abyssal marine sediment. Barents Sea. Arctic Ocean	*Aspergillus protuberus* MUT 3638	*S. aureus*, *K. pneumoniae*, *A. baumanii* and *B. metallica*	Bisvertinolone	$C_{28}H_{33}O_9$	[87]
Solar saltern, Phetchaburi, Thailand	*Aspergillus flavus*, *Aspergillus gracilis*, and *Aspergillus penicillioids*	Antibacterial and antioxidant	Crude extracellular compounds	NR	[102]
Putian saltern of Fujian, China	*Aspergillus flocculosus* PT05-1	*E. aerogenes*, *P. aeruginosa*, and *C. albicans*	Ergosteroids: (22*R*,23*S*)-epoxy-3b,11a,14b,16b-tetrahydr-oxyergosta-5,7-dien-12-one	$C_{28}H_{42}O_6$	[100]
			Pyrrole derivates: 6-(1H-pyrrol-2-yl) hexa-1,3,5-trienyl-4-methoxy-2H-pyran-2-one	$C_{16}H_{15}NO_3$	
Putian saltern of Fujian, China	*Aspergillus terreus* PT06-2	*E. aerogenes*, *P. aeruginosa*, and *C. albicans*	Terremide A	$C_{21}H_{17}N_3O_5$	[101]
			Terremide B	$C_{21}H_{15}N_3O_4$	
			Terrelactone A	$C_{24}H_{26}O_8$	
Semiarid saltpans in Botwana	*Aspergillus terreus* Tsp22	*B. megaterium* and *S. aureus*	Crude extracellular compounds	NR	[103]

Abbreviations: Not reported (NR). Microorganisms: *Acinetobacter* (*A.*): *A. baumanii. Bacillus* (*B.*): *B. megaterium. Burkholderia* (*B.*): *B. metallica. Candida* (*C.*): *C. albicans. Enterobacter* (*E.*): *E. aerogenes. Escherchia* (*E.*): *E. coli. Haemophilus* (*H.*): *H. influenzae. Klebsiella* (*K.*): *K. pneumonia. Pseudomonas* (*P.*): *P. aeruginosa. Staphylococcus* (*S.*): *S. aureus.*

4. Anticancer Compounds

Natural products are relevant anticancer drugs, which are also called bioactive molecules, produced by organisms. Although, earlier and the well-established anticancer natural products have been obtained from plant cells originally, microorganisms are an excellent alternative, due to the diversity of the microbial world, their easy manipulation, and they can be screened physiologically to discover new natural products with antitumor activity. Although bacterial cells have different communication methods with tumor cells other than metabolites experimentally, bacterial metabolites have been considered the most conventional way against cancer cells viability. Today, more attention is focused on extremophiles as a new source of novel biomolecules [104,105]. Among extremophiles, halophilic and halotolerant microorganisms, which inhabit hypersaline environments, are considered as reliable sources of antitumor metabolites with fewer side effects. In recent years, several studies have been focused on the importance of metabolites from halophilic microorganisms on cancer treatment. The halophilic bacteria, archaea, and fungi involved on the production of anti-cancer biomolecules are summarized in Table 4.

4.1. Bacteria

Since the last two decades, halophilic bacteria have attracted the interests of researchers due to their adaptability to a wide range of salinities. Some studies have been carried out to determine the role of halophilic bacteria in cancer treatment. In one of these studies, Chen et al. (2010) assayed fourteen crude extracts from 45 halophilic bacterial strains and showed cytotoxic activity against human liver cancer cell line Bel 7402 with a half maximal inhibitory concentration (IC_{50}) of 500 µg/mL and five of them showed remarkable activities with IC50 lower than 40 µg/mL [106]. The antineoplastic antibiotic known as tubercidin, was isolated from the halophilic actinobacterium *Actinopolyspora erythraea* YIM 90600, this compound exhibited the capability to stabilize the tumor suppressor Programmed Cell Death Protein 4 (Pdcd4), which is known to antagonize critical events in oncogenic pathways. Tubercidin, significantly inhibited proteasomal degradation of a model Pdcd4-luciferase fusion protein, with an IC_{50} of 0.88 ± 0.09 µM, unveiling a novel biological activity for this well-studied natural product [107].

In two studies on different extracts of halophilic and halotolerant bacteria isolated from brine-seawater interface of the Red Sea, Sagar et al. (2013) tested the cytotoxic and apoptotic activity of their extracts against three human cancer cell lines, including HeLa (cervical carcinoma), MCF-7 (breast adenocarcinoma) and DU145 (prostate carcinoma). In one of their studies, a total of 20 lipophilic (chloroform) and hydrophilic (70% ethanol) extracts from twelve different strains were assessed. Among these, twelve extracts were found to be very active after 24 h of treatment, which were further evaluated for their cytotoxic and apoptotic effects at 48 h. The extracts from the isolates *Halomonas* sp. P1-37B, *Halomonas* sp. P3-37A, and *Sulfitobacter* sp. P1-17B were found to be the most potent against tested cancer cell lines [108]. In the other study, ethyl acetate extracts of 24 strains were assayed and the results showed that most extracts were cytotoxic against one or more cancer cell lines. Out of the thirteen most active microbial extracts, six extracts induced significantly higher apoptosis (>70%) in cancer cells. Molecular studies revealed that extracts from *Chromohalobacter salexigens* strains P3-86A and P3-86B followed the sequence of events of apoptotic pathway involving matrix metalloproteinases (MMP) disruption, Caspase-3/7 activity, Caspase-8 cleavage, polymeric adenosine diphosphate ribose polymerase 1 (PARP-1) cleavage, and phosphatidylserine exposure, whereas the extracts from another *Chromohalobacter salexigens* strain K30 induced Caspase-9 mediated apoptosis. The extracts from *Halomonas meridiana* strain P3-37B and *Idiomarina loihiensis* strain P3-37C were unable to induce any change in MMP in HeLa cancer cells and thus suggested a mitochondria-independent apoptosis induction. However, further detection of a PARP-1 cleavage product and the observed changes in Caspase-8 and Caspase-9 suggested the involvement of caspase-mediated apoptotic pathways [109]. An ethyl acetate extract from *Streptomyces* sp. WH26 showed significant cellular toxicity. Two new compounds, 8-*O*-methyltetrangulol and naphthomycin A, were isolated from this extract via silica gel column chromatography and high-pressure liquid chromatography (HPLC). These two compounds showed potent cytotoxic activity against several human cancer cell lines including A549, HeLa, BEL-7402, and HT-29 [110]. Novel anticancer molecules, Salternamide A–D, were isolated from a halophilic *Streptomyces* sp. isolated from a saltern on Shinui Island, in the Republic of Korea, and exhibited an extensive viability reduction in several cancer cell lines [111]. Among these molecules, Salternamide A inhibited the hypoxia-induced accumulation of HIF-1α in several cancer cell lines and suppressed the HIF-1α by downregulation of its upstream signaling pathways such as PI3K/Akt/mTOR, p42/p44 MAPK, and STAT3. Moreover, in human colorectal cancer cell lines, salternamide A caused cell death by arresting the cells in the G2/M phase and lead to apoptosis [112]. A halophilic bacterium, *Vibrio* sp. strain A1SM3-36-8, isolated from Manaure solar saltern in Colombia, showed a high potential to inhibit methicillin-resistant *Staphylococcus aureus* and causing a slight inhibition of lung cancer cell lines [51]. In another study, among nine moderately halophilic bacteria isolated from saline environments of Iran, the supernatant of four strains showed ability to reduce the viability of HUVEC cancer cell line while one of these supernatants induced the proliferation of adipose-derived mesenchymal stem cells [113]. The actinobacterium *Nocardiopsis lucentensis* DSM 44048 isolated from Salt marsh soil in Alicante, Spain produces a new benzoxazole derivatives, Nocarbenzoxazole G. The compound showed cytotoxic activity against liver carcinoma cells (HepG2) and HeLa cancer cells with IC50 values of 3 and 1 μM, respectively [114]. A halotolerant *Bacillus* sp. KCB14S006, which was isolated from a saltern, produced three new lipopeptides with cytotoxic activity. These new lipopeptides lead to a ~30% decrease in the viability of HeLa and src(ts)-NRK cells [115]. In another study, the methanolic extracts of *Bacillus* sp. VITPS14 and *Bacillus* sp. VITPS16 showed cytotoxicity against HeLa cancer cell line but not against A549 cells. These halophilic strains were isolated from soil samples of Marakkanam saltern and Pichavaram mangrove forest, India, respectively. Another halophilic strain, *Bacillus* sp. VITPS7, isolated from this area showed significant antioxidant activity. The presence of β-carotene and flavonoids was confirmed in these extracts [116]. In another study, twenty-four novel halophilic bacteria isolated from the surrounding of active volcanic Barren Island Andaman and the Nicobar Islands in India were examined for their cytotoxic activity against MDA-MB-231 breast cancer cell line. About 65% of these bacterial strains decreased the viability of this cell line to 50% or lower [117]. Metabolites from *Piscibacillus* sp. C12A1 isolated from Sambhar Lake, India, decreased the viability of MDA-MB-231 breast cancer cell line with downregulation of Bcl-xL and CDK-2 expression. Furthermore, cell migration and colony formation of the cells were inhibited in the presence of these metabolites [118].

Biosurfactants produced by microorganisms are active molecules that create an amphipathic surface containing hydrophilic and hydrophobic moieties. In recent years, these biomolecules were also found to possess several interesting properties of therapeutic and biomedical importance. Biosurfactants from the halophilic bacteria *Bacillus* sp. BS3 and *Halomonas* sp. BS4 had the ability to reduce the viability of mammary epithelial carcinoma cells to 24.8% and to 46.8 significantly ($p < 0.05$) at 0.25 μg/mL and 2.5 μg/mL concentrations, respectively [53,119].

Extracellular polymeric substances (EPS) have recently been attracting considerable attention because of their potential applications in many fields, including biomedicine. EPSs are heterogeneous polymers that contain a wide range of homo- or hetero-carbohydrates as well as organic and inorganic substituents. EPSs produced by both halophilic bacteria and archaea showed remarkable anticancer activity. Also, these polysaccharide polymers have been introduced as important agents for developing nanocarrier systems for anti-cancer drugs. For example, in 2011, Ruiz-Ruiz et al. showed that at a concentration of 500 μg/mL, the over sulfated exopolysaccharide of the halophilic bacterium *Halomonas stenophila* strain B100 completely blocked the proliferation of the human T leukemia cells (Jurkat cells) in a dose-response manner. Also, they revealed the positive effect of sulfate groups in viability reduction of Jurkat cells [120]. Moreover, in another study, the anti-cancer activity of the polysaccharide levan and its aldehyde-activated derivatives was reported. This polysaccharide was isolated from *Halomonas smyrnensis* AAD6 and its anticancer activity against human cancer cell lines such as lung (A549), liver (HepG2/C3A), gastric (AGS), and breast (MCF-7) cancer cells (Table 4) has been investigated. In this study, all evaluated cells were treated with levan samples at a broad concentration ranging from 10 to 1000 μg/mL. All samples were found to display growth inhibition against cancer cell lines at the highest dose (1000 μg/mL). Unmodified levan showed higher anti-cancer effect against AGS cells against other cancer cell lines. Aldehyde-activated levan showed higher anti-tumor activity than unmodified levan against all cancer cell lines. Oxidized levan samples showed higher anticancer activity against A549 and HepG2/C3A cells. By increasing the oxidation degree, the anti-cancer activity also increased. Therefore, it was clearly demonstrated that the introduction of the chemically modified group, aldehydes, into the linear levan molecule could significantly enhance the antitumor activity of levan polysaccharide [121].

Recent preclinical and medicinal studies have shown an inverse relationship between dietary uptake of carotenoids and cancer occurrence. It was reported that the extracted carotenoid from the halotolerant bacterium *Kocuria* sp. QWT-12, isolated from industrial tannery wastewater in Qom, in Iran, had the ability to reduce the viability of human breast cancer cell lines MCF-7, MDA-MB-468, and MDA-MB-231 with an IC50 of 1, 4, and 8 mg/mL, respectively. Also, this carotenoid decreased the viability of human lung cancer cell line A549, with IC50 of 4 mg/mL. This carotenoid did not reduce the viability of normal fibroblast cell line at these concentrations [122].

Among all anticancer enzymes, L-asparaginase and L-glutaminase are enzymes with the ability to inhibit acute lymphoblastic leukemia and other cancer cells. Halophilic and halotolerant bacteria are novel sources of these anticancer enzymes. For example, a screening from 85 halophilic strains from the hypersaline Urmia Lake in Iran revealed that 16 (19%) and three strains (3.5%) showed L-asparaginase and L-glutaminase activity, respectively. It was shown that L-asparaginase was produced mainly by strains belonging to the genus *Bacillus*, while L-glutaminase was produced mainly by strains of the genus *Salicola* [27]. In another study, it was reported that from 110 halophilic strains isolated from different saline environments of Iran, a total of 29, four, and two strains produced anticancer enzymes including L-asparaginase, L-glutaminase, and L-arginase, respectively. These strains belonged to the genera *Bacillus*, *Dietzia*, *Halobacillus*, *Rhodococcus*, *Paenibacillus*, and *Planococcus*, as Gram-positive bacteria, and *Pseudomonas*, *Marinobacter*, *Halomonas*, *Idiomarina*, *Vibrio*, and *Stappia* as Gram-negative bacteria [123]. From these strains, the anti-cancer activity of a novel recombinant L-asparaginase enzyme produced by *Halomonas elongata* strain IBRC M10216 was assayed against human lymphoblastic and myeloid leukemia cell lines, Jurkat and U937 (Table 4). This enzyme enhanced the viability of these cancer cell lines with IC50 values of 2 and 1 U/mL, respectively, but at these concentrations had no effect on the viability of normal HUVEC cell line [124].

Table 4. Halophilic bacteria, archaea, and fungi and their relation to cancer treatment.

Anticancer Activity of:	Isolation Source	Halophilic Strain	Cancer Cell Lines	Molecule	Formula	Reference
			Bacteria			
Metabolite	Marakkanam saltern and Pichavaram mangroveForest in India	*Bacillus* sp. VITPS16	Cervical carcinoma	Squalene	$C_{30}H_{50}$	[116]
				3-Methyl-2-(2-oxopropyl) furan	$C_8H_{10}O_2$	
				Methyl hexadeconate	$C_{17}H_{34}O_2$	
	Topsoil saltern in Jeungdo, Jeollanam-do, Republic of Korea	*Nocardiopsis* sp. HYJ128	Stomach and Leukemia carcinoma	Borrelidin C	$C_{28}H_{43}NO_7$	[42]
				Borrelidin D	$C_{28}H_{43}NO_7$	
	Saltern in Incheon in Korea	*Bacillus* sp. KCB14S006	Cervical carcinoma Myeloid leukemia	Iturin F_1	$C_{51}H_{80}N_{12}O_{15}Na$	[115]
				Iturin F_2	$C_{51}H_{80}N_{12}O_{15}Na$	
				Iturin A_8	$C_{51}H_{80}N_{12}O_{14}Na$	
				Iturin A_9	$C_{51}H_{80}N_{12}O_{14}Na$	
	A saltern on Shinui Island in Korea	*Streptomyces* sp.	Colorectal cancer Gastric cancer	Salternamide A	$C_{23}H_{32}ClNO_5$	[111]
	Salt marsh soil, Alicante, Spain	*Nocardiopsis lucentensis* DSM 44048	Liver cancer Cervical cancer cells	Nocarbenzoxazole G	$C_{15}H_{13}NO_4$	[114]
-	Brine-seawater interface of the Red Sea	12 halophilic marine strains	Breast adenocarcinoma Cervical carcinoma Prostate carcinoma	Crude extract	NR	[108]
-	Deep-sea brine pools of the Red Sea	24 halophilic marine strains	Breast adenocarcinoma Cervical carcinoma Prostate carcinoma	Crude extract	NR	[109]
-	Weihai Solar Saltern in China	*Streptomyces* sp. WH26	Lung adenocarcinoma Liver hepatocellular adenocarcinoma	8-*O*-Methyltetrangulol	$C_{20}H_{14}O_4$	[110]
-			Cervical carcinoma	Naphthomycin A	$C_{40}H_{46}ClNO_9$	
-	Baicheng salt field, Xingjiang Province, China	*Actinopolyspora erythraea* YIM 90600	Colorectal cancer Tumor suppressor Programmed Cell Death Protein 4 (Pdcd4)	Actinopolysporins A	$C_{15}H_{28}O_4$	[107]
				Actinopolysporins B	$C_{16}H_{30}O_4$	
				Actinopolysporins C	$C_{16}H_{30}O_2$	
	Weihai Solar Saltern in China	45 moderately halophilic strains	Liver hepatocellular adenocarcinoma	Crude extracts	NR	[106]

Table 4. *Cont.*

Anticancer Activity of:	Isolation Source	Halophilic Strain	Cancer Cell Lines	Molecule	Formula	Reference
Supernatant metabolite	Sambhar Lake in India	*Piscibacillus* sp. C12A1	Breast adenocarcinoma	Crude extract	NR	[118]
	Brine and sediment of the Manaure solar saltern in Colombia	*Vibrio* sp. A1SM3-36-8	Lung adenocarcinoma	13-*cis*-docosenamide	$C_{22}H_{43}NO$	[51]
	Different hypersaline lakes in Iran	9 moderately halophilic strains	Umbilical vein endothelial cancer cell	Crude extract	NR	[113]
Biosurfactant	Thamaraikulam solar salt works in India	*Halomonas* sp. BS4	Mammary epithelial carcinoma	1,2-Ethanediamine, *N,N,N′,N′*-tetra	$C_6H_{16}N_2$	[119]
				8-Methyl-6-nonenamide	$C_{10}H_{19}NO$	
				9-Octadecenamide, (*Z*)	$C_{18}H_{35}NO$	
	Solar salt works in India	*Bacillus* sp. BS3	Mammary epithelial carcinoma	13-Docosenamide, (*Z*)	$CH_3(CH_2)_7CH{=}CH(CH_2)_{11}CONH_2$	[53]
				Mannosamine	$C_6H_{13}NO_5{\cdot}HCl$	
				9-Octadecenamide, (*Z*)	$C_{18}H_{35}NO$	
				2-Octanol,2-methyl-6-methylene	$C_{12}H_{22}O_2$	
				Cylohex-1,4,5-triol-3-one-1-carbo	$C_5H_8FN_3$	
				2-Butanamine, 2-methyl-	$C_5H_{13}N$	
				1,2-Ethanediamine, *N,N,N′,N′*-tetramethyl-	$C_6H_{16}N_2$	
Exopolysaccharide	Çamalti saltern area in Turkey	*Halomonas smyrnensis* strain AAD6	Breast adenocarcinoma Lung adenocarcinoma Liver hepatocellular adenocarcinoma Gastric adenocarcinoma	Levan	$C_{18}H_{32}O_{16}$	[121]
	Sabinar saline wetland in Spain	*Halomonas stenophila* strain B100	Lymphoblastic leukemia	Single acidic exopolysaccharide with glucose, mannose and galactose	NR	[120]
Carotenoid	Industrial tannery wastewater in Iran	*Kocuria* sp. MA-2	Prostate carcinoma	Neurosporene	$C_{40}H_{58}$	[122]
Enzyme	Hypersaline soil in Iran	*Halomonas elongata* IBRC-M 10216	Lymphoblastic leukemia Myeloid leukemia	L-asparaginase	$C_{1377}H_{2208}N_{382}O_{442S17}$	[124]

Table 4. *Cont.*

Anticancer Activity of:	Isolation Source	Halophilic Strain	Cancer Cell Lines	Molecule	Formula	Reference
Archaea						
Supernatant metabolite	Aran Bidgol hypersaline lake in Iran	*Halobacterium salinarum* IBRC-M 10715	Prostate carcinoma	Crude extract	NR	[105]
Exopolysaccharide	Urmia Lake in Iran	*Halorubrum* sp. TBZ112	Gastric adenocarcinoma	Monosaccharide composition mainly composed of mannose, glucosamine, galacturonic acid, arabinose, and glucuronic acid	NR	[125]
Carotenoid	Marine solar saltern in eastern China	*Halogeometricum limi* strain RO1-6 *Haloplanus vescus* strain RO5-8	Liver hepatocellular adenocarcinoma	Bacterioruberin	$C_{50}H_{76}O_4$	[127]
	Tunisian solar saltern	*Halobacterium halobium*	Liver hepatocellular adenocarcinoma	Bacterioruberin	$C_{50}H_{76}O_4$	[126]
Fungi						
Metabolite	Weihai Solar Saltern in China	*Aspergillus* sp. F1	Lung adenocarcinoma Liver hepatocellular adenocarcinoma Cervical carcinoma Colorectal cancer	Cytochalasin E	$C_{28}H_{33}NO_7$	[128]
				Ergosterol	$C_{28}H_{44}O$	
				Rosellichalasin	$C_{28}H_{33}NO_5$	

Abbreviations: Not reported (NR).

4.2. *Archaea*

Although most studies in this field have been focused on halophilic bacteria, some studies investigated the potentials of haloarchaea. In one of these studies, among nine haloarchaeal strains isolated from Aran-Bidgol Salt Lake, in Iran, supernatant metabolites from *Halobacterium salinarum* IBRC M10715 had the most potent cytotoxic effect on prostate cancer cell lines (DU145 and PC3, IC50 = 0.5 mg/mL) without any effects on normal fibroblast cells (HFF-5). Moreover, the selective metabolite significantly increased both early and late apoptosis (about 11% and 9%, respectively) in the androgen-dependent PC3 cell line and reduced sphere formation ability of both cancer cell lines with down-regulation of SOX2 gene expression. Furthermore, prostate cancer cell tumors developed in nude mice significantly shrank post intratumor injection of the metabolite from *Halobacterium salinarum* IBRC M10715 [105]. *Halorubrum* sp. TBZ112 is a haloarchaeal species isolated from the Urmia Lake, Iran. It was reported that this strain could produce EPSs. The isolated EPSs possess a relatively low molecular weight in comparison with those EPSs isolated from other extreme environments (5 vs. ≥100 kDa, respectively) and the absence of sulfate functional groups in their structure was reported. The anticancer activity of the EPSs from *Halorubrum* sp. TBZ112 was examined and the results did not show any significant changes in the viability of gastric cancer cells (MKN-45) and normal human dermal fibroblast cells (HDF) at concentrations of 100, 250, 500, and 1000 μg/mL after 24 and 48 h of treatment. As the existence of sulfate functional groups and the EPSs bioactivities are directly related, the low cytotoxicity potential of the EPSs from *Halorubrum* sp. TBZ112 was not unexpected [125].

Both in vivo and in vitro studies confirm chemoprevention effects of some carotenoids anticancer activity. Halophilic microorganisms showed great potential toward the production of various carotenoids such as β-carotene, bacterioruberin, and xanthophylls. In recent years, some investigations were carried out to determine the role of carotenoids or other bioactive molecules produced by halophiles on cancer treatment. The effects of *Halobacterium halobium* carotenoid extract on the viability of human hepatoma, HepG2, have been analyzed. This haloarchaeal strain was isolated from a Tunisian solar saltern and the results emphasized that increasing concentrations of the carotenoid extract of this halophilic archaeon decreased significantly the viability of the HepG2 cancer cell line [126]. Carotenoids from the haloarchaea *Halogeometricum limi* strain RO1-6 and *Haloplanus vescus* strain RO5-8 showed a potent antioxidant activity in comparison with β-carotene. In addition, these carotenoid extracts inhibited HepG2 cells in vitro, in a dose-dependent manner. Bacterioruberin was the predominant carotenoid extracted from these haloarchaea [127].

4.3. *Fungi*

The biotechnological applications of halophilic fungi are remarkedly less studied in comparison with halophilic bacteria. There is only one study focused on the cytotoxic effect of metabolites from a moderately halophilic fungal strain, *Aspergillus* sp. F1 [128]. Based on this publication, this strain produced three compounds with anticancer activity including cytochalasin E, ergosterol, and rosellichalasin, and higher salt concentrations increased the production of these compounds. All isolated compounds decreased the viability of A549, Hela, BEL-7402, and RKO human cancer cell lines and the inhibition effect of ergosterol on human colon cancer cell line, RKO, was the most potent cytotoxic report in this study.

Table 4 summarize all the mentioned reports in Section 4, which are related to the anticancer effect of halophilic bacteria, archaea, and fungi isolated from different saline and hypersaline environments in the world.

The following table (Table 5) gathers the most promising new compounds derived from halophilic microorganisms. The minimum inhibitory concentration (MIC) and the half maximal inhibitory concentration (IC_{50}) are shown, based on their in vitro bioactivity. The results suggest that these compounds could be candidates for preclinical trials.

Table 5. Promising new compounds derived from halophilic microorganisms candidates for preclinical trials.

Compound	Structure	Antibiotic Activity		Anticancer Activity		Reference
		Microorganism	MIC (μM)	Cell Lines	IC_{50} (μM)	
Borrelidin C, D	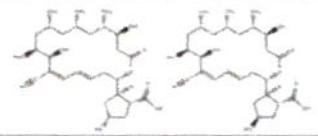	*S. enterica*	16–63	Stomach	5.5	[42]
				Leukemia	5.7	
				Leukemia	6.7	
Angucyclinone: *N*-(4-aminocyclooctyl)-3,5-dinitrobenzamide	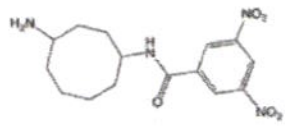	*S. aureus*, *S. epidermis*, *B. subtilis*, *B. megaterium*, *P. aeruginosa*	16	Breast, cervical, ovarian cyst, adenocarcinoma	10 nM	[50]
		S. mutans	4			
		X. malvacearum, *S. typhi*, *E. coli*	32			
		B. cereus	8			
		C. albicans	16			
Streptomonomicin STM	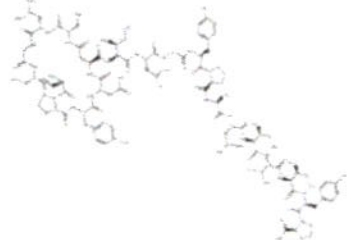	*B. anthracis*	2–4	NR	NR	[48]
		B. halodurans	4			
		B. cereus	4–7			
		Bacillus sp.	7			
		B. subtilis	29			
		L. monocytogenes	14			
		E. faecalis	29			
		S. aureus	57			
4-oxo-1,4-dihydroquinoline-3-carboxamide	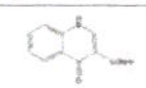	*S. aureus*	64	NR	NR	[43]
		B. subtilis	64			
6′-Hydroxy-4,2′,3′,4″-tetramethoxy-p-terphenyl	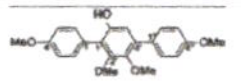	*B. subtilis*	64	NR	NR	[44]
		C. albicans	32			
Lynamicin A, B, C, and D	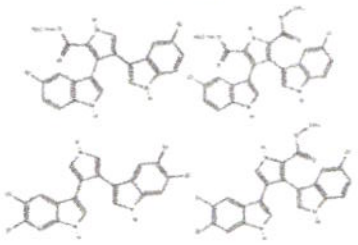	*S. aureus*	1.8–6.2	NR	NR	[57]
		S. epidermidis	2.2–9.5			
		S. pneumoniae	18–57			
		E. faecalis	3.3–19			
		E. faecium	4.4–19			
		H. influenzae	4.4–38			
		E. coli	13–16			

Table 5. *Cont.*

Compound	Structure	Antibiotic Activity		Anticancer Activity		Reference
		Microorganism	MIC (μM)	Cell Lines	IC_{50} (μM)	
Essramycin	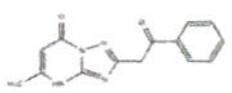	*E. coli*	8	NR	NR	[58]
		P. aeruginosa	3.5			
		B. subtilis, S. aureus	1			
		M. luteus	1.5			
Resistomycin 1-hydroxy-1-Norresistomycin	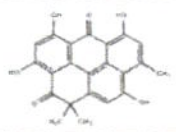	*E. coli*	40	NR	NR	[60]
		S. aureus				
		S. viridochromogenes				
Resistoflavin methyl ether	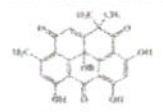 R=Me	*B. subtilis*	3.1	NR	NR	
		E. coli, S. aureus, C. albicans	10			
Lajollamycin	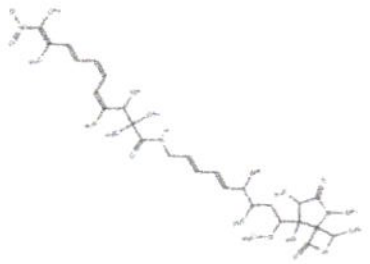	*MSSA*	4	Murine melanoma cell line B16-F10	9.6	[61]
		MRSA	5			
		SPPS	2			
		PRSP	1.5			
		VSEF	14			
		VREF	20			
		E. coli	12			

Note: Not reported (NR). Microorganisms: *Bacillus (B.): B. cereus, B. halodurans, B. megaterium, B. subtilis, B. anthracis. Candida (C.): C. albicans. Enterococcus (E.): E. faecalis, E. faecium,* Vancomycin resistant *Enterococcus faecium (VREF)*, Vancomycin sensitive *Enterococcus faecalis (VSEF), Vancomycin resistant enterococci (VRE). Escherichia (E.): E. coli. Haemophilus (H.): H. influenzae. Listeria (L.): L. monocytogenes. Micrococcus (M.): M. luteus. Pseudomonas (P.): P. aeruginosa. Salmonella (S.): S. typhi, S. enterica. Staphylococcus (S.): S. aureus, S. epidermidis, S. mutans*, Methicillin Sensitive *Staphylococcus aureus (MSSA), Methicillin-resistant Staphylococcus aureus (MRSA). Streptococcus (S.): S. pneumoniae*, Penicillin resistant *Streptococcus pneumoniae (PRSP)*, Penicillin sensitive *Streptococcus pneumoniae (SPPS). Streptomyces (S.): S. viridochromogenes. Xanthomonas (X.): X. malvacearum.*

5. Future Perspectives

As the prevalence of antimicrobial resistance increases, researchers are developing new technologies and strategies to find alternatives that reduce the morbidity and mortality caused by the MDR bacteria. Categorizing the need for obtaining new molecules, the most requested by the public health are antimicrobial and anticancer compounds according to the data annually reported by the World Health Organization (WHO). The current and future of natural product discovery is the application of a combination of multi-omics approaches. Depending on the phase of the study, it is foreseen genomics, metagenomics, transcriptomics, proteomics, and metabolomics to reveal the biosynthetic capabilities of a single microorganism or microbial communities in hypersaline environments.

The discovery of novel lead compounds requires more that in silico predicted genes and large promising data. The current problem with massive approaches is precisely the lack of concrete results traduced in novel lead compound derived of "meta-omics" studies. The heterologous expression of biosynthetic genes is the bottleneck since in several cases the recombinant product and its expression is totally different from what was expected. However, it is important to emphasize that the cultivation of hidden and uncultivable microbiota is improving with the assessment of metagenomic studies [129,130].

Genome mining has been implemented as a mandatory tool widely used to characterize the genetic basis of secondary metabolite biosynthesis based on the features of secondary metabolites organized as biosynthetic gene clusters (BGCs), especially the profile of gene encoding key signature enzymes [131–133]. The application of Next Generation Sequencing (NGS) allows the study of microbial diversity every day more accessible and affordable that allows the prediction of cryptic metabolic pathways and genes involved in the activity. The genome-guided discovery relies on sophisticated methods for identification of knew gene families related clusters. The accurate prediction and analysis of relevant genes for secondary metabolite biosynthetic pathways in microbes is performed through the tool based on the Antibiotics and Secondary Metabolites Analysis Shell (antiSMASH) [134].

Due to the high rate of rediscovery of known compounds, the dereplication is an essential approach that allows the identification of duplicate molecules. Dereplication is relying on finding a matching of mass spectra with those present in the mass spectrometry data repository. The development of new computational tools like the algorithm searching spectral, DEREPLICATOR+ is helping to identifying in one order of magnitude peptidic natural products (PNPs) that include nonribosomal peptides (NRPs), and ribosomally synthesized and post-translationally modified peptides (RiPPs). The matching is extended to the identification of polyketides, terpenes, benzenoids, alkaloids, flavonoids, and other classes of natural products. One of the utilities of DEREPLICATOR+ is the enabling of cross-validation of genome-mining and peptidogenomics/glycogenomics results [135].

Several laboratories working in microbial bioprospecting keep their private collection once the antimicrobial, anticancer, antifungal, etc. activity is detected. In many cases, these positive isolates derived from primary screenings are not further studied by genome sequencing and dereplication. A common issue is the obtaining of the purified active compound under laboratory conditions with limited facilities and handling large data with a proper analysis. Moreover, it is important to consider the dereplication costs and time-consuming interpreting. The mentioned facts delay the biodiscovery attempts and constitute the reasonable causing of keeping a stored library of potential compounds. The projection of drug discovery product research is the simplification and accessibility to all these tools faster and with less effort. The power of genome mining in studying natural product biosynthesis by showing the widespread distribution of NRPS/PKS gene clusters and by the elicitation of previously unidentified pathways has been demonstrated. It is clear that coupling genome mining and dereplication will accelerate the biodiscovery at initial steps. The integration and linking of computational approaches are certainly the future of natural product research.

In this review, we have focused in all anticancer molecules reported from halophilic microorganisms. According to the cellular lines used, the focus of primary screenings is addressed to the leading cancer types that affect the global population. However, it is important that further screenings should include cellular lines with intrinsic chemoresistance, like sarcoma and glioblastoma, characterized by aggressive overproliferation. The future of novel anticancer agents seems to be a combination of high-throughput screening assessed by predictive biomarkers.

Author Contributions: A.V. and P.C. designed the review article. P.C., M.A.A., and A.V. prepared and edited the manuscript. P.C. and M.A.A. prepared the tables. All authors revised and contributed to the preparation of the manuscript. All authors have read and agreed to the published version of the manuscript.

Funding: This study was supported by the Italian Foundation with the South (Fondazione CON IL SUD) project 2018-PDR-00533 (to P.C.), the Spanish Ministry of Economy and Competitiveness (MINECO) through project CGL2017-83385-P, which included European (FEDER) funds, and Junta de Andalucía (Spain) (to A.V.), and the Iranian National Science Foundation (INSF) (to M.A.A.).

Conflicts of Interest: The authors declare that there are no conflicts of interest.

References

1. Oren, A. Microbial life at high salt concentrations: Phylogenetic and metabolic diversity. *Saline Syst.* **2008**, *4*, 2. [CrossRef]
2. Kushner, D.J. Life in high salt and solute concentrations: Halophilic bacteria. In *Microbial Life in Extreme Environments*; Kushner, D.J., Ed.; Academic Press: London, UK, 1978; p. 318.
3. Kushner, D.; Kamekura, M. Physiology of halophilic eubacteria. In *Halophilic Bacteria*; Rodriguez-Valera, F., Ed.; CRC Press: Boca Raton, FL, USA, 1988; Volume 1, pp. 109–138.
4. Rodriguez-Valera, F.; Ruiz-Berraquero, F.; Ramos-Cormenzana, A. Characteristics of the heterotrophic bacterial populations in hypersaline environments of different salt concentrations. *Microb. Ecol.* **1981**, *7*, 235–243. [CrossRef] [PubMed]
5. Seckbach, J.; Oren, A.; Stan-Lotter, H. (Eds.) *Polyextremophiles: Life Under Multiple Forms of Stress*; Springer: Heidelberg, Germany, 2013.
6. Bowers, K.J.; Mesbah, N.M.; Wiegel, J. Biodiversity of poly-extremophilic bacteria: Does combining the extremes of high salt, alkaline pH and elevated temperature approach a physico-chemical boundary for life? *Saline Syst.* **2009**, *5*, 9. [CrossRef] [PubMed]
7. Mesbah, N.M.; Wiegel, J. Life under multiple extreme conditions: Diversity and physiology of the halophilic alkalithermophiles. *Appl. Environ. Microbiol.* **2012**, *78*, 4074–4082. [CrossRef] [PubMed]
8. Ventosa, A.; Nieto, J.J.; Oren, A. Biology of moderately halophilic aerobic bacteria. *Microbiol. Mol. Biol. Rev.* **1998**, *62*, 504–544.
9. Bremer, E.; Krämer, R. Responses of microorganisms to osmotic stress. *Annu. Rev. Microbiol.* **2019**, *73*, 313–334. [CrossRef]
10. De la Haba, R.R.; Sánchez-Porro, C.; Marquez, M.C.; Ventosa, A. Taxonomy of halophiles. In *Extremophiles Handbook*; Horikoshi, K., Ed.; Springer Japan: Tokyo, Japan, 2011; pp. 255–308.
11. Andrei, A.-Ş.; Banciu, H.L.; Oren, A. Living with salt: Metabolic and phylogenetic diversity of archaea inhabiting saline ecosystems. *FEMS Microbiol. Lett.* **2012**, *330*, 1–9. [CrossRef]
12. Ventosa, A.; Oren, A.; Ma, Y. (Eds.) *Halophiles and Hypersaline Environments*; Springer: Berlin/Heidelberg, Germany, 2011.
13. Akpolat, C.; Ventosa, A.; Birbir, M.; Sánchez-Porro, C.; Caglayan, P. Molecular identification of moderately halophilic bacteria and extremely halophilic archaea isolated from salted sheep skins containing red and yellow discolorations. *J. Am. Leather Chem. Assoc.* **2015**, *110*, 211–220.
14. Ventosa, A. Unusual micro-organisms from unusual habitats: Hypersaline environments. In *Prokaryotic Diversity*; Logan, N.A., Lappin-Scott, H.M., Oyston, P.C.F., Eds.; Cambridge University Press: Cambridge, UK, 2006; pp. 223–254.
15. Ventosa, A.; Fernández, A.B.; León, M.J.; Sánchez-Porro, C.; Rodriguez-Valera, F. The Santa Pola saltern as a model for studying the microbiota of hypersaline environments. *Extremophiles* **2014**, *18*, 811–824. [CrossRef]
16. Ventosa, A.; de la Haba, R.R.; Sánchez-Porro, C.; Papke, R.T. Microbial diversity of hypersaline environments: A metagenomic approach. *Curr. Opin. Microbiol.* **2015**, *25*, 80–87. [CrossRef]
17. Samylina, O.S.; Namsaraev, Z.B.; Grouzdev, D.S.; Slobodova, N.V.; Zelenev, V.V.; Borisenko, G.V.; Sorokin, D.Y. The patterns of nitrogen fixation in haloalkaliphilic phototrophic communities of Kulunda Steppe soda lakes (Altai, Russia). *FEMS Microbiol. Ecol.* **2019**, *95*, fiz174. [CrossRef] [PubMed]

18. Naghoni, A.; Emtiazi, G.; Amoozegar, M.A.; Cretoiu, M.S.; Stal, L.J.; Etemadifar, Z.; Shahzadeh Fazeli, S.A.; Bolhuis, H. Microbial diversity in the hypersaline Lake Meyghan, Iran. *Sci. Rep.* **2017**, *7*, 11522. [CrossRef] [PubMed]
19. Amoozegar, M.A.; Siroosi, M.; Atashgahi, S.; Smidt, H.; Ventosa, A. Systematics of haloarchaea and biotechnological potential of their hydrolytic enzymes. *Microbiology* **2017**, *163*, 623–645. [CrossRef] [PubMed]
20. Oren, A.; Rodriguez-Valera, F. The contribution of halophilic bacteria to the red coloration of saltern crystallizer ponds. *FEMS Microbiol. Ecol.* **2001**, *36*, 123–130. [CrossRef]
21. Charlesworth, J.C.; Burns, B.P. Untapped resources: Biotechnological potential of peptides and secondary metabolites in archaea. *Archaea* **2015**, *2015*, 1–7. [CrossRef]
22. Chen, Y.-H.; Lu, C.-W.; Shyu, Y.-T.; Lin, S.-S. Revealing the saline adaptation strategies of the halophilic bacterium *Halomonas beimenensis* through high-throughput omics and transposon mutagenesis approaches. *Sci. Rep.* **2017**, *7*, 13037. [CrossRef]
23. Das, S.; Dash, H.R. (Eds.) *Microbial Diversity in the Genomic Era*; Academic Press: Cambridge, MA, USA; Elsevier: Amsterdam, The Netherlands, 2018.
24. Vavourakis, C.D.; Mehrshad, M.; Balkema, C.; van Hall, R.; Andrei, A.-Ş.; Ghai, R.; Sorokin, D.Y.; Muyzer, G. Metagenomes and metatranscriptomes shed new light on the microbial-mediated sulfur cycle in a Siberian soda lake. *BMC Biol.* **2019**, *17*, 69. [CrossRef]
25. DasSarma, P.; Coker, J.A.; Huse, V.; DasSarma, S. Halophiles, industrial applications. In *Encyclopedia of Industrial Biotechnology*; American Cancer Society: Atlanta, GA, USA, 2010; pp. 1–43.
26. Yin, J.; Chen, J.-C.; Wu, Q.; Chen, G.-Q. Halophiles, coming stars for industrial biotechnology. *Biotechnol. Adv.* **2015**, *33*, 1433–1442. [CrossRef]
27. Shirazian, P.; Asad, S.; Amoozegar, M.A. The potential of halophilic and halotolerant bacteria for the production of antineoplastic enzymes: L-asparaginase and L-glutaminase. *EXCLI J.* **2016**, *15*, 268–279.
28. Kiadehi, M.S.H.; Amoozegar, M.A.; Asad, S.; Siroosi, M. Exploring the potential of halophilic archaea for the decolorization of azo dyes. *Water Sci. Technol.* **2018**, *77*, 1602–1611. [CrossRef]
29. Giani, M.; Garbayo, I.; Vílchez, C.; Martínez-Espinosa, R.M. Haloarchaeal carotenoids: Healthy novel compounds from extreme environments. *Mar. Drugs* **2019**, *17*, 524. [CrossRef] [PubMed]
30. Amoozegar, M.A.; Safarpour, A.; Noghabi, K.A.; Bakhtiary, T.; Ventosa, A. Halophiles and their vast potential in biofuel production. *Front. Microbiol.* **2019**, *10*, 1895. [CrossRef] [PubMed]
31. Jin, M.; Gai, Y.; Guo, X.; Hou, Y.; Zeng, R. Properties and applications of extremozymes from deep-sea extremophilic microorganisms: A mini review. *Mar. Drugs* **2019**, *17*, 656. [CrossRef] [PubMed]
32. Tseng, W.-P.; Chen, Y.-C.; Chen, S.-Y.; Chen, S.-Y.; Chang, S.-C. Risk for subsequent infection and mortality after hospitalization among patients with multidrug-resistant Gram-negative bacteria colonization or infection. *Antimicrob. Resist. Infect. Control* **2018**, *7*, 93. [CrossRef] [PubMed]
33. Peters, L.; Olson, L.; Khu, D.T.K.; Linnros, S.; Le, N.K.; Hanberger, H.; Hoang, N.T.B.; Tran, D.M.; Larsson, M. Multiple antibiotic resistance as a risk factor for mortality and prolonged hospital stay: A cohort study among neonatal intensive care patients with hospital-acquired infections caused by gram-negative bacteria in Vietnam. *PLoS ONE* **2019**, *14*, e0215666. [CrossRef]
34. Cassini, A.; Högberg, L.D.; Plachouras, D.; Quattrocchi, A.; Hoxha, A.; Simonsen, G.S.; Colomb-Cotinat, M.; Kretzschmar, M.E.; Devleesschauwer, B.; Cecchini, M.; et al. Attributable deaths and disability-adjusted life-years caused by infections with antibiotic-resistant bacteria in the EU and the European Economic Area in 2015: A population-level modelling analysis. *Lancet Infect. Dis.* **2019**, *19*, 56–66. [CrossRef]
35. Rodriguez-Valera, F.; Juez, G.; Kushner, D.J. Halocins: Salt-dependent bacteriocins produced by extremely halophilic rods. *Can. J. Microbiol.* **1982**, *28*, 151–154. [CrossRef]
36. Gohel, S.D.; Sharma, A.K.; Dangar, K.G.; Thakrar, F.J.; Singh, S.P. Antimicrobial and biocatalytic potential of haloalkaliphilic actinobacteria. In *Halophiles*; Maheshwari, D.K., Saraf, M., Eds.; Springer: Heidelberg, Germany, 2015; Volume 6, pp. 29–55.
37. Ventosa, A.; Mellado, E.; Sanchez-Porro, C.; Marquez, M.C. Halophilic and halotolerant microorganisms from soils. In *Microbiology of Extreme Soils*; Dion, P., Nautiyal, C.S., Eds.; Springer: Berlin/Heidelberg, Germany, 2008; pp. 87–115.
38. Hamedi, J.; Mohammadipanah, F.; Ventosa, A. Systematic and biotechnological aspects of halophilic and halotolerant actinomycetes. *Extremophiles* **2013**, *17*, 1–13. [CrossRef]

39. Manteca, Á.; Yagüe, P. Streptomyces as a source of antimicrobials: Novel approaches to activate cryptic secondary metabolite pathways. In *Antimicrobial, Antibiotic Resistant, Antibiofilm Strategies and Activity Methods*; Intechopen: London, UK, 2019; pp. 1–21.
40. Adlin Jenifer, J.S.C.; Michaelbabu, M.; Eswaramoorthy Thirumalaikumar, C.L.; Jeraldin Nisha, S.R.; Uma, G.; Citarasu, T. Antimicrobial potential of haloalkaliphilic *Nocardiopsis* sp. AJ1 isolated from solar salterns in India. *J. Basic Microbiol.* **2019**, *59*, 288–301. [CrossRef]
41. Hadj Rabia-Boukhalfa, Y.; Eveno, Y.; Karama, S.; Selama, O.; Lauga, B.; Duran, R.; Hacène, H.; Eparvier, V. Isolation, purification and chemical characterization of a new angucyclinone compound produced by a new halotolerant *Nocardiopsis* sp. HR-4 strain. *World J. Microbiol. Biotechnol.* **2017**, *33*, 126. [CrossRef]
42. Kim, J.; Shin, D.; Kim, S.-H.; Park, W.; Shin, Y.; Kim, W.K.; Lee, S.K.; Oh, K.-B.; Shin, J.; Oh, D.-C. Borrelidins C–E: New Antibacterial macrolides from a saltern-derived halophilic *Nocardiopsis* sp. *Mar. Drugs* **2017**, *15*, 166. [CrossRef] [PubMed]
43. Tian, S.; Yang, Y.; Liu, K.; Xiong, Z.; Xu, L.; Zhao, L. Antimicrobial metabolites from a novel halophilic actinomycete *Nocardiopsis terrae* YIM 90022. *Nat. Prod. Res.* **2014**, *28*, 344–346. [CrossRef] [PubMed]
44. Tian, S.-Z.; Pu, X.; Luo, G.; Zhao, L.-X.; Xu, L.-H.; Li, W.-J.; Luo, Y. Isolation and characterization of new *p*-terphenyls with antifungal, antibacterial, and antioxidant activities from halophilic actinomycete *Nocardiopsis gilva* YIM 90087. *J. Agric. Food Chem.* **2013**, *61*, 3006–3012. [CrossRef] [PubMed]
45. Gorajana, A.; Vinjamuri, S.; Poluri, E.; Zeeck, A. 1-Hydroxy-1-norresistomycin, a new cytotoxic compound from a marine actinomycete, *Streptomyces chibaensis*. *J. Antibiot.* **2005**, *8*, 526–529. [CrossRef] [PubMed]
46. Maskey, R.P.; Helmke, E.; Laatsch, H. Himalomycin A and B: Isolation and structure elucidation of new fridamycin type antibiotics from a marine *Streptomyces* isolate. *J. Antibiot.* **2003**, *56*, 942–949. [CrossRef] [PubMed]
47. Parthasarathi, S.; Sathya, S.; Bupesh, G.; Samy, R.D.; Mohan, M.R.; Kumar, G.S.; Manikandan, M.; Kim, C.J.; Balakrishnan, K. Isolation and characterization of antimicrobial compound from marine *Streptomyces hygroscopicus* BDUS 49. *World J. Fish Mar. Sci.* **2012**, *4*, 268–277.
48. Metelev, M.; Tietz, J.I.; Melby, J.O.; Blair, P.M.; Zhu, L.; Livnat, I.; Severinov, K.; Mitchell, D.A. Structure, bioactivity, and resistance mechanism of Streptomonomicin, an unusual lasso peptide from an understudied halophilic actinomycete. *Chem. Biol.* **2015**, *22*, 241–250. [CrossRef]
49. Frikha Dammak, D.; Zarai, Z.; Najah, S.; Abdennabi, R.; Belbahri, L.; Rateb, M.E.; Mejdoub, H.; Maalej, S. Antagonistic properties of some halophilic thermoactinomycetes isolated from superficial sediment of a solar saltern and production of cyclic antimicrobial peptides by the novel isolate *Paludifilum halophilum*. *BioMed Res. Int.* **2017**, *2017*, 1–13. [CrossRef]
50. Mangamuri, U.K.; Vijayalakshmi, M.; Poda, S.; Manavathi, B.; Chitturi, B.; Yenamandra, V. Isolation and biological evaluation of N-(4-aminocyclooctyl)-3,5-dinitrobenzamide, a new semisynthetic derivative from the mangrove-associated actinomycete *Pseudonocardia endophytica* VUK-10. *3 Biotech* **2016**, *6*, 158. [CrossRef]
51. Conde-Martínez, N.; Acosta-González, A.; Díaz, L.E.; Tello, E. Use of a mixed culture strategy to isolate halophilic bacteria with antibacterial and cytotoxic activity from the Manaure solar saltern in Colombia. *BMC Microbiol.* **2017**, *17*, 230. [CrossRef]
52. Bell, R.; Carmeli, S.; Sar, N. Vibrindole A, a Metabolite of the marine bacterium, *Vibrio parahaemolyticus*, isolated from the toxic mucus of the boxfish *Ostracion cubicus*. *J. Nat. Prod.* **1994**, *57*, 1587–1590. [CrossRef] [PubMed]
53. Donio, M.; Ronica, S.; Viji, V.T.; Velmurugan, S.; Jenifer, J.A.; Michaelbabu, M.; Citarasu, T. Isolation and characterization of halophilic *Bacillus* sp. BS3 able to produce pharmacologically important biosurfactants. *Asian Pac. J. Trop. Med.* **2013**, *6*, 876–883. [CrossRef]
54. Velmurugan, S.; Raman, K.; Thanga Viji, V.; Donio, M.B.S.; Adlin Jenifer, J.; Babu, M.M.; Citarasu, T. Screening and characterization of antimicrobial secondary metabolites from *Halomonas salifodinae* MPM-TC and its in vivo antiviral influence on Indian white shrimp *Fenneropenaeus indicus* against WSSV challenge. *J. King Saud Univ. Sci.* **2013**, *25*, 181–190. [CrossRef]
55. Wang, H.; Fewer, D.P.; Holm, L.; Rouhiainen, L.; Sivonen, K. Atlas of nonribosomal peptide and polyketide biosynthetic pathways reveals common occurrence of nonmodular enzymes. *Proc. Natl. Acad. Sci. USA* **2014**, *111*, 9259–9264. [CrossRef]

56. Bose, U.; Hewavitharana, A.; Ng, Y.; Shaw, P.; Fuerst, J.; Hodson, M. LC-MS-based metabolomics study of marine bacterial secondary metabolite and antibiotic production in *Salinispora arenicola*. *Mar. Drugs* **2015**, *13*, 249–266. [CrossRef]
57. McArthur, K.A.; Mitchell, S.S.; Tsueng, G.; Rheingold, A.; White, D.J.; Grodberg, J.; Lam, K.S.; Potts, B.C.M. Lynamicins A−E, chlorinated bisindole pyrrole antibiotics from a novel marine actinomycete. *J. Nat. Prod.* **2008**, *71*, 1732–1737. [CrossRef]
58. El-Gendy, M.M.A.; Shaaban, M.; Shaaban, K.A.; El-Bondkly, A.M.; Laatsch, H. Essramycin: A first triazolopyrimidine antibiotic isolated from nature. *J. Antibiot.* **2008**, *61*, 149–157. [CrossRef]
59. Hughes, C.C.; Prieto-Davo, A.; Jensen, P.R.; Fenical, W. The Marinopyrroles, antibiotics of an unprecedented structure class from a marine *Streptomyces* sp. *Org. Lett.* **2008**, *10*, 629–631. [CrossRef]
60. Kock, I.; Maskey, R.P.; Biabani, M.A.F.; Helmke, E.; Laatsch, H. 1-Hydroxy-1-norresistomycin and resistoflavin methyl ether: New antibiotics from marine-derived streptomycetes. *J. Antibiot.* **2005**, *58*, 530–534. [CrossRef] [PubMed]
61. Manam, R.R.; Teisan, S.; White, D.J.; Nicholson, B.; Grodberg, J.; Neuteboom, S.T.C.; Lam, K.S.; Mosca, D.A.; Lloyd, G.K.; Potts, B.C.M. Lajollamycin, a nitro-tetraene spiro-β-lactone-γ-lactam antibiotic from the marine actinomycete *Streptomyces nodosus*. *J. Nat. Prod.* **2005**, *68*, 240–243. [CrossRef] [PubMed]
62. Maskey, R.P.; Li, F.C.; Qin, S.; Fiebig, H.H.; Laatsch, H. Chandrananimycins A-C: Production of novel anticancer antibiotics from a marine *Actinomadura* sp. isolate M048 by variation of medium composition and growth conditions. *J. Antibiot.* **2003**, *56*, 622–629. [CrossRef]
63. Fariq, A.; Yasmin, A.; Jamil, M. Production, characterization and antimicrobial activities of bio-pigments by *Aquisalibacillus elongatus* MB592, *Salinicoccus sesuvii* MB597, and *Halomonas aquamarina* MB598 isolated from Khewra Salt Range, Pakistan. *Extremophiles* **2019**, *23*, 435–449. [CrossRef]
64. Trenozhnikova, L.; Azizan, A. Discovery of actinomycetes from extreme environments with potential to produce novel antibiotics. *Cent. Asian J. Glob. Health* **2018**, *7*, 337. [CrossRef]
65. Kumar, R.R.; Jadeja, V.J. Characterization and partial purification of an antibacterial agent from halophilic actinomycete *Kocuria* sp. strain rsk4. *BioImpacts* **2018**, *8*, 253–261. [CrossRef]
66. Ballav, S.; Kerkar, S.; Thomas, S.; Augustine, N. Halophilic and halotolerant actinomycetes from a marine saltern of Goa, India producing anti-bacterial metabolites. *J. Biosci. Bioeng.* **2015**, *119*, 323–330. [CrossRef]
67. Ray, L.; Suar, M.; Pattnaik, A.K.; Raina, V. *Streptomyces chilikensis* sp. nov., a halophilic streptomycete isolated from brackish water sediment. *Int. J. Syst. Evol. Microbiol.* **2013**, *63*, 2757–2764. [CrossRef]
68. Rao, K.V.R. Isolation and characterization of antagonistic actinobacteria from mangrove soil. *J. Biochem. Tech.* **2012**, *3*, 361–365.
69. Mangamuri, U.K.; Vijayalakshmi Muvva, V.; Poda, S.; Kamma, S. Isolation, identification and molecular characterization of rare actinomycetes from mangrove ecosystem of Nizampatnam. *Malays. J. Microbiol.* **2012**, *8*, 83–91. [CrossRef]
70. Kamat, T.; Kerkar, S. Bacteria from salt pans: A potential resource of antibacterial metabolites. *RRST-Biotech.* **2011**, *3*, 46–52.
71. Gayathri, A.; Madhanraj, P.; Panneerselvam, A. Diversity, antibacterial activity and molecular characterization of actinomycetes isolated from salt pan region of Kodiakarai, Nagapattinam DT. *Asian J. Pharm. Technol.* **2011**, *1*, 79–81.
72. Meklat, A.; Sabaou, N.; Zitouni, A.; Mathieu, F.; Lebrihi, A. Isolation, taxonomy, and antagonistic properties of halophilic actinomycetes in Saharan soils of Algeria. *Appl. Environ. Microbiol.* **2011**, *77*, 6710–6714. [CrossRef] [PubMed]
73. Jose, A.; Santhi, S.; Solomon, R.D.J. In vitro antimicrobial potential and growth characteristics of *Nocardiopsis* sp. JAJ16 isolated from crystallizer pond. *Int. J. Curr. Res.* **2010**, *3*, 024–026.
74. Saurav, K. Diversity and optimization of process parameters for the growth of *Streptomyces* VITSVK9 spp. isolated from Bay of Bengal, India. *J. Nat. Environ. Sci.* **2010**, *1*, 56–65.
75. Suthindhir, K.; Kannabiran, K. Cytotoxic and antimicrobial potential of actinomycete species *Saccharopolyspora salina* VITSDK4 isolated from the Bay of Bengal coast of India. *Am. J. Infect. Dis.* **2009**, *5*, 90–98. [CrossRef]
76. Suthindhiran, K.; Kannabiran, K. Hemolytic activity of *Streptomyces* VITSDK1 spp. isolated from marine sediments in Southern India. *J. Mycol. Médicale* **2009**, *19*, 77–86. [CrossRef]
77. Cao, L.; Yun, W.; Tang, S.; Zhang, P.; Mao, P.; Jing, X.; Wang, C.; Lou, K. Biodiversity and enzyme screening of actinomycetes from Hami lake. *Wei Sheng Wu Xue Bao* **2009**, *49*, 287–293.

78. Ramesh, S.; Mathivanan, N. Screening of marine actinomycetes isolated from the Bay of Bengal, India for antimicrobial activity and industrial enzymes. *World J. Microbiol. Biotechnol.* **2009**, *25*, 2103–2111. [CrossRef]
79. Hakvåg, S.; Fjærvik, E.; Josefsen, K.; Ian, E.; Ellingsen, T.; Zotchev, S. Characterization of *Streptomyces* spp. isolated from the sea surface microlayer in the Trondheim Fjord, Norway. *Mar. Drugs* **2008**, *6*, 620–635. [CrossRef]
80. Dhanasekaran, D.; Rajakumar, G.; Sivamani, P.; Selvamani, S.; Panneerselvam, A.; Thajuddin, N. Screening of salt pans actinomycetes for antibacterial agents. *Internet J. Microbiol.* **2004**, *1*, 1–4.
81. Magarvey, N.A.; Keller, J.M.; Bernan, V.; Dworkin, M.; Sherman, D.H. Isolation and characterization of novel marine-derived actinomycete taxa rich in bioactive metabolites. *Appl. Environ. Microbiol.* **2004**, *70*, 7520–7529. [CrossRef]
82. Kokare, C.R.; Mahadik, K.R.; Kadam, S.S.; Chopade, B.A. Isolation, characterization and antimicrobial activity of marine halophilic *Actinopolyspora* species AH1 from the west coast of India. *Curr. Sci.* **2004**, *86*, 5.
83. Meseguer, I.; Rodríguez-Valera, F.; Ventosa, A. Antagonistic interactions among halobacteria due to halocin production. *FEMS Microbiol. Lett.* **1986**, *36*, 177–182. [CrossRef]
84. Torreblanca, M.; Meseguer, I.; Ventosa, A. Production of halocins is a practically universal feature of archaeal halophilic rods. *Lett. Appl. Microbiol.* **1994**, *19*, 201–205. [CrossRef]
85. Shand, R.F.; Leyva, K.J. Peptide and protein antibiotics from the domain Archaea: Halocins and sulfolobicins. In *Bacteriocins: Ecology and Evolution*; Riley, M.A., Chavan, M.A., Eds.; Springer: Berlin/Heidelberg, Germany, 2007; pp. 93–109.
86. Atanasova, N.S.; Pietilä, M.K.; Oksanen, H.M. Diverse antimicrobial interactions of halophilic archaea and bacteria extend over geographical distances and cross the domain barrier. *MicrobiologyOpen* **2013**, *2*, 811–825. [CrossRef]
87. Corral, P.; Esposito, F.P.; Tedesco, P.; Falco, A.; Tortorella, E.; Tartaglione, L.; Festa, C.; D'Auria, M.V.; Gnavi, G.; Varese, G.C.; et al. Identification of a Sorbicillinoid-producing *Aspergillus* strain with antimicrobial activity against *Staphylococcus aureus*: A new polyextremophilic marine fungus from Barents Sea. *Mar. Biotechnol.* **2018**, *20*, 502–511. [CrossRef]
88. Besse, A. Antimicrobial peptides and proteins in the face of extremes: Lessons from archaeocins. *Biochimie* **2015**, *118*, 344–355. [CrossRef]
89. Quadri, I.; Hassani, I.I.; l'Haridon, S.; Chalopin, M.; Hacène, H.; Jebbar, M. Characterization and antimicrobial potential of extremely halophilic archaea isolated from hypersaline environments of the Algerian Sahara. *Microbiol. Res.* **2016**, *186–187*, 119–131. [CrossRef]
90. Pi, B.; Yu, D.; Dai, F.; Song, X.; Zhu, C.; Li, H.; Yu, Y. A Genomics based discovery of secondary metabolite biosynthetic gene clusters in *Aspergillus ustus*. *PLoS ONE* **2015**, *10*, e0116089. [CrossRef]
91. Kjærbølling, I.; Vesth, T.C.; Frisvad, J.C.; Nybo, J.L.; Theobald, S.; Kuo, A.; Bowyer, P.; Matsuda, Y.; Mondo, S.; Lyhne, E.K.; et al. Linking secondary metabolites to gene clusters through genome sequencing of six diverse *Aspergillus* species. *Proc. Natl. Acad. Sci. USA* **2018**, *115*, E753–E761. [CrossRef]
92. Wolfender, J.-L.; Litaudon, M.; Touboul, D.; Queiroz, E.F. Innovative omics-based approaches for prioritisation and targeted isolation of natural products—New strategies for drug discovery. *Nat. Prod. Rep.* **2019**, *36*, 855–868. [CrossRef]
93. Metcalf, J.A.; Funkhouser-Jones, L.J.; Brileya, K.; Reysenbach, A.-L.; Bordenstein, S.R. Antibacterial gene transfer across the tree of life. *eLife* **2014**, *25*, 3. [CrossRef] [PubMed]
94. Plemenitaš, A.; Lenassi, M.; Konte, T.; Kejžar, A.; Zajc, J.; Gostinčar, C.; Gunde-Cimerman, N. Adaptation to high salt concentrations in halotolerant/halophilic fungi: A molecular perspective. *Front. Microbiol.* **2014**, *5*, 199. [CrossRef] [PubMed]
95. Gunde-Cimerman, N.; Plemenitaš, A.; Oren, A. Strategies of adaptation of microorganisms of the three domains of life to high salt concentrations. *FEMS Microbiol. Rev.* **2018**, *42*, 353–375. [CrossRef] [PubMed]
96. Plemenitaš, A.; Vaupotič, T.; Lenassi, M.; Kogej, T.; Gunde-Cimerman, N. Adaptation of extremely halotolerant black yeast *Hortaea werneckii* to increased osmolarity: A molecular perspective at a glance. *Stud. Mycol.* **2008**, *61*, 67–75. [CrossRef]
97. Moubasher, A.-A.H.; Abdel-Sater, M.A.; Soliman, Z.S.M. Yeasts and filamentous fungi associated with some dairy products in Egypt. *J. Mycol. Médicale* **2018**, *28*, 76–86. [CrossRef]

98. Chamekh, R.; Deniel, F.; Donot, C.; Jany, J.-L.; Nodet, P.; Belabid, L. Isolation, identification and enzymatic activity of halotolerant and halophilic fungi from the Great Sebkha of Oran in Northwestern of Algeria. *Mycobiology* **2019**, *47*, 230–241. [CrossRef]
99. Chung, D.; Kim, H.; Choi, H.S. Fungi in salterns. *J. Microbiol.* **2019**, *57*, 717–724. [CrossRef]
100. Zheng, J.; Wang, Y.; Wang, J.; Liu, P.; Li, J.; Zhu, W. Antimicrobial ergosteroids and pyrrole derivatives from halotolerant *Aspergillus flocculosus* PT05-1 cultured in a hypersaline medium. *Extremophiles* **2013**, *17*, 963–971. [CrossRef]
101. Wang, Y.; Zheng, J.; Liu, P.; Wang, W.; Zhu, W. Three new compounds from *Aspergillus terreus* PT06-2 grown in a high salt medium. *Mar. Drugs* **2011**, *9*, 1368–1378. [CrossRef]
102. Ali, I.; Siwarungson, N.; Punnapayak, H.; Lotrakul, P.; Prasongsuk, S.; Bankeeree, W.; Rakshit, S.K. Screening of potential biotechnological applications from obligate halophilic fungi, isolated from a man-made solar saltern located in Phetchaburi province, Thailand. *Pak. J. Bot.* **2014**, *46*, 983–988.
103. Lebogang, L.; Taylor, J.E.; Mubyana-John, T. A preliminary study of the fungi associated with saltpans in Botswana and their anti-microbial properties. *Bioremediation Biodivers. Bioavailab.* **2009**, *3*, 61–71.
104. Safarpour, A.; Amoozegar, M.A.; Ventosa, A. Hypersaline environments of Iran: Prokaryotic biodiversity and their potentials in microbial biotechnology. In *Extremophiles in Eurasian Ecosystems: Ecology, Diversity, and Applications*; Egamberdieva, D., Birkeland, N.-K., Panosyan, H., Li, W.-J., Eds.; Springer: Singapore, 2018; Volume 8, pp. 265–298.
105. Safarpour, A.; Ebrahimi, M.; Shahzadeh Fazeli, S.A.; Amoozegar, M.A. Supernatant metabolites from halophilic archaea to reduce tumorigenesis in prostate cancer in-vitro and in-vivo. *Iran. J. Pharm. Res.* **2019**, *18*, 241–253. [PubMed]
106. Chen, L.; Wang, G.; Bu, T.; Zhang, Y.; Wang, Y.; Liu, M.; Lin, X. Phylogenetic analysis and screening of antimicrobial and cytotoxic activities of moderately halophilic bacteria isolated from the Weihai Solar Saltern (China). *World J. Microbiol. Biotechnol.* **2010**, *26*, 879–888. [CrossRef]
107. Zhao, L.-X.; Huang, S.-X.; Tang, S.-K.; Jiang, C.-L.; Duan, Y.; Beutler, J.A.; Henrich, C.J.; McMahon, J.B.; Schmid, T.; Blees, J.S.; et al. Actinopolysporins A–C and tubercidin as a Pdcd4 stabilizer from the halophilic actinomycete *Actinopolyspora erythraea* YIM 90600. *J. Nat. Prod.* **2011**, *74*, 1990–1995. [CrossRef] [PubMed]
108. Sagar, S.; Esau, L.; Hikmawan, T.; Antunes, A.; Holtermann, K.; Stingl, U.; Bajic, V.B.; Kaur, M. Cytotoxic and apoptotic evaluations of marine bacteria isolated from brine-seawater interface of the Red Sea. *BMC Complement. Altern. Med.* **2013**, *13*, 29. [CrossRef] [PubMed]
109. Sagar, S.; Esau, L.; Holtermann, K.; Hikmawan, T.; Zhang, G.; Stingl, U.; Bajic, V.B.; Kaur, M. Induction of apoptosis in cancer cell lines by the Red Sea brine pool bacterial extracts. *BMC Complement. Altern. Med.* **2013**, *13*, 344. [CrossRef]
110. Liu, H.; Xiao, L.; Wei, J.; Schmitz, J.C.; Liu, M.; Wang, C.; Cheng, L.; Wu, N.; Chen, L.; Zhang, Y.; et al. Identification of *Streptomyces* sp. nov. WH26 producing cytotoxic compounds isolated from marine solar saltern in China. *World J. Microbiol. Biotechnol.* **2013**, *29*, 1271–1278. [CrossRef]
111. Kim, S.-H.; Shin, Y.; Lee, S.-H.; Oh, K.-B.; Lee, S.K.; Shin, J.; Oh, D.-C. Salternamides A–D from a halophilic *Streptomyces* sp. actinobacterium. *J. Nat. Prod.* **2015**, *78*, 836–843. [CrossRef]
112. Bach, D.-H.; Kim, S.-H.; Hong, J.-Y.; Park, H.J.; Oh, D.-C.; Lee, S.K. Salternamide A suppresses hypoxia-induced accumulation of HIF-1α and induces apoptosis in human colorectal cancer cells. *Mar. Drugs* **2015**, *13*, 6962–6976. [CrossRef]
113. Sarvari, S.; Seyedjafari, E.; Amoozgar, M.A.; Bakhshandeh, B. The effect of moderately halophilic bacteria supernatant on proliferation and apoptosis of cancer cells and mesenchymal stem cells. *Cell. Mol. Biol. Noisy Gd. Fr.* **2015**, *61*, 30–34.
114. Sun, M.; Zhang, X.; Hao, H.; Li, W.; Lu, C. Nocarbenzoxazoles A–G, benzoxazoles produced by halophilic *Nocardiopsis lucentensis* DSM 44048. *J. Nat. Prod.* **2015**, *78*, 2123–2127. [CrossRef] [PubMed]
115. Son, S.; Ko, S.-K.; Jang, M.; Kim, J.; Kim, G.; Lee, J.; Jeon, E.; Futamura, Y.; Ryoo, I.-J.; Lee, J.-S.; et al. New cyclic lipopeptides of the iturin class produced by saltern-derived *Bacillus* sp. KCB14S006. *Mar. Drugs* **2016**, *14*, 72. [CrossRef] [PubMed]
116. Prathiba, S.; Jayaraman, G. Evaluation of the anti-oxidant property and cytotoxic potential of the metabolites extracted from the bacterial isolates from mangrove forest and saltern regions of South India. *Prep. Biochem. Biotechnol.* **2018**, *48*, 750–758. [CrossRef] [PubMed]

117. Lawrance, A.; Balakrishnan, M.; Gunasekaran, R.; Srinivasan, R.; Valsalan, V.N.; Gopal, D.; Ramalingam, K. Unexplored deep sea habitats in active volcanic Barren Island, Andaman and Nicobar Islands are sources of novel halophilic eubacteria. *Infect. Genet. Evol.* **2018**, *65*, 1–5. [CrossRef]
118. Neelam, D.K.; Agrawal, A.; Tomer, A.K.; Bandyopadhayaya, S.; Sharma, A.; Jagannadham, M.V.; Mandal, C.C.; Dadheech, P.K. A *Piscibacillus* sp. isolated from a soda lake exhibits anticancer activity against breast cancer MDA-MB-231 cells. *Microorganisms* **2019**, *7*, 34. [CrossRef]
119. Donio, M.B.S.; Ronica, F.A.; Viji, V.T.; Velmurugan, S.; Jenifer, J.S.C.A.; Michaelbabu, M.; Dhar, P.; Citarasu, T. *Halomonas* sp. BS4, a biosurfactant producing halophilic bacterium isolated from solar salt works in India and their biomedical importance. *SpringerPlus* **2013**, *2*, 149. [CrossRef]
120. Ruiz-Ruiz, C.; Srivastava, G.K.; Carranza, D.; Mata, J.A.; Llamas, I.; Santamaría, M.; Quesada, E.; Molina, I.J. An exopolysaccharide produced by the novel halophilic bacterium *Halomonas stenophila* strain B100 selectively induces apoptosis in human T leukaemia cells. *Appl. Microbiol. Biotechnol.* **2011**, *89*, 345–355. [CrossRef]
121. Sarilmiser, H.K.; Ozlem, A.; Gonca, O.; Arga, K.Y.; Toksoy Oner, E. Effective stimulating factors for microbial levan production by *Halomonas smyrnensis* AAD6T. *J. Biosci. Bioeng.* **2015**, *119*, 455–463. [CrossRef]
122. Rezaeeyan, Z.; Safarpour, A.; Amoozegar, M.A.; Babavalian, H.; Tebyanian, H.; Shakeri, F. High carotenoid production by a halotolerant bacterium, *Kocuria* sp. strain QWT-12 and anticancer activity of its carotenoid. *EXCLI J.* **2017**, *16*, 840–851.
123. Zolfaghar, M.; Amoozegar, M.A.; Khajeh, K.; Babavalian, H.; Tebyanian, H. Isolation and screening of extracellular anticancer enzymes from halophilic and halotolerant bacteria from different saline environments in Iran. *Mol. Biol. Rep.* **2019**, *46*, 3275–3286. [CrossRef]
124. Ghasemi, A.; Asad, S.; Kabiri, M.; Dabirmanesh, B. Cloning and characterization of *Halomonas elongata* L-asparaginase, a promising chemotherapeutic agent. *Appl. Microbiol. Biotechnol.* **2017**, *101*, 7227–7238. [CrossRef] [PubMed]
125. Hamidi, M.; Mirzaei, R.; Delattre, C.; Khanaki, K.; Pierre, G.; Gardarin, C.; Petit, E.; Karimitabar, F.; Faezi, S. Characterization of a new exopolysaccharide produced by *Halorubrum* sp. TBZ112 and evaluation of its anti-proliferative effect on gastric cancer cells. *3 Biotech* **2019**, *9*, 1. [CrossRef] [PubMed]
126. Abbes, M.; Baati, H.; Guermazi, S.; Messina, C.; Santulli, A.; Gharsallah, N.; Ammar, E. Biological properties of carotenoids extracted from *Halobacterium halobium* isolated from a Tunisian solar saltern. *BMC Complement. Altern. Med.* **2013**, *13*, 255. [CrossRef] [PubMed]
127. Hou, J.; Cui, H.-L. *In vitro* antioxidant, antihemolytic, and anticancer activity of the carotenoids from halophilic archaea. *Curr. Microbiol.* **2018**, *75*, 266–271. [CrossRef]
128. Xiao, L.; Liu, H.; Wu, N.; Liu, M.; Wei, J.; Zhang, Y.; Lin, X. Characterization of the high cytochalasin E and rosellichalasin producing *Aspergillus* sp. nov. F1 isolated from marine solar saltern in China. *World J. Microbiol. Biotechnol.* **2013**, *29*, 11–17. [CrossRef]
129. León, M.J.; Fernández, A.B.; Ghai, R.; Sánchez-Porro, C.; Rodriguez-Valera, F.; Ventosa, A. From metagenomics to pure culture: Isolation and characterization of the moderately halophilic bacterium *Spiribacter salinus* gen. nov., sp. nov. *Appl. Environ. Microbiol.* **2014**, *80*, 3850–3857. [CrossRef]
130. Hamm, J.N.; Erdmann, S.; Eloe-Fadrosh, E.A.; Angeloni, A.; Zhong, L.; Brownlee, C.; Williams, T.J.; Barton, K.; Carswell, S.; Smith, M.A.; et al. Unexpected host dependency of *Antarctic nanohaloarchaeota*. *Proc. Natl. Acad. Sci. USA* **2019**, *116*, 14661–14670. [CrossRef]
131. Blin, K.; Kim, H.U.; Medema, M.H.; Weber, T. Recent development of antiSMASH and other computational approaches to mine secondary metabolite biosynthetic gene clusters. *Brief. Bioinform.* **2019**, *20*, 1103–1113. [CrossRef]
132. Wang, S.; Zheng, Z.; Zou, H.; Li, N.; Wu, M. Characterization of the secondary metabolite biosynthetic gene clusters in archaea. *Comput. Biol. Chem.* **2019**, *78*, 165–169. [CrossRef]
133. Zheng, Y.; Saitou, A.; Wang, C.-M.; Toyoda, A.; Minakuchi, Y.; Sekiguchi, Y.; Ueda, K.; Takano, H.; Sakai, Y.; Abe, K.; et al. Genome features and secondary metabolites biosynthetic potential of the class *Ktedonobacteria*. *Front. Microbiol.* **2019**, *10*, 893. [CrossRef]

134. Weber, T.; Blin, K.; Duddela, S.; Krug, D.; Kim, H.U.; Bruccoleri, R.; Lee, S.Y.; Fischbach, M.A.; Müller, R.; Wohlleben, W.; et al. antiSMASH 3.0—A comprehensive resource for the genome mining of biosynthetic gene clusters. *Nucleic Acids Res.* **2015**, *43*, W237–W243. [CrossRef] [PubMed]
135. Mohimani, H.; Gurevich, A.; Shlemov, A.; Mikheenko, A.; Korobeynikov, A.; Cao, L.; Shcherbin, E.; Nothias, L.-F.; Dorrestein, P.C.; Pevzner, P.A. Dereplication of microbial metabolites through database search of mass spectra. *Nat. Commun.* **2018**, *9*, 4035. [CrossRef] [PubMed]

marine drugs

MDPI

Article

Characterization of Carotenoid Biosynthesis in Newly Isolated *Deinococcus* sp. AJ005 and Investigation of the Effects of Environmental Conditions on Cell Growth and Carotenoid Biosynthesis

Jun Young Choi, Kunjoong Lee and Pyung Cheon Lee *

Department of Molecular Science and Technology and Department of Applied Chemistry and Biological Engineering, Ajou University, Woncheon-dong, Yeongtong-gu, Suwon 16499, Korea; custum@ajou.ac.kr (J.Y.C.); digh0724@ajou.ac.kr (K.L.)

* Correspondence: pclee@ajou.ac.kr; Tel.: +82-31-219-2461

Received: 29 November 2019; Accepted: 11 December 2019; Published: 14 December 2019

Abstract: Our purpose was to characterize the structures of deinoxanthin from *Deinococcus* sp. AJ005. The latter is a novel reddish strain and was found to synthesize two main acyclic carotenoids: deinoxanthin and its derivative. The derivative (2-keto-deinoxanthin) contains a 2-keto functional group instead of a 2-hydroxyl group on a β-ionone ring. A deinoxanthin biosynthesis pathway of *Deinococcus* sp. AJ005 involving eight putative enzymes was proposed according to genome annotation analysis and chemical identification of deinoxanthin. Optimal culture pH and temperature for *Deinococcus* sp. AJ005 growth were pH 7.4 and 20 °C. Sucrose as a carbon source significantly enhanced the cell growth in comparison with glucose, glycerol, maltose, lactose, and galactose. When batch fermentation was performed in a bioreactor containing 40g/L sucrose, total carotenoid production was 650% higher than that in a medium without sucrose supplementation. The culture conditions found in this study should provide the basis for the development of fermentation strategies for the production of deinoxanthin and of its derivative by means of *Deinococcus* sp. AJ005.

Keywords: *Deinococcus*; deinoxanthin; carotenoid

1. Introduction

Deinococcus strains are Gram-positive bacteria having a variety of metabolic pathways. Their habitats range from common environments, such as air, soils, and seas [1–3], to extremes such as high altitudes: stratosphere and alpine conditions [4–6]. Novel *Deinococcus* strains have been continuously isolated from Antarctic and marine fishes in extreme environments [7,8]. Notably, *Deinococcus* strains are known for their survival under strong γ-rays or UV radiation and desiccation conditions [9]. Several studies have shown that, to withstand these extreme environments, *Deinococcus* strains have unique metabolic capabilities including redundant DNA repair systems and biosynthesis of antioxidants such as the carotenoid deinoxanthin [10,11].

The latter is a major monocyclic carotenoid present in many *Deinococcus* strains, and its chemical structure was first characterized using deinoxanthin from *D. radiodurans* featuring high resistance to radiation [12,13]. Deinoxanthin has been reported to be more effective in scavenging very reactive singlet oxygen species (which fatally damage cellular metabolic pathways) than β-carotene, lutein, and lycopene [14,15]. Furthermore, deinoxanthin has anticancer activity [16] and can serve as a biomarker of a living organism in space research [17]. Given that carotenoids, including deinoxanthin, are being used as antioxidants, cosmetic ingredients, and food or feed additives [18,19], carotenoid-producing *Deinococcus* strains have aroused interest as microbial producers of bioactive carotenoids.

Recently, a novel reddish *Deinococcus* strain, AJ005, was isolated from seawater near King George Island, and the AJ005 genome was completely sequenced and made publicly available [20]. *Deinococcus* sp. AJ005 synthesizes red carotenoids, and its complete genome consists of a single circular chromosome (3.3 Mbp) and four circular plasmids (p380k, p115k, p96k, and p17k; Figure 1).

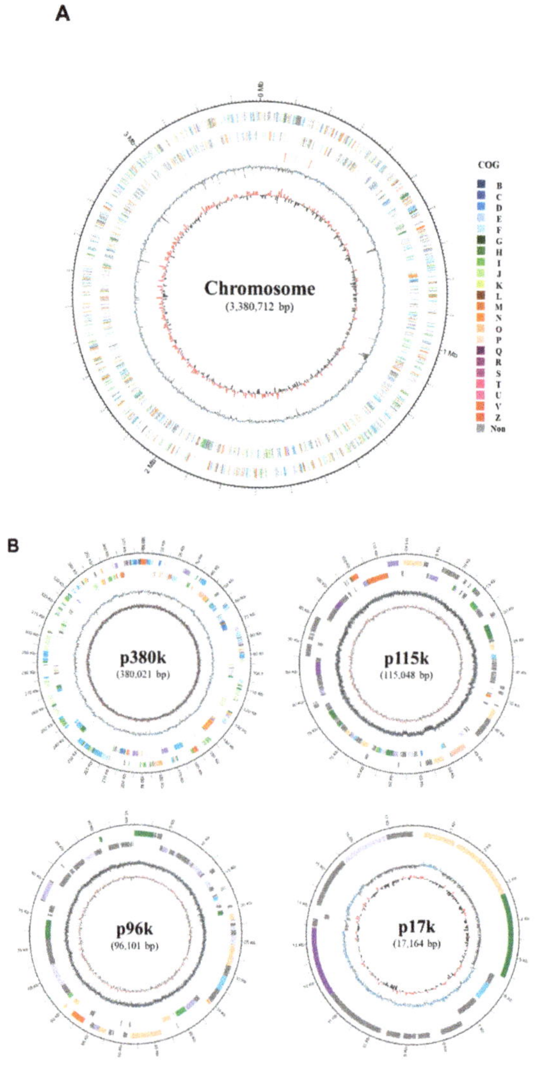

Figure 1. Circular representation of the chromosome and four plasmids of *Deinococcus* sp. AJ005. (**A**) From the outer to inner circle: predicted protein-coding sequences (colored according to Clusters of Orthologous Groups (COGs) categories) on the plus strand, predicted protein-coding sequences (colored by COGs categories) on the minus strand, RNA genes (transfer RNAs (tRNAs): blue, ribosomal RNAs (rRNAs): red), GC content (blue/black), and a GC skew (red/black). (**B**). From the outer to inner circle: predicted protein-coding sequences (colored by COGs categories) on the plus strand, predicted protein-coding sequences (colored by COGs categories) on the minus strand, GC content (blue/black), and a GC skew (red/black).

In this study, our purpose was to characterize the structures of deinoxanthin from *Deinococcus* sp. AJ005. We proposed that a deinoxanthin biosynthetic pathway exists in *Deinococcus* sp. AJ005 on the basis of genome annotation analysis and chemical identification of isolated carotenoids. In addition, we investigated the effects of culture conditions on the deinoxanthin biosynthesis in this strain.

2. Results and Discussion

2.1. Characterization of Carotenoids of Deinococcus Sp. AJ005

To identify carotenoids of *Deinococcus* sp. AJ005, total carotenoids were extracted and analyzed by C18 reverse-phase high-performance liquid chromatography (HPLC). The HPLC analysis of the carotenoid profile yielded two main polar peaks (Figure 2A). After purification by silica chromatography, the two polar carotenoids were analyzed by liquid chromatography with mass spectrometry (MS) in positive APCI (atmospheric-pressure chemical ionization) mode. According to our analysis of mass spectra and UV/Vis spectra, a carotenoid corresponding to peak 1 had a molecular ion $(M+H)^+$ with m/z 581.4 and λ_{max} = 453 (shoulder), 475, and 492 (shoulder) nm (Figure 2B), whereas the carotenoid corresponding to peak 2 had a molecular ion $(M+H)^+$ of m/z 583.4 and λ_{max} = 453 (shoulder), 475, and 492 (shoulder) nm (Figure 2C). The mass fragmentation pattern of peak 2 was similar to the reported pattern of deinoxanthin [21,22]: 565.3 ($(M+H)^+ - 18$; loss of H_2O), 547.4 ($(M+H)^+ - 18 - 18$; loss of 2 molecules of H_2O), and 523.3 ($(M+H)^+ - 60$; loss of the acyclic end containing a hydroxyl group). On the basis of the molecular ion, UV/Vis spectra, and the mass fragmentation pattern, the carotenoid corresponding to peak 2 is proposed to be deinoxanthin. The carotenoid corresponding to peak 1 had the same UV/Vis spectrum as that of deinoxanthin and a mass fragmentation pattern similar to that of deinoxanthin with a difference of −2 m/z: 561.3 ($(M+H)^+ - 18$) in peak 1 versus 565.3 ($(M+H)^+ - 18$) in peak 2 and 521.3 ($(M+H)^+ - 60$) in peak 1 versus 523.3 ($(M+H)^+ - 60$) in peak 2. Therefore, the carotenoid corresponding to peak 1 is proposed to be a deinoxanthin derivative (2-keto-deinoxanthin) containing a 2-keto functional group instead of a 2-hydroxyl functional group in the ring structure. The 2-keto group in 2-keto-deinoxanthin did not significantly influence the shape of the UV/Vis spectrum, resulting in the same UV/Vis spectrum of deinoxanthin.

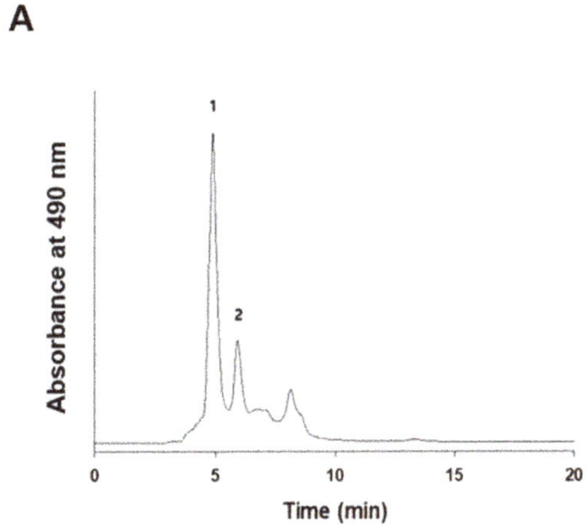

Figure 2. *Cont.*

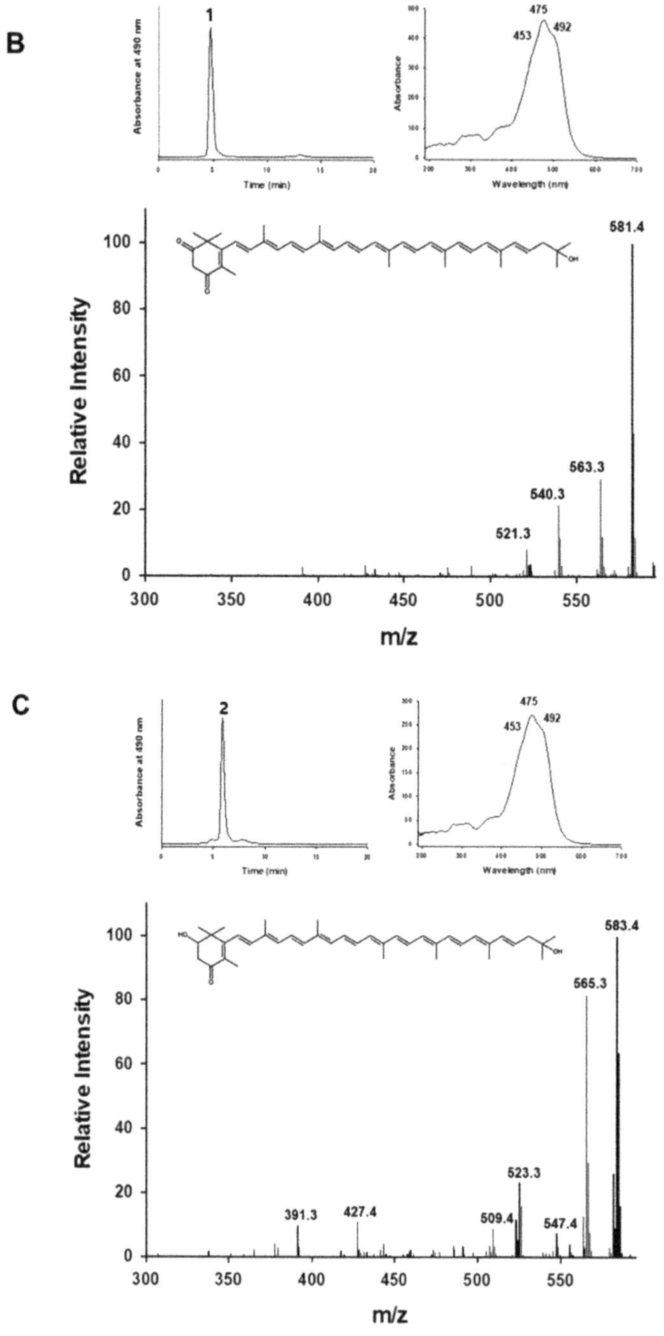

Figure 2. The carotenoid profile of *Deinococcus* sp. AJ005 and MS analysis of the carotenoids. (**A**) The high-performance liquid chromatography (HPLC) profile of a crude carotenoid extract; (**B**) HPLC/mass spectrometry (MS) chromatograms and the UV/Vis spectrum of the isolated deinoxanthin derivative; (**C**) HPLC/MS chromatograms and a UV/Vis spectrum of isolated deinoxanthin.

2.2. The Proposed Carotenoid Biosynthetic Pathway and Genes Encoding Putative Carotenogenic Enzymes in Deinococcus Sp. AJ005

Genome annotation analysis predicted seven genes encoding the putative deinoxanthin pathway enzymes on the chromosome of *Deinococcus* sp. AJ005: GGPP synthase (*crtE*), phytoene synthase (*crtB*), phytoene desaturase (*crtI*), lycopene cyclase (*crtLm*), β-carotene 4-ketolase (*crtO*), C-1′,2′ hydratase (*cruF*), and C-3′,4′ desaturase (*crtD*). Unfortunately, a gene encoding 2-β-ionone ring hydroxylase for the deinoxanthin biosynthesis and a gene encoding 2-β-ionone ring oxygenase for the biosynthesis of the deinoxanthin derivative (2-keto-deinoxanthin) were not found. Nonetheless, there was a gene encoding a putative cytochrome P450 (which might be a 2-β-ionone ring hydroxylase) on the chromosome of *Deinococcus* sp. AJ005. A recent study [22] showed that the cytochrome P450 CYP287A1 of *D. radiodurans* R1 is a novel 2-β-ionone ring hydroxylase in the deinoxanthin pathway. The BLASTp analysis revealed that there is a 70% amino acid identity between the putative cytochrome P450 of *Deinococcus* sp. AJ005 and the cytochrome P450 CYP287A1 of *D. radiodurans* R1. In addition to the above eight genes, one gene coding for a putative lycopene elongase (*crtEb*), two genes encoding a putative phytoene dehydrogenase, two genes encoding a putative cytochrome P450 hydroxylase, and one gene encoding a possible cytochrome P450 were predicted on the chromosome of *Deinococcus* sp. AJ005. According to the chemical identification of deinoxanthin and of the deinoxanthin derivative from the crude carotenoid extract of *Deinococcus* sp. AJ005 and according to the putative carotenogenic enzymes, a carotenoid pathway of *Deinococcus* sp. AJ005 was proposed (Figure 3). Functional analysis of the putative enzymes (in particular three cytochrome P450s) needs to be performed to elucidate the proposed carotenoid pathway.

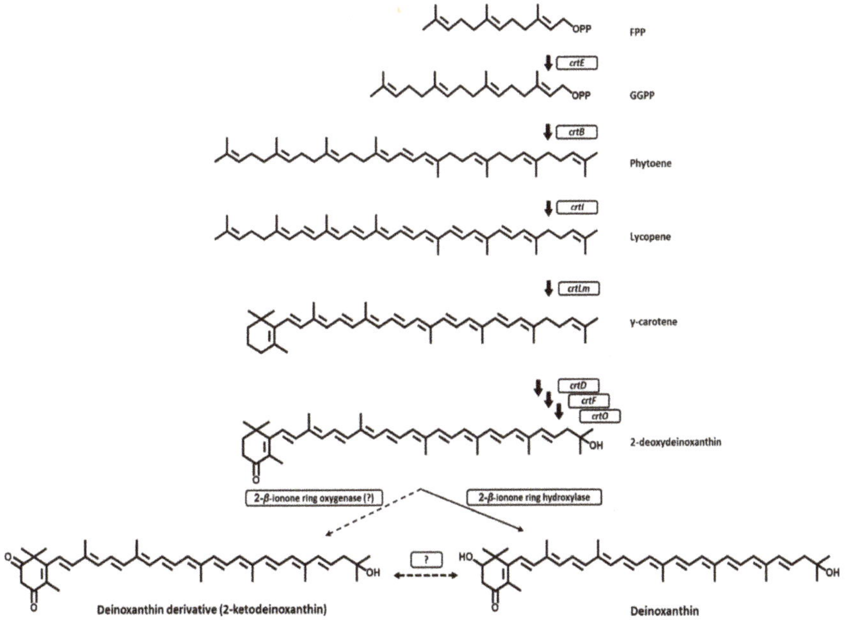

Figure 3. Proposed biosynthetic pathways for deinoxanthin and for its derivative in *Deinococcus* sp. AJ005[T]. The following enzymes are involved in these biosynthetic pathways: CrtE, GGPP synthase; CrtB, phytoene synthase; CrtI, phytoene desaturase; CrtLm, lycopene cyclase; CrtO, β-carotene 4-ketolase; CruF, C-1′,2′ hydratase; CrtD, C-3′,4′ desaturase; 2-β-ionone ring hydroxylase; and 2-β-ionone ring oxygenase (unidentified). The ? mark represents the possibility of oxido-reduction catalyzed by an unknown enzyme.

2.3. *Effects of Culture Media, Culture pH, and Temperature on Cell Growth*

To investigate the effects of culture media, culture pH, temperature, and a carbon source on the growth of *Deinococcus* sp. AJ005 cells, 100 mL flask cultures were carried out. Among several media (Luria–Bertani (LB), Terrific Broth (TB), Marine Broth 2216 (MB), and Tryptone-Glucose-Yeast extract (TGY) broth) containing 1 g/L glucose and with pH adjusted to 7.5, the growth of *Deinococcus* sp. AJ005 cells reached the highest OD_{600} of 4.3 ± 0.1 in the TGY medium at 20 °C, followed by the TB, LB, and MB media (Figure 4A). Next, the effects of culture pH and temperature on the growth of *Deinococcus* sp. AJ005 cells were studied in the TGY medium containing 1 g/L glucose. An initial culture pH of 7.4 at 20 °C was found to be optimal for cell growth (OD_{600} of 6.4 ± 0.1), and pH values above 7.6 or below 6.8 significantly reduced the cell growth (Figure 4B). At culture temperatures of 18 °C and 20 °C, the cell growth reached the highest OD_{600} of 5.5 ± 0.3 in the TGY medium containing 1 g/L glucose and with pH adjusted to 7.4. No growth was observed below 4 °C or above 28 °C (Figure 4C). Carbon sources significantly affected the growth of *Deinococcus* sp. AJ005 cells. When *Deinococcus* sp. AJ005 was grown in the TGY medium containing 10 g/L one of six carbon sources (i.e., glucose, glycerol, maltose, lactose, galactose, or sucrose); the greatest cell growth (OD_{600} of 5.3 ± 0.2) was observed in the TGY medium containing sucrose, followed by glycerol, maltose, galactose, lactose, and glucose (Figure 4D).

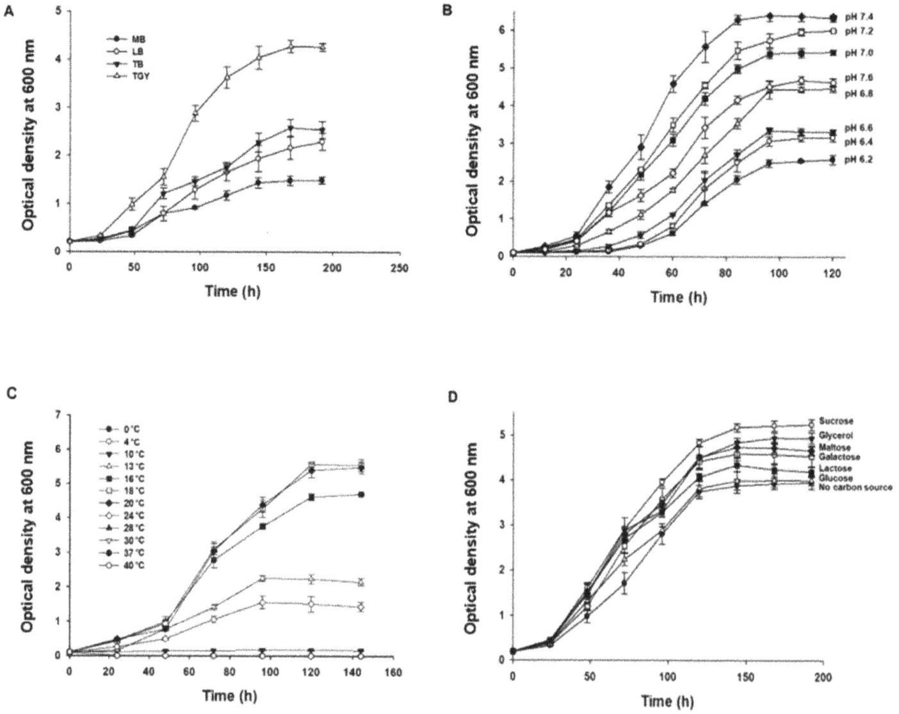

Figure 4. Cell growth of *Deinococcus* sp. AJ005^T in flask cultures under different culture conditions. (**A**) Four culture media (pH 7.5 and 20 °C); (**B**) eight culture pH values (20 °C); (**C**) 12 culture temperatures (pH 7.4); and (**D**) six carbon sources (10 g/L, 20 °C, and pH 7.4).

2.4. *Batch Fermentation Involving Deinococcus sp. AJ005 for Carotenoid Production*

To achieve high production of deinoxanthin and of the deinoxanthin derivative, bioreactor fermentation with *Deinococcus* sp. AJ005 was performed at 20 °C and pH 7.4 in the TGY medium containing 0, 20, or 40 g/L sucrose. In the TGY medium containing 0 g/L sucrose, the cell growth reached an OD_{600} of 7.3 ± 0.3, and the maximum specific growth rate was 0.085 h^{-1} (Figure 5A). In the TGY medium containing 20 g/L sucrose, the cell growth reached an OD_{600} of 11.2 ± 0.7, and the maximum specific growth rate was 0.12 h^{-1} (Figure 5B). We noticed that 20 g/L sucrose was completely consumed in 72 h. In the TGY medium containing 40 g/L sucrose, the cell growth reached an OD_{600} of 16.1 ± 0.6, and the maximum specific growth rate was 0.18 h^{-1} (Figure 5C), whereas 40 g/L sucrose was completely consumed in 90 h. Total carotenoid production was proportional to the cell growth (Figure 5D). Total carotenoid production in the TGY medium containing 40 g/L sucrose was 650% higher than that in the TGY medium containing 0 g/L sucrose and 80% higher than that in the TGY medium containing 20 g/L sucrose.

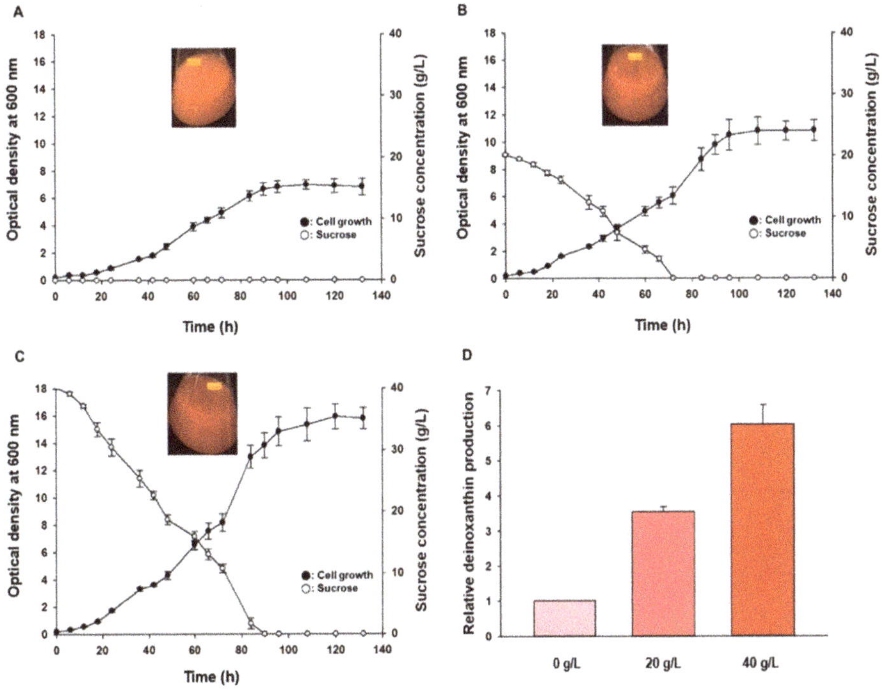

Figure 5. Bioreactor batch fermentation of the TGY(medium (containing different concentrations of sucrose) by *Deinococcus* sp. AJ005. (**A**) 0 g/L sucrose (**B**); 20 g/L sucrose; (**C**) 40 g/L sucrose; (**D**) relative carotenoid production in the medium containing 0, 20, or 40 g/L sucrose.

3. Materials and Methods

3.1. Flask Fermentation Involving Deinococcus Sp. AJ005

Deinococcus sp. AJ005, isolated from seawater near King George Island, was grown in 100 mL of a culture medium in a 500 mL baffled flask with rotary shaking at 250 rpm at various pH levels and temperatures as described below. Luria-bertani, TB, MB, and TGY media containing 1 g/L glucose were used for growing *Deinococcus* sp. AJ005 at 20 °C and pH 7.5. To investigate the influence of culture pH on the cell growth, *Deinococcus* sp. AJ005 was grown in 100 mL of the TGY medium containing 1 g/L glucose and with pH adjusted to 6.2–7.6 in increments of 0.2 by means of the phosphate buffer system. To investigate the impact of culture temperature on the cell growth, *Deinococcus* sp. AJ005 was grown at 0, 2, 4, 10, 13, 16, 18, 20, 24, 28, 30, 37, or 40 °C in 100 mL of the TGY medium containing 1 g/L glucose and with pH adjusted to 7.4. Glucose, glycerol, maltose, lactose, galactose, and sucrose (Sigma–Aldrich) served as a carbon source (10 g/L) in the TGY medium with pH adjusted to 7.4.

3.2. Bioreactor Fermentation by Deinococcus Sp. AJ005

Bioreactor batch fermentation was carried out with 1.5 L of the TGY medium containing sucrose (0, 20, or 40 g/L) as a carbon source in 5 L jar BioFlo 320 (Eppendorf, Hamburg, Germany). Pre-cultures (100 mL) were grown in the TGY medium at 20 °C for 1 day and inoculated into a bioreactor. The temperature was maintained at 20 °C, and pH was automatically maintained at 7.4 by adding 2.0 N HCl or 2.0 N NaOH. The dissolved oxygen level was maintained at 30% by supplying air and by adjusting agitation between 200 and 500 rpm.

3.3. Extraction and Analysis of Carotenoids

Deinococcus sp. AJ005 was grown in 1 L of the TGY medium. Carotenoids were repeatedly extracted from cell pellets of *Deinococcus* sp. AJ005 by means of 10 mL of methanol. The colored supernatants were concentrated to 10 mL in an EZ-2 Plus centrifugal evaporator (Genevac Inc., Ipswich, United Kingdom), and an equal volume of ethyl acetate and of a 5N NaCl solution was added. The upper colored phase was collected, washed with distilled water, passed through an anhydrous magnesium sulfate column, and completely dried with nitrogen gas. Carotenoids were purified from the crude carotenoid extract by silica chromatography (10 × 50 cm) based on silica gel 60 (Merck, Darmstadt, Germany). Elution was performed with hexane:acetone (6.5:3.5 *v*/*v*). Each purified carotenoid was completely dried and dissolved in methanol. Next, 10 μL of a carotenoid was injected into an Agilent 1200 HPLC system equipped with a ZORBAX SB-C18 column (4.6 × 250 mm, 5-micron, Agilent Technologies, Santa Clara, California, USA) and with a photodiode array detector (Agilent Technologies, USA). Each carotenoid was subjected to diode array detection at 480 nm wavelength. The HPLC conditions were as follows: 23 °C column temperature, a 0.8 mL/min flow rate, and an isocratic mobile phase of acetonitrile, methanol, and isopropyl alcohol (40:50:10 *v*/*v*/*v*). The mass fragmentation spectra of carotenoids were monitored in the positive ion mode of an Agilent LC/MS 6150 Quadrupole system equipped with an atmospheric-pressure chemical ionization interface (Agilent Technologies). The MS conditions were as follows: 3 kV capillary voltage, 4.0 μA corona current, 12 L/min drying gas flow, 35 psi_g nebulizer pressure, and 350 °C drying gas temperature and vaporizer temperature.

3.4. Monitoring Cell Growth and Quantification of Carbohydrates and Carotenoids

Cell growth was monitored by measuring the absorbance at 600 nm (OD_{600}) with a SPECTRAmax Plus384 spectrophotometer (Molecular Devices, San Jose, California, USA). The concentrations of glucose, glycerol, maltose, lactose, galactose, and sucrose were determined using an Agilent 1100 HPLC system equipped with a refractive index detector (Agilent, Santa Clara, California, USA) and an Aminex HPX-87H column (Bio-Rad, Hercules, California, USA) at a flow rate of 0.7 mL/min and column temperature of 50 °C, with 4 mM H_2SO_4 as the mobile phase. The total-carotenoid amount was measured via the absorbance of the methanol extract at a wavelength of 475 nm on the SPECTRAmax Plus384 spectrophotometer.

4. Conclusions

Deinococcus sp. AJ005 synthesizes two main types of acyclic carotenoids: deinoxanthin and a deinoxanthin derivative (2-keto-deinoxanthin). Genome sequence analysis of deinoxanthin-producing *Deinococcus* sp. AJ005 uncovered eight genes encoding putative deinoxanthin biosynthesis enzymes. The culture conditions found in this study should provide the basis for the development of fermentation strategies for the production of deinoxanthin and of its derivative by means of *Deinococcus* sp. AJ005.

Author Contributions: J.Y.C., K.L., and P.C.L. planned and designed the experiments. J.Y.C. and K.L. performed the experiments and analyzed data. P.C.L. drafted the manuscript. P.C.L. coordinated the study and finalized the manuscript. All authors read and approved the final manuscript.

Funding: This research was funded by the National Research Foundation of Korea, grant number 2012M1A2A2026562, and by the Priority Research Centers Program through the National Research Foundation of Korea, grant number 2019R1A6A11051471.

Conflicts of Interest: The authors declare no conflict of interest. The funders had no role in the design of the study; in the collection, analyses, or interpretation of data; in the writing of the manuscript, or in the decision to publish the results.

References

1. Yoo, S.H.; Weon, H.Y.; Kim, S.J.; Kim, Y.S.; Kim, B.Y.; Kwon, S.W. *Deinococcus aerolatus* sp. nov. and *Deinococcus aerophilus* sp. nov., isolated from air samples. *Int. J. Syst. Evol. Microbiol.* **2010**, *60*, 1191–1195. [CrossRef] [PubMed]
2. Dong, N.; Li, H.R.; Yuan, M.; Zhang, X.H.; Yu, Y. *Deinococcus antarcticus* sp. nov., isolated from soil. *Int. J. Syst. Evol. Microbiol.* **2015**, *65*, 331–335. [CrossRef] [PubMed]
3. Rainey, F.A.; Ray, K.; Ferreira, M.; Gatz, B.Z.; Nobre, F.; Bagaley, D.; Rash, B.A.; Park, M.J.; Earl, A.M.; Shank, N.C.; et al. Extensive Diversity of Ionizing-Radiation-Resistant Bacteria Recovered from Sonoran Desert Soil and Description of Nine New Species of the Genus *Deinococcus* Obtained from a Single Soil Sample. *Appl. Environ. Microbiol.* **2005**, *71*, 5225–5235. [CrossRef] [PubMed]
4. Yang, Y.; Itoh, T.; Yokobori, S.; Itahashi, S.; Shimada, H.; Satoh, K.; Ohba, H.; Narumi, I.; Yamagishi, A. *Deinococcus aerius* sp. nov., isolated from the high atmosphere. *Int. J. Syst. Evol. Microbiol.* **2009**, *59*, 1862–1866. [CrossRef]
5. Yang, Y.; Itoh, T.; Yokobori, S.; Shimada, H.; Itahashi, S.; Satoh, K.; Ohba, H.; Narumi, I.; Yamagishi, A. *Deinococcus aetherius* sp. nov., isolated from the stratosphere. *Int. J. Syst. Evol. Microbiol.* **2010**, *60*, 776–779. [CrossRef]
6. Callegan, R.P.; Nobre, M.F.; McTernan, P.M.; Battista, J.R.; Navarro-Gonzalez, R.; McKay, C.P.; da Costa, M.S.; Rainey, F.A. Description of four novel psychrophilic, ionizing radiation-sensitive *Deinococcus* species from alpine environments. *Int. J. Syst. Evol. Microbiol.* **2008**, *58*, 1252–1258. [CrossRef]
7. Shashidhar, R.; Bandekar, J.R. *Deinococcus piscis* sp. nov., a radiation-resistant bacterium isolated from a marine fish. *Int. J. Syst. Evol. Microbiol.* **2009**, *59*, 2714–2717. [CrossRef]
8. Hirsch, P.; Gallikowski, C.A.; Siebert, J.; Peissl, K.; Kroppenstedt, R.; Schumann, P.; Stackebrandt, E.; Anderson, R. *Deinococcus frigens* sp. nov., *Deinococcus saxicola* sp. nov., and *Deinococcus marmoris* sp. nov., low temperature and draught-tolerating, UV-resistant bacteria from continental Antarctica. *Int. J. Syst. Evol. Microbiol.* **2004**, *27*, 636–645. [CrossRef]
9. Cox, M.M.; Keck, J.L.; Battista, J.R. Rising from the Ashes: DNA Repair in *Deinococcus radiodurans*. *PLoS Genet.* **2010**, *6*, e1000815. [CrossRef]
10. Lange, C.C.; Wackett, L.P.; Minton, K.W.; Daly, M.J. Engineering a recombinant *Deinococcus radiodurans* for organopollutant degradation in radioactive mixed waste environments. *Netw. Address Transl.* **1998**, *16*, 929–933. [CrossRef]
11. Brim, H.; Osborne, J.P.; Kostandarithes, H.M.; Fredrickson, J.K.; Wackett, L.P.; Daly, M.J. *Deinococcus radiodurans* engineered for complete toluene degradation facilitates Cr(VI) reduction. *Microbiology* **2006**, *152*, 2469–2477. [CrossRef] [PubMed]
12. Lemee, L.; Peuchant, E.; Clerc, M.; Brunner, M.; Pfander, H. Deinoxanthin: A new carotenoid isolated from *Deinococcus Radiodurans*. *Tetrahedron Lett.* **1997**, *53*, 919–926. [CrossRef]
13. Bamji, M.S.; Krinsky, N.I. The carotenoid pigments of a radiation-resistant *Micrococcus* species. *Biochim. Biophys. Acta* **1966**, *115*, 276–284. [CrossRef]
14. Ji, H.F. Insight into the strong antioxidant activity of deinoxanthin, a unique carotenoid in *Deinococcus radiodurans*. *Int. J. Mol. Sci.* **2010**, *11*, 4506–4510. [CrossRef] [PubMed]
15. Tian, B.; Xu, Z.; Sun, Z.; Lin, J.; Hua, Y. Evaluation of the antioxidant effects of carotenoids from *Deinococcus radiodurans* through targeted mutagenesis, chemiluminescence, and DNA damage analyses. *Biochim. Biophys. Acta* **2007**, *1770*, 902–911. [CrossRef] [PubMed]
16. Choi, Y.J.; Hur, J.M.; Lim, S.; Jo, M.; Kim, D.H.; Choi, J.I. Induction of apoptosis by deinoxanthin in human cancer cells. *Anticancer Res.* **2014**, *34*, 1829–1835. [PubMed]

17. Leuko, S.; Bohmeier, M.; Hanke, F.; Boettger, U.; Rabbow, E.; Parpart, A.; Rettberg, P.; de Vera, J.P. On the Stability of Deinoxanthin Exposed to Mars Conditions during a Long-Term Space Mission and Implications for Biomarker Detection on Other Planets. *Front. Microbiol.* **2017**, *8*, 1680. [CrossRef]
18. Schmidt, R. Deactivation of O2(1Δg) Singlet Oxygen by Carotenoids: Internal Conversion of Excited Encounter Complexes. *J. Phys. Chem. A* **2004**, *108*, 5509–5513. [CrossRef]
19. Mayne, S.T. Beta-carotene, carotenoids, and disease prevention in humans. *FASEB J.* **1996**, *10*, 690–701. [CrossRef]
20. Choi, J.Y.; Lee, K.; Lee, P.C. Complete genome sequence of the carotenoid-producing *Deinococcus* sp. strain AJ005. *Microbiol. Resour. Announc.* **2019**, *8*, e01245-19. [CrossRef]
21. Hansler, A.; Chen, Q.; Ma, Y.; Gross, S.S. Untargeted metabolite profiling reveals that nitric oxide bioynthesis is an endogenous modulator of carotenoid biosynthesis in *Deinococcus radiodurans* and is required for extreme ionizing radiation resistance. *Arch. Biochem.* **2016**, *589*, 38–52. [CrossRef] [PubMed]
22. Zhou, Z.; Zhang, W.; Su, S.; Chen, M.; Lu, W.; Lin, M.; Molnar, I.; Xu, Y. CYP287A1 is a carotenoid 2-beta-hydroxylase required for deinoxanthin biosynthesis in *Deinococcus radiodurans* R1. *Appl. Microbiol. Biotechnol.* **2015**, *99*, 10539–10546. [CrossRef] [PubMed]

marine drugs

Article

Synthesis of Bioactive Silver Nanoparticles by a *Pseudomonas* Strain Associated with the Antarctic Psychrophilic Protozoon *Euplotes focardii*

Maria Sindhura John [1], Joseph Amruthraj Nagoth [1], Kesava Priyan Ramasamy [1], Alessio Mancini [1], Gabriele Giuli [2], Antonino Natalello [3], Patrizia Ballarini [1], Cristina Miceli [1] and Sandra Pucciarelli [1,*]

1 School of Biosciences and Veterinary Medicine, University of Camerino, 62032 Camerino, Italy; sindhuramaria@gmail.com (M.S.J.); amruthjon@gmail.com (J.A.N.); kesavanlife@gmail.com (K.P.R.); alessio.mancini@unicam.it (A.M.); patrizia.ballarini@unicam.it (P.B.); cristina.miceli@unicam.it (C.M.)
2 School of Sciences and Technology, University of Camerino, 62032 Camerino, Italy; gabriele.giuli@unicam.it
3 Department of Biotechnology and Biosciences, University of Milano-Bicocca, 20126 Milano, Italy; antonino.natalello@unimib.it
* Correspondence: sandra.pucciarelli@unicam.it; Tel.: +39-0737-403231

Received: 30 November 2019; Accepted: 31 December 2019; Published: 3 January 2020

Abstract: The synthesis of silver nanoparticles (AgNPs) by microorganisms recently gained a greater interest due to its potential to produce them in various sizes and morphologies. In this study, for AgNP biosynthesis, we used a new *Pseudomonas* strain isolated from a consortium associated with the Antarctic marine ciliate *Euplotes focardii*. After incubation of *Pseudomonas* cultures with 1 mM of $AgNO_3$ at 22 °C, we obtained AgNPs within 24 h. Scanning electron (SEM) and transmission electron microscopy (TEM) revealed spherical polydispersed AgNPs in the size range of 20–70 nm. The average size was approximately 50 nm. Energy dispersive X-ray spectroscopy (EDS) showed the presence of a high intensity absorption peak at 3 keV, a distinctive property of nanocrystalline silver products. Fourier transform infrared (FTIR) spectroscopy found the presence of a high amount of AgNP-stabilizing proteins and other secondary metabolites. X-ray diffraction (XRD) revealed a face-centred cubic (fcc) diffraction spectrum with a crystalline nature. A comparative study between the chemically synthesized and *Pseudomonas* AgNPs revealed a higher antibacterial activity of the latter against common nosocomial pathogen microorganisms, including *Escherichia coli, Staphylococcus aureus* and *Candida albicans*. This study reports an efficient, rapid synthesis of stable AgNPs by a new *Pseudomonas* strain with high antimicrobial activity.

Keywords: green synthesis biomaterials; silver nitrate; antibiotics; nanotechnology

1. Introduction

Nanotechnology has become an emerging field in the area of biotechnology, dealing with the synthesis, design and manipulation of particles with approximate sizes from 1 to 100 nm. Nanoparticles (NPs) are used in biomedical sciences, healthcare, drug–gene delivery, space industries, cosmetics, chemical industries, optoelectronics, etc. [1]. Various physiochemical methods have been used for AgNP synthesis, including microwave, biochemical and electrochemical synthesis, chemical reduction (aqueous and non-aqueous), irradiation, ultrasonic-associated, photo-induced, photo-catalytic and microemulsion methods. However, these methodologies have various disadvantages because they imply high energy consumption and the use of toxic reagents with the generation of hazardous waste, which causes potential risks to the environment and human health [2,3]. In these days, there is a growing need to develop simple, cost-effective, reliable, bio-compatible and eco-friendly approaches for the synthesis of nanomaterials, which do not contain toxic chemicals in the synthesis protocols. For mining the metallic nanomaterials, microbial-mediated green synthesis has recently been considered as a promising source [4]. Green synthesis of nanoparticles represents a cost-effective and environmentally friendly method with advantages over conventional methods that involve chemical, potentially toxic solvents. For green NP synthesis, the most important issues are the solvent medium combined with the selection of ecologically nontoxic, reducing and stabilizing agents [5]. There are different green methods for nanoparticle synthesis, but the most commonly appreciated is through bacteria, because bacteria are usually easy to grow [6]. Capping agents are considered fundamental for nanoparticles stabilization. Capped AgNPs are known to exhibit better antibacterial activity with respect to uncapped AgNPs [7]. Biologically synthesized nanoparticles have remarkable potential since they can be easily coated with a lipid/protein layer, which confers physiological solubility and stability useful for applications in biomedicine [8].

AgNPs possess general antibacterial and bactericidal properties. These are mostly against methicillin-resistant strains [9]. Gram-negative and Gram-positive bacteria are relevant causes of numerous infections in hospitals. Due to the increased microbial resistance to multiple antibiotics [10], many researchers are interested in developing novel and effective antimicrobial agents [11]. Furthermore, AgNPs exhibit anti-biofilm activities [12] and synergistic activities with diverse antibiotics, such as β-lactams, macrolides and lincosamides [13]. The use of silver-coated antiseptics shows a broad-spectrum activity and a far lower chance than antibiotics in inducing the typical microbial resistance [14].

The mechanism at the basis of the extracellular synthesis of nanoparticles using microbes appears based on enzymes such as the secreted nitrate reductase that helps in the production of metal nanoparticles from metal ions [15]. Such mechanism was shown in *Bacillus licheniformis* [16]. The biosynthesis and stabilization of nanoparticles in *Stenotrophomonas maltophilia* via charge capping, involving the electron shuttle enzymatic metal reduction process produced by the Nicotinamide Adenine Dinucleotide Phosphate (NADPH)-dependent reductase enzyme, has also been reported [17]. In *Pseudomonas* spp., a possible process for the biosynthesis of AgNPs is described, to be performed by a Nicotinamide Adenine Dinucleotide (NADH)-dependent nitrate reductase [18,19]. The enzyme may be responsible for the reduction of Ag^+ to Ag^0 and the subsequent formation of AgNPs, where the NADH-dependent reductase is expected to act as a carrier while the bioreduction occurs by means of the electrons from NADH [18,19].

The aim of this study is to develop a simple and low-cost approach for AgNP intracellular synthesis using a new Pseudomonas strain isolated from a consortium associated with the psychrophilic marine ciliated protozoon Euplotes focardii [20], which we named Pseudomonas sp. ef1 [21]. E. focardii is a free-swimming ciliate endemic of the oligotrophic coastal sediments of the Antarctic Terra Nova Bay [22]. It has been maintained in cultures for more than 20 years after the first isolation. E. focardii's optimal growing temperature is about 4–5 °C, with a drop at 8–10 °C and not surviving if exposed to temperatures over 10 °C [22]. We showed that the AgNPs produced by Pseudomonas sp. ef1 possess higher antimicrobial activity with respect to those chemically synthesized, which could be used against common pathogenic microorganisms.

2. Results and Discussion

2.1. Biosynthesis of AgNPs and UV–Vis Spectroscopy Characterization

We primarily investigated the biosynthesis of AgNPs by *Pseudomonas* sp. ef1 through the observation of the culture medium colour change by incubation of the bacterial biomass with 1 mM $AgNO_3$ at 22 °C (the optimal growing temperature of *Pseudomonas* sp. ef1). A change in colour from white to brown occurred within 24 h in the presence of light (Figure S1). The change to a brown colour of the culture was maintained for 72 h (Figure S1A,B). No colour change was observed in the control culture containing the heat-killed bacterial biomass with 1 mM $AgNO_3$ (data not shown).

Medium colour change related to extracellular synthesis of AgNPs has been previously reported in another *Pseudomonas* culture [23], as well as in *Bacillus methylotrophicus* [24] and *Actinobacteria* SL19 and SL24 strains, and in fungi as Fusarium semitectum, *Aspergillus fumigatus* [25] and Streptomyces sp. The culture medium colour change is attributed to the excitation of the surface plasmon resonance of AgNPs [26,27].

Pseudomonas sp. ef1 AgNPs formation was confirmed by UV–vis spectroscopy, considered one of the most valuable methods for the characterization of the optical response of metal nanoparticles, including AgNPs. This method has been demonstrated to be appropriately sensitive to check AgNPs' intense surface plasmon resonances (SPRs) [28] in the range of 350–600 nm [29–31]. A 0.1 mL aliquot of the *Pseudomonas* sp. ef1 culture was diluted with 0.9 mL of ddH2O and UV–visible spectra was recorded from 300 to 800 nm wavelength at room temperature: A relevant peak at about 420 nm was found (Figure S1C), as also reported for AgNPs produced by *Pseudomonas* putida NCIM 2650 [32] and Pseudomonas sp. (JQ989348) [33]. By contrast, *Pseudomonas* sp. "ram bt-1" AgNPs showed absorbance spectra at 430 nm [34]. The presence of a single SPR peak suggests AgNPs of spherical shape [35].

2.2. Morphology and Chemical Composition of Pseudomonas sp. ef1 AgNPs

We performed scanning electron microscopy (SEM) to define the size and shape of the AgNPs synthesized by *Pseudomonas* sp. ef1. SEM images (Figure S2A,A') revealed polydispersed (i.e., non-uniform in size) AgNPs of spherical shape. Their size ranged from 20 to about 100 nm.

To better understand the surface morphology and for getting additional information on the size, a TEM investigation was conducted (Figure 1). Aliquots of AgNP solution were placed onto a nitrocellulose- and Formvar-coated copper grid and maintained to dry under room conditions. TEM micrographs suggested particle sizes around 10 nm (clearly visible in Figure 1A) to 70 nm (Figure 1B), with the average size being 50 nm. The particles showed a spherical shape, well separated from each other even when these formed aggregates, suggesting the presence of capping peptides around each particle, whose role is to stabilize the nanoparticles.

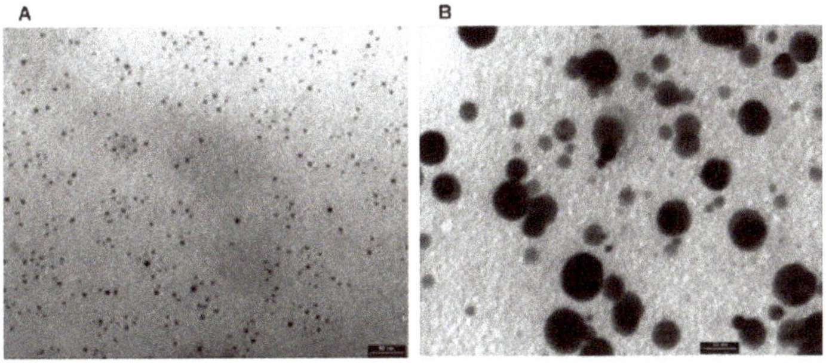

Figure 1. Transmission electron microscopy (TEM) micrographs of *Pseudomonas* sp. ef1 silver nanoparticles (AgNPs). The particles show a spherical shape with size from 10 nm (**A**) to 70 nm (**B**), with the average size being 50 nm. Bars: 50 nm

Pseudomonas sp. ef1 AgNPs appear similar to those produced by other *Pseudomonas* [36–42]. The TEM grid analysis of *Pseudomonas* sp. ef1 bio-AgNPs revealed smooth-surfaced polydispersed particles, approximately spherical in shape with the size ranging from 12.5 to 100 nm. By contrast, bio-AgNPs from Pseudomonas putida were monodispersed and smaller in size (6 to 16 nm) [43].

The chemical composition of the *Pseudomonas* sp. ef1 AgNPs was obtained by energy dispersive X-ray (EDX) spectrum analysis (Figure 2). We observed an intense signal of Ag at 3 keV, which confirmed the presence of AgNPs. Metallic AgNPs are typically reported to show a strong signal peak at 3 keV, due to surface plasmon resonance [44,45]. However, other element (C, N and O) signals were detected at normal mode (Figure 2 and Table 1). These elements probably derive from the emissions of the capping proteins. The EDX spectrum analysis of Pseudomonas fluorescens CA 417 AgNPS also showed the presence of a high intensity absorption peak at 3 keV [46].

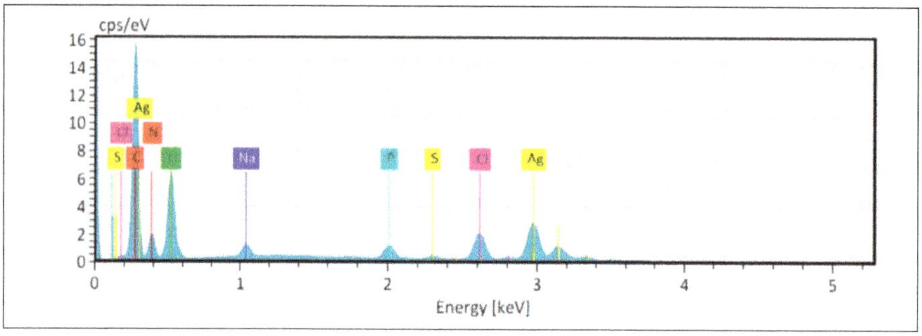

Figure 2. EDAX investigation of *Pseudomonas* sp. ef1 AgNPs. A: EDAX spectrum of AgNPs; Ag, C, N and O indicate the silver (the highest peak, recorded at 3 keV), carbon, nitrogen and oxygen signals (the relative amounts are reported in Table 1).

Table 1. Quantitative EDAX results of *Pseudomonas* sp. ef1 AgNPs.

Element	At.No	Netto	Mass [%]	Mass Norm [%]	Atom [%]	Abs. err [%] 1 sigma	rel err [%] 1 sigma
Carbon	6	197121	22.22	29.78	48.86	2.45	11.01
Nitrogen	7	27658	7.08	9.49	13.35	0.90	12.76
Oxygen	8	90933	15.84	21.22	26.15	1.82	11.48
Sodium	11	16435	1.20	1.61	1.38	0.10	8.09
Phosphorus	15	22015	1.45	1.95	1.24	0.08	5.60
Sulfur	16	4429	0.32	0.43	0.26	0.04	11.83
Chlorine	17	51613	4.53	6.07	3.38	0.18	4.02
Silver	47	127532	21.98	29.46	5.38	0.76	3.45
Sum			**74.64**	**100.00**	**100.00**		

2.3. *Capping Proteins and Crystalline Structure of Pseudomonas sp. AgNPs*

To confirm the potential interactions between the silver salts and the capping proteins, which could account for the reduction of Ag^{+} ions with consequent stabilization of AgNPs, we performed FTIR measurements (Figure 3A). The amide linkages between the amino acid residues in proteins produce a typical signature in the infrared spectral region [47].

The FTIR spectrum of *Pseudomonas* sp. ef1 AgNPs is characterized by the protein Amide A, B, I, II and III bands (Figure 3). In particular, the peaks around 3280 cm^{-1} (Amide A) and 3070 cm^{-1} (Amide B) are mainly assigned to the NH vibrations. The absorption maximum of the Amide I band, due to the C=O stretching of the peptide bond, occurs around 1632 cm^{-1}. The Amide II band, mainly due to the amide NH bending, peaked around 1538 cm^{-1}. The complex absorption in the 1200–950 cm^{-1} spectral region can be tentatively assigned to carbohydrate absorption. The 1740 cm^{-1} peak is characteristic of C=O carbonyl groups [48].

The overall FTIR pattern confirms that capping proteins are present in the AgNPs and that these proteins are not extensively aggregated. Protein–nanoparticle interactions are produced either through free amine groups or cysteine residues and through the electrostatic attraction of negatively charged carboxylate groups, specifically in enzymes [49]. The free amine and carbonyl groups of bacterial proteins could possibly be responsible for the formation and stabilization of AgNPs [50,51].

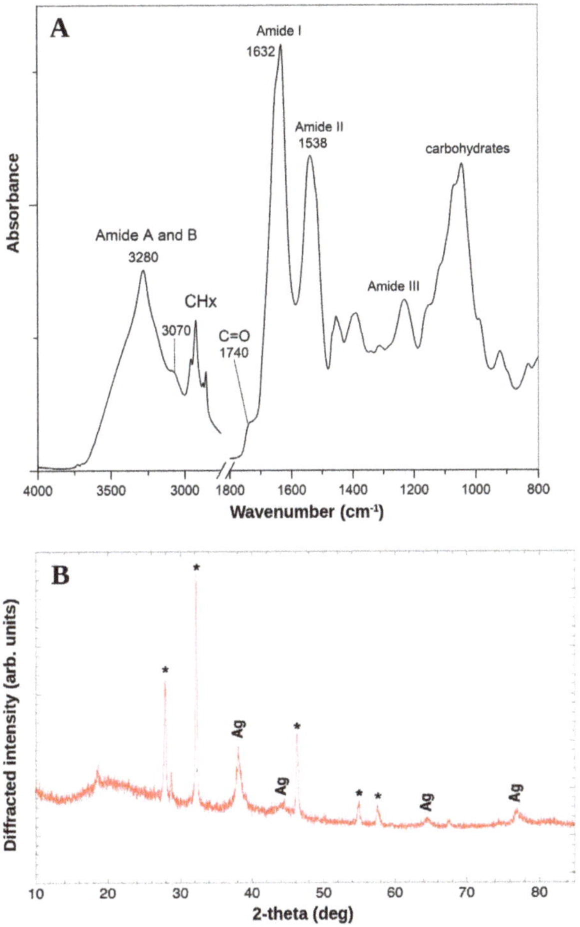

Figure 3. (**A**) FTIR absorption spectrum of *Pseudomonas* sp. ef1 AgNPs. The peak position and the assignment of the main components are reported. (**B**) XRD spectrum recorded for *Pseudomonas* sp. ef1 AgNPs. Four intense peaks at 38.95°, 45.12°, 65.39° and 78.12° correspond to plane values of (1 1 1), (2 0 0), (2 2 0) and (3 1 1) at the 2θ angle, which were consistent with the standard data JCPDS file no. 01-087-0717, indicated by asterisks.

The capping proteins prevent aggregation and provide nanoparticle stability [52]. Fourier transform infrared spectrum applied to the deep-sea bacterium Pseudomonas sp. JQ989348 AgNPs showed the presence of proteins in large amounts, as well as other secondary metabolites [33].

The crystalline structure of Pseudomonas sp. ef1 AgNPs was confirmed by XRD analysis (Figure 3B). The AgNPs diffraction spectrum showed a face-centred cubic (fcc) crystalline nature, including peaks at 38.95°, 45.12°, 65.39° and 78.12° (labelled as Ag in Figure 3B), which corresponded to plane values of (1 1 1), (2 0 0), (2 2 0) and (3 1 1) at the 2θ angle. These were consistent with the standard data JCPDS file no. 01-087-0717. Peaks indicated by asterisks in Figure 3B probably correspond to the crystallization of the bio-organic phase occurring on the AgNPs surface, as also reported in [53–57]. Alternatively, these peaks may be due to AgNO3, which has not been reduced by Pseudomonas sp. ef1.

X-ray diffraction (XRD) analysis of *Pseudomonas* fluorescens CA 417 AgNPs also revealed well-defined peaks at 38° 44°, 64° and 78°, thus showing the face-centred cubic (fcc) metallic crystal corresponding to the (111), (200), (220) and (311) facets of the crystal planes at the 2θ angle [46]. The crystalline structure of biogenic AgNPs of Pseudomonas putida MVP2 was also confirmed by XRD [43].

2.4. *Pseudomonas sp. ef1* AgNPs Antimicrobial Activity

The antibacterial activity of *Pseudomonas* sp. ef1 AgNPs was tested against pathogenic Gram-positive and Gram-negative bacteria, as well as fungi, and compared with that of chemically synthesized AgNPs and $AgNO_3$ (Table S1 and Figure 4). In the comparative study, the biosynthesized AgNPs exhibited a stronger antibacterial property than the chemically synthesized AgNPs and $AgNO_3$ (Figure 4). Among Gram-negative bacteria, the larger inhibition zone (Ø 19.0 mm) was against *Escherichia coli* and the smallest (Ø 14.0 mm) was against *Pseudomonas aeruginosa* and *Serratia marcescens*. Among Gram-positive bacteria, the highest zone of 15 mm was formed against *Staphylococcus aureus*. Among fungi, the larger zone was against *Candida albicans* (Ø 15.0 mm).

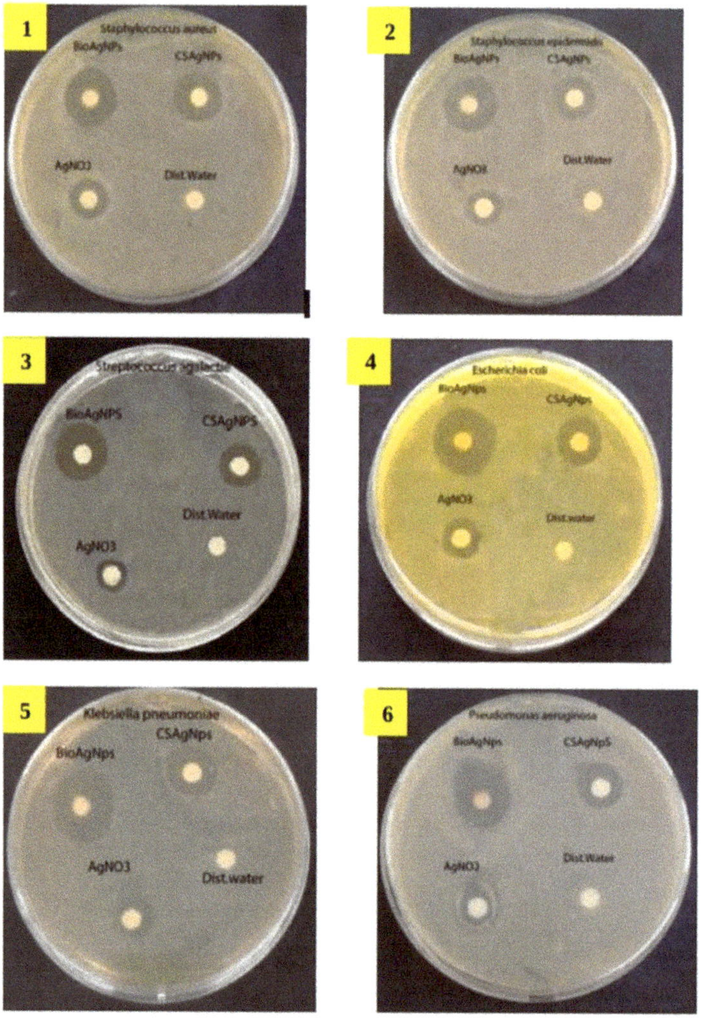

Figure 4. *Cont.*

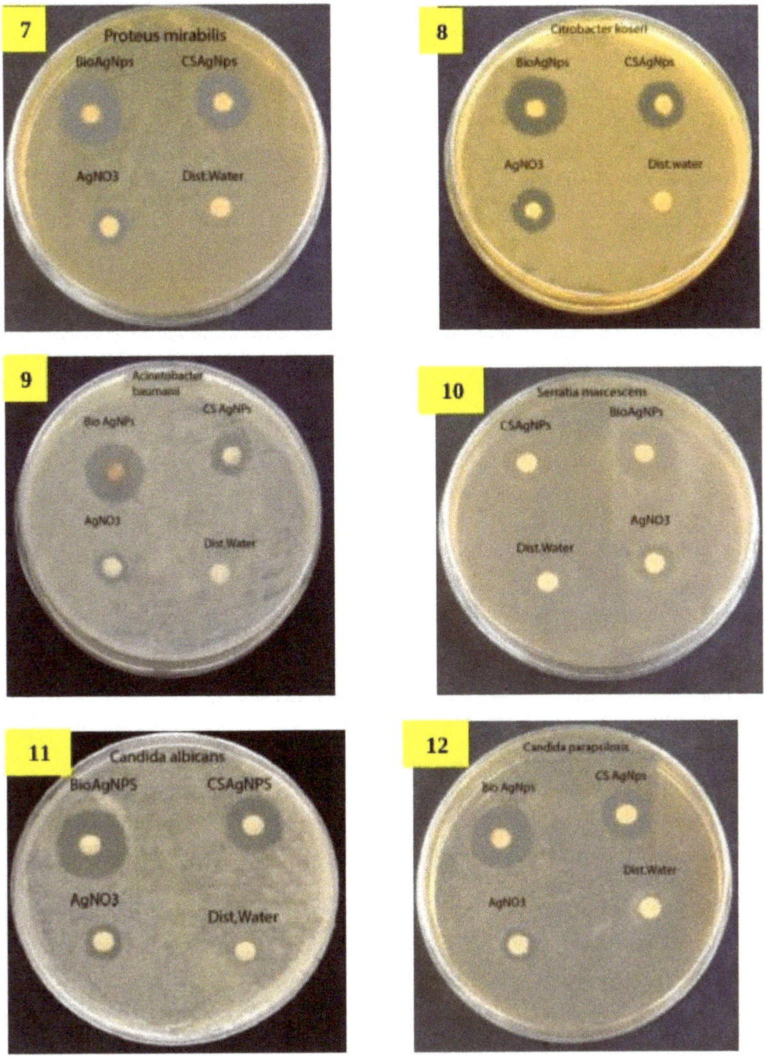

Figure 4. Antimicrobial activity of *Pseudomonas* sp. ef1 AgNPs tested against twelve human pathogens. The bio AgNPs disks were compared with chemically synthesized AgNPs disks. $AgNO_3$ disks and distilled water disks were used as control. The human pathogens are: 1. *Staphylococcus aureus*, 2. *Staphylococcus epidermidis*, 3. *Streptococcus agalactie*, 4. *Escherichia coli*, 5. *Klebsiella pneumonia*, 6. *Pseudomonas aeruginosa*, 7. *Proteus mirabilis*, 8. *Citrobacter koseri*, 9. *Acinetobacter baumanii*, 10. *Serratia marcescens*, 11. *Candida albicans*, 12. *Candida parapsilosis*.

It has been reported that *E. coli* showed a greater sensitivity by comparison with that of *Bacillus cereus* and *Streptococcus pyogene*, probably due to the narrow cell walls of Gram-negative bacteria with respect to Gram-positive bacteria [58].

The use of the biosynthesized AgNPs may be one of the promising approaches to overcome bacterial resistance and could also play a new key role in pharmacotherapeutics. The mechanism of the AgNP-mediated bactericidal property is still to be understood. A mechanism proposed by other studies is that AgNPs attach to the cell wall, thus modifying the membrane integrity and disturbing its permeability and cell respiration functions [59,60]. Most likely, the antibacterial activity of AgNPs is size dependent. This means that smaller AgNPs that have a large surface area available for interactions function as more efficient antimicrobial agents than larger ones. It is also possible that AgNPs can penetrate inside the bacteria and not only interact with the membrane of the cell [60]. Another possible process responsible of AgNPs antimicrobial activity may be the release of Ag^+ ions, since they may play a partial but relevant role in the bactericidal effect [60].

3. Materials and Methods

3.1. Synthesis of AgNPs by *Pseudomonas sp. ef1*

The bacterial biomass was produced by inoculating *Pseudomonas* sp. ef1 into Luria-Bertani (LB) medium (10 g of Tryptone, 10 g of NaCl and 5 g of yeast extract, dissolved in 1 L of ddH_20). The culture flasks were incubated on an orbital shaker set at 220 rpm, at 22 °C. After 24 h the biomass was harvested by centrifuging at 5000 rpm for 30 min. After removal of the supernatant, approximately 2 mg of the bacterial biomass was transferred into an Erlenmeyer flask containing a solution of 1 mM $AgNO_3$. The mixture was placed in the orbital shaker set at 200 rpm for 24 h at 22 °C. The heat-killed biomasses incubated with silver nitrate were maintained as control. Biosynthesis was carried out in bright condition as visible light irradiation is known to increase the biosynthetic rate of AgNPs formation. The bioreduction of Ag^+ ions were monitored by changes in colour of the bacterial biomass reaction mixture containing the $AgNO_3$ (Figure S1) and by UV–visible spectroscopy (UV-1800, Shimadzu): a 0.1 mL aliquot of the sample was diluted with 0.9 mL of ddH_2O and UV–visible spectra was recorded from 300 to 800 nm wavelength. ddH_2O was used as blank.

3.2. Purification of AgNPs

Bacterial biomass was collected by centrifugation at 5000 rpm for 30 min. The resulting pellet was then suspended in ddH_2O and ultra-sonicated at a pulse rate of 6V at intervals of 30 s for ten cycles. Afterwards, the solution was centrifuged again at 5000 rpm for 30 min and the supernatant loaded on a Sephadex G-50 resin equilibrated in 10 mM Tris buffer (pH 7.0) to remove contaminating debris and proteins. AgNPs were finally extracted from the buffered solution by adding 3 volumes of isopropanol to the obtained nanoparticle solution. Isopropyl alcohol is known to dissolve a wide range of non-polar compounds and to evaporate quickly compared to ethanol. The mixture was rotated on the orbital shaker overnight and subjected to evaporation to obtain a purified powdered highly enriched in NPs.

3.3. Chemical Synthesis of AgNPs

A solution of 1 mM of $AgNO_3$ was heated to boil. As the solution started to boil, a sodium citrate solution was added drop-by-drop until the solution turned into a greyish-yellow color, indicating Ag^+ ion formation. Heating was continued for 60 s. The solution was then chilled to room temperature.

3.4. Scanning Electron Microscopy (SEM), Transmission Electron Microscopy (TEM) and Energy Dispersive X-ray Analysis (EDAX)

For SEM (ZIESSA, Sigma 300) analysis, purified AgNPs were sonicated for 15 min to reach a uniform distribution. A drop of the solution was loaded on carbon-coated copper grids and allowed to evaporate under infrared light for 30 min.

TEM (PHILIPS EM208S) analysis was performed using an acceleration voltage of 100 kV. Drops of an AgNP solution were loaded on nitrocellulose- and Formvar-coated copper TEM grids. After 2 min, the extra solution was removed, and the grids were allowed to dry at room temperature. The acquired data were analysed by Statistical Software (StatSoft, Tulsa, Okla., United States) using the variability plot of average methods. After 100 measurements the size distribution of the AgNPs was estimated using TEM imaging and analysis software (TIA).

EDAX analysis of AgNPs was performed using Field Emission Scanning Electron Microscope (FESEM) equipped with an EDAX attachment.

3.5. Fourier Transform Infrared Spectroscopy (FTIR) Analysis

AgNPs were deposed on the single reflection diamond element of the attenuated total reflection (ATR) device (Quest, Specac) and dried at room temperature. The ATR/FTIR spectrum was collected by the Varian 670-IR spectrometer, equipped with a nitrogen-cooled Mercury Cadmium Telluride detector, under the following conditions: triangular apodization, scan speed of 25 kHz, resolution of 2 cm^{-1} and 512 scan co-additions [61].

3.6. X-ray Diffraction Analysis (XRD)

X-ray Diffraction measurements were performed by scanning drop-coated films of AgNps in a wide range of Bragg angle 2θ at a rate of 2 min^{-1}. A Philips PW 1830 instrument was used, and it was operated at a voltage of 40 kV with a current of 30 mA using monochromatic Cu Kα radiation (λ = 1.5405 Å). The diffracted intensities were recorded in the 2θ range of 10°–80°. To elucidate the crystalline structure, the resulting images were compared with the Joint Committee on Powder Diffraction Standards (JCPDS) library.

3.7. Screening of Antimicrobial Activity of Biosynthesized AgNps

The evaluation of the biosynthesized AgNPs antibacterial activity was carried out by the Kirby–Bauer disc diffusion method on the following twelve stains: Staphylococcus aureus, Staphylococcus epidermidis, Streptococcus agalactiae (Gram-positive bacteria); *Escherichia coli, Klebsiella pneumonia, Pseudomonas* sp., *Proteus mirabilis, Citrobacter koseri, Acinetobacter baumanii, Serratia marcescens* (Gram-negative bacteria); and *Candida albicans* and *Candida parapsilosis* (fungi).

The biosynthesized AgNPs were tested for antibacterial activity by the Kirby–Bauer disc diffusion method. The pathogenic cultures were subcultured into peptone broth and incubated at 37 °C to reach 10^5–10^6 CFU ml^{-1}. The fresh cultures of pathogens were plated using a sterile cotton swab on Petri dishes containing Muller Hinton Agar. Six millimetre filter paper disks impregnated with 25 μL of biosynthesized AgNPs using a sterile micropipette were placed on the pathogen-plated agar. Bio-AgNPs disks were compared with chemically synthesized AgNPs disks. $AgNO_3$ disks and distilled water disks were used as control. The plates were incubated at 37 °C for 18–24 h to measure the zone of inhibition.

4. Conclusions

In this study we reported an easy and efficient biological method to synthesize AgNPs using the biomass of a novel *Pseudomonas* strain isolated from a bacterial consortium found in association with the Antarctic ciliate *E. focardii*. We also characterized these AgNPs. Their stability makes the present method a viable alternative to chemical synthesis methods. Due to the lesser specificity of the reaction parameters, this process can be explored for large-scale synthesis of AgNPs. The study highlights an efficient strategy to obtain bionanomaterial that can be used against a large number of drug resistant pathogenic bacteria, thus contributing to solve this globally serious concern, especially given there being a limited choice of antibiotic treatment [62]. Furthermore, these AgNPs show the highest antimicrobial activity with respect to those that are chemically synthesized. The *Pseudomonas* strain here used can also be exploited to remove silver nitrate contamination from the environment, allowing to associate its potential in bioremediation and in antibiotics production.

5. Patents

The results of this paper are related to the patent number 102019000014121 deposited in 06/08/2019.

Supplementary Materials: The following are available online at http://www.mdpi.com/1660-3397/18/1/38/s1, Figure S1: AgNP synthesis by *Pseudomonas* sp. ef1. Table S1: Antimicrobial activity of AgNPs synthesized by *Pseudomonas* sp. against various pathogenic organisms. Supplementary references.

Author Contributions: All authors contributed to the conception and design of this study; material preparation, collection and analysis of data were performed by M.S.J., J.A.N. and K.P.R.; The draft of the manuscript was prepared by M.S.J., J.A.N. and A.M.; all authors contributed to the improvement of the previous versions of the manuscript; all authors read and approved the final version. All authors have read and agreed to the published version of the manuscript.

Funding: This work was supported by the EC MSCA H2020 RISE Metable-645693.

Acknowledgments: We thanks Laura Petetta (University of Camerino) for the support in SEM analysis.

Conflicts of Interest: The authors declare no conflict of interest.

References

1. Khan, I.; Saeed, K.; Khan, I. Nanoparticles: Properties, applications and toxicities. *Arab. J. Chem.* **2019**, *12*, 908–931. [CrossRef]
2. Iravani, S.; Korbekandi, H.; Mirmohammadi, S.V.; Zolfaghari, B. Synthesis of silver nanoparticles: Chemical, physical and biological methods. *Res. Pharm. Sci.* **2014**, *9*, 385–406. [PubMed]
3. Gandhi, H.; Khan, S. Biological Synthesis of Silver Nanoparticles and Its Antibacterial Activity. *J. Nanomed. Nanotechnol.* **2016**, *7*, 1–3. [CrossRef]
4. Gurunathan, K.; Kalishwaralal, R.; Vaidyanathan, V.; Deepak, S.R.K.; Pandian, J.; Muniyandi, N.; Hariharan, S.H.E. Biosynthesis, purification and characterization of silver nanoparticles using *Escherichia coli*. *Colloids Surf.* **2009**, *74*, 328–335. [CrossRef] [PubMed]
5. Badr, Y.; Wahed, E.; Mahmoud, M.G. Photo catalytic degradation of methyl red dye by silica nanoparticles. *J. Hazard. Mater.* **2008**, *154*, 245–253. [CrossRef] [PubMed]
6. Parikh, R.Y.; Singh, S.; Prasad, B.L.V.; Patole, M.S.; Sastry, M.; Shouche, Y.S. Extracellular synthesis of crystalline silver nanoparticles and molecular evidence of silver resistance from *Morganella* sp.: Towards understanding biochemical synthesis mechanism. *Chembiochem* **2008**, *9*, 1415–1422. [CrossRef] [PubMed]
7. Abdel-Mohsen, A.M.; Hrdina, R.; Burgert, L.; Abdel, R.M.; Rahman, M.; Hasova, D.; Smejkalova, M.; Kolar, M.; Pekar, A.S. Antibacterial activity and cell viability of hyaluronan fiber with silver nanoparticles. *Carbohydr. Polym.* **2013**, *92*, 1177–1187. [CrossRef] [PubMed]
8. Emerich, D.F.; Thanos, C.G. The pinpoint promise of nanoparticle-based drug delivery and molecular diagnosis. *Biomol. Eng.* **2006**, *23*, 171–184. [CrossRef]
9. Shahverdi, A.R.; Fakhimi, A.; Shahverdi, H. Synthesis and effect of silver nanoparticles on the antibacterial activity of different antibiotics against Staphylococcus aureus and *Escherichia coli*. *Nanomed. Nanotechnol.* **2007**, *3*, 168–171. [CrossRef]
10. Criswell, D. The "evolution of antibiotic resistance". *Act Facts* **2004**, *33*, 1–4.
11. Fayaz, A.M.; Balaji, K.; Girilal, M.; Yadav, R.; Kalaichelvan, P.T.; Venketesan, R. Biogenic synthesis of silver nanoparticles and their synergistic effect with antibiotics: A study against Gram-positive and Gram-negative bacteria. *Nanomed. Nanotechnol.* **2010**, *6*, 103–109. [CrossRef] [PubMed]
12. Kalishwaralal, K.; Barath Mani Kanth, S.; Pandian, S.R.K.; Deepak, V.; Gurunathan, S. Silver nanoparticles impede the biofilm formation by *Pseudomonas* sp and *Staphylococcus epidermidis*. *Colloids Surf.* **2010**, *79*, 340–344. [CrossRef] [PubMed]
13. Panacek, A.; Kvitek, L.; Prucek, R.; Kolar, M.; Vecerova, R.; Pizurova, N.; Sharma, V.K.; Nevecna, T.; Zboril, R. Silver colloid nanoparticles: Synthesis, characterization, and their antibacterial activity. *J. Phys. Chem.* **2006**, *110*, 6248–16253. [CrossRef] [PubMed]
14. Jones, S.A.; Bowler, P.G.; Walker, M.; Parsons, D. Controlling wound bio burden with a novel silver containing hydrofiber dressing. *Wound Repair Regen.* **2004**, *12*, 288–294. [CrossRef] [PubMed]
15. Duran, N.; Marcato, D.P.; Alves, L.O.; de Souza, G.; Esposito, E. Mechanical aspect of biosynthesis of silver nanoparticles by several *Fusarium oxysporum* strains. *J. Nanobiotechnol.* **2005**, *3*, 8–15. [CrossRef] [PubMed]
16. Kalimuthu, K.; Babu, R.S.; Venkataraman, D.; Bilal, M.; Gurunathan, S. Biosynthesis of silver nanocrystals by *Bacillus licheniformis*. *Colloids Surf.* **2008**, *65*, 150–153. [CrossRef]

17. Nangia, Y.; Wangoo, N.; Goyal, N.; Shekhawat, G.; Suri, C.R. A novel bacterial isolate *Stenotrophomonas maltophilia* as living factory for synthesis of gold nanoparticles. *Microb. Cell Factories* **2009**, *8*, 39. [CrossRef]
18. Eckhardt, S.; Brunetto, P.S.; Gagnon, J.; Priebe, M.; Giese, B.; Fromm, K.M. Nanobio silver: Its interactions with peptides and bacteria, and its uses in medicine. *Chem. Rev.* **2013**, *113*, 4708–4754. [CrossRef]
19. Hulkoti, N.I.; Taranath, T.C. Biosynthesis of nanoparticles using microbes—A review. *Colloids Surf. Biointerfaces* **2014**, *121*, 474–483. [CrossRef]
20. Pucciarelli, S.; Devaraj, R.R.; Mancini, A.; Ballarini, P.; Castelli, M.; Schrallhammer, M.; Petroni, G.; Miceli, C. Microbial Consortium Associated with the Antarctic Marine Ciliate Euplotes focardii: An Investigation from Genomic Sequences. *Microb. Ecol.* **2015**, *70*, 484–497. [CrossRef]
21. Ramasamy, K.P.; Telatin, A.; Mozzicafreddo, M.; Miceli, C.; Pucciarelli, S. Draft Genome Sequence of a New *Pseudomonas* sp. Strain, ef1, Associated with the Psychrophilic Antarctic Ciliate *Euplotes Focardii*. *Microbiol. Resour. Announc.* **2019**, *10*, 8. [CrossRef] [PubMed]
22. Pucciarelli, S.; La Terza, A.; Ballarini, P.; Barchetta, S.; Yu, T.; Marziale, F.; Passini, V.; Methé, B.; Detrich, H.W., 3rd; Miceli, C. Molecular cold-adaptation of protein function and gene regulation: The case for comparative genomic analyses in marine ciliated protozoa. *Mar. Genom.* **2009**, *2*, 57–66. [CrossRef] [PubMed]
23. Quinteros, M.A.; Aiassa Martínez, I.M.; Dalmasso, P.R.; Páez, L.R. Silver Nanoparticles: Biosynthesis Using an ATCC Reference Strain of *Pseudomonas* sp and Activity as Broad Spectrum Clinical Antibacterial Agents. *Int. J. Biomater.* **2016**, *2016*, 1–7. [CrossRef] [PubMed]
24. Wang, C.; Kim, Y.J.; Singh, P.; Mathiyalagan, R.; Jin, Y.; Yang, D.C. Green synthesis of silver nanoparticles by *Bacillus methylotrophicus*, and their antimicrobial activity. *Artif. Cells Nanomed. Biotechnol.* **2015**, *6*, 1–6.
25. Alani, F.; Moo-Young, M.; Anderson, W. Biosynthesis of silver nanoparticles by a new strain of Streptomyces sp. compared with *Aspergillus fumigatus*. *World J. Microbiol. Biotechnol.* **2012**, *28*, 1081–1086. [CrossRef]
26. Ahmad, A.; Mukherjee, P.; Senapati, S.; Mandal, D.; Khan, M.I.; Kumar, R. Extracellular biosynthesis of silver nanoparticles using the fungus *Fusarium oxysporum*. *Colloids Surf.* **2003**, *28*, 313–318. [CrossRef]
27. Duran, N.; Marcato, P.D.; Souza, G.; Alves, G.O.L.; Esposito, E. Antibacterial Effect of Silver Nanoparticles Produced by Fungal Process on Textile Fabrics and Their Effluent Treatment. *J. Biomed. Nanotechnol.* **2007**, *3*, 203–208. [CrossRef]
28. Mulvaney, P. Surface plasmon spectroscopy of nanosized metal particles. *Langmuir* **1996**, *12*, 788–800. [CrossRef]
29. Sastry, M.; Patil, V.; Sainkar, S.R. Electrostatically controlled diffusion of carboxylic acid derivatized silver colloidal particles in thermally evaporated fatty amine films. *J. Phys. Chem.* **1998**, *102*, 1404–1410. [CrossRef]
30. Henglein, A. Physicochemical properties of small metal particles in solution: "Microelectrode" reactions, chemisorption, composite metal particles, and the atom-to-metal transition. *J. Phys. Chem.* **1993**, *97*, 5457–5471. [CrossRef]
31. Ravindra, B.K.; Rajasab, A.H. A comparative study on biosynthesis of silver nanoparticles using four different fungal species. *Int. J. Pharm. Pharm. Sci.* **2014**, *6*, 372–376.
32. Thamilselvi, V.; Radha, K.V. Synthesis of silver nanoparticles from *Pseudomonas putida* ncim 2650 in silver nitrate supplemented growth medium and optimization using response surface methodology. *Dig. J. Nanomater. Biostruct.* **2013**, *8*, 1101–1111.
33. Ramalingam, V.; Rajaram, R.; Prem Kumar, C.; Santhanam, P.; Dhinesh, P.; Vinothkumar, S.; Kaleshkumar, K. Biosynthesis of silver nanoparticles from deep sea bacterium Pseudomonas sp JQ989348 for antimicrobial, antibiofilm, and cytotoxic activity. *J. Basic Microbiol.* **2014**, *54*, 928–936. [CrossRef] [PubMed]
34. Rammohan, M.; Balakrishnan, K. Rapid Synthesis and Characterization of Silver Nano Particles by Novel Pseudomonas sp."ram bt-1". *J. Ecobiotechnol.* **2011**, *3*, 24–28.
35. Kanchana, A.; Agarwal, I.; Sunkar, S.; Nellore, J.; Namasivayam, K. Biogenic silver nanoparticles from *Spinacia oleracea* and *Lactuca sativa* and their potential antimicrobial activity. *Dig. J. Nanomater. Biostruct.* **2011**, *6*, 1741–1750.
36. Shivakrishna, P.; Ram Prasad, M.; Krishna, G.; Singara Charya, M.A. Synthesis of Silver Nano Particles from Marine Bacteria *Pseudomonas aerogenosa*. *Octa J. Biosci.* **2013**, *1*, 108–114.
37. Busi, S.; Rajkumari, J.; Ranjan, B.; Karuganti, S. Green rapid biogenic synthesis of bioactive silver nanoparticles (AgNPs) using *Pseudomonas* sp. ET. *Nanobiotechnol.* **2014**, *8*, 267–274. [CrossRef]

38. Shahverdi, A.R.; Minaeian, S.; Shahverdi, H.R.; Jamalifar, H.; Nohi, A.A. Rapid synthesis of silver nanoparticles using culture supernatants of Enterobacteria: A novel biological approach. *Process. Biochem.* **2007**, *42*, 919–923. [CrossRef]
39. Das, V.L.; Thomas, R.; Varghese, R.T.; Soniya, E.V.; Mathew, J.; Radhakrishnan, E.K. Extracellular synthesis of silver nanoparticles by the *Bacillus* strain CS 11 isolated from industrialized area. *Biotech* **2014**, *4*, 121–126. [CrossRef]
40. Dipak, P.; Narayan Sinha, S. Extracellular Synthesis of Silver Nanoparticles Using Pseudomonas sp KUPSB12 and Its Antibacterial Activity. *Jordan J. Biol. Sci.* **2014**, *7*, 245–250.
41. Klaus, T.; Joerger, R.; Olsson, E.; Granquist, C.G. Silver based crystalline nanoparticles, microbially fabricated. *Proc. Natl. Acad. Sci. USA* **1999**, *96*, 13611–13614. [CrossRef] [PubMed]
42. Nair, B.; Pradeep, T. Coalescence of nanoclusters and formation of sub-micron crystallites assisted by Lactobacillus strains. *Cryst. Growth Des.* **2002**, *4*, 295–298.
43. Gopinath, V.; Priyadarshini, S.; FaiLoke, M.; Arunkumar, J.; Marsili, E.; Mubarak, D.; Vadivelu, A.J. Biogenic synthesis, characterization of antibacterial silver nanoparticles and its cell cytotoxicity. *Arab. J. Chem.* **2017**, *10*, 1107–1117. [CrossRef]
44. Magudapatty, P.; Gangopadhgayrans, P.; Panigrahi, B.K.; Nair, K.G.M.; Dhara, S. Electrical transport studies of Ag nanoclusters embedded in glass matrix. *Phys. B Condens. Matter* **2001**, *299*, 142–146. [CrossRef]
45. Kaviya, S.; Santhanalaksnmi, J.; Viswanathan, B.; Muthumany, J.; Srinivasan, K. Biosynthesis of silver nanoparticles using citrus sinensis peel extract and its antibacterial activity. *Spectrochim. Acta Part A* **2011**, *79*, 594–598. [CrossRef]
46. Syed, B.; Prasad, N.; Dhananjaya, M.N.; Mohan, B.L.; Kumar, K.; Yallappa, S.; Satish, S. Synthesis of silver nanoparticles by endosymbiont Pseudomonas fluorescens CA 417 and their bactericidal activity. *Enzym. Microb. Technol.* **2016**, *95*, 128–136. [CrossRef]
47. Barth, A. Infrared spectroscopy of proteins. *BBA- Bioenerg.* **2007**, *1767*, 1073–1101. [CrossRef]
48. Baker, M.J.; Hussain, S.R.; Lovergne, L.; Untereiner, V.; Hughes, C.; Lukaszewski, R.A.; Thiéfin, G.; Sockalingum, G.D. Developing and understanding biofluid vibrational spectroscopy: A critical review. *Chem. Soc. Rev.* **2017**, *45*, 1803–1818. [CrossRef]
49. Gole, A.; Dash, C.; Ramakrishnan, V.; Sainkar, S.R.; Mandale, A.B.; Rao, M.; Sastry, M. Pepsin—Gold Colloid Conjugates: Preparation, Characterization, and Enzymatic Activity. *Langmuir* **2001**, *17*, 1674–1679. [CrossRef]
50. Babu, M.M.G.; Gunasekaran, P. Production and structural characterization of crystalline silver nanoparticles from *Bacillus cereus* isolate. *Colloids Surf.* **2009**, *74*, 191–195. [CrossRef]
51. Balaji, D.S.; Basavaraja, S.; Deshpande, R.; Mahesh, D.; Prabhakar, B.K.; Venkataraman, A. Extracellular biosynthesis of functionalized silver nanoparticles by strains of *Cladosporium cladosporioides* fungus. *Colloids Surf. B* **2009**, *68*, 88–92. [CrossRef] [PubMed]
52. Afreen, R.V.; Rathod, V.; Ranganath, E. Synthesis of monodispersed silver nanoparticles by Rhizopus stolonifer and its antibacterial activity against MDR strains of Pseudomonas sp from burnt patients. *Int. J. Environ. Sci.* **2011**, *1*, 1582–1592.
53. Sathyavathi, R.; Krishna, M.B.M.; Rao, S.V.; Saritha, R.; Rao, D.N. Biosynthesis of silver nanoparticles using coriandrum sativum leaf extract and their application in nonlinear optics. *Adv. Sci. Lett.* **2010**, *3*, 1–6. [CrossRef]
54. Mickymaray, S. One-step Synthesis of Silver Nanoparticles Using Saudi Arabian Desert Seasonal Plant *Sisymbrium irio* and Antibacterial Activity Against Multidrug-Resistant Bacterial Strains. *Biomolecules* **2019**, *9*, 662. [CrossRef]
55. Shaik, M.R.; Khan, M.; Kuniyil, M.; Al-Warthan, A.; Alkhathlan, H.Z.; Siddiqui, M.R.H.; Shaik, J.P.; Ahamed, A.; Mahmood, A.; Khan, M.; et al. Plant-Extract-Assisted Green Synthesis of Silver Nanoparticles Using *Origanum vulgare* L. Extract and Their Microbicidal Activities. *Sustainability* **2018**, *10*, 913.
56. Das, G.; Patra, J.K.; Debnath, T.; Ansari, A.; Shin, H.-S. Investigation of antioxidant, antibacterial, antidiabetic, and cytotoxicity potential of silver nanoparticles synthesized using the outer peel extract of *Ananas comosus* (L.). *PLoS ONE* **2019**, *14*, e0220950. [CrossRef]
57. Bibi, N.; Ali, Q.; Tanveer, Z.I.; Rahman, H.; Anees, M. Antibacterial efficacy of silver nanoparticles prepared using *Fagonia cretica* L. leaf extract. *Inorgan. Nano-Met. Chem.* **2019**, *49*, 260–266. [CrossRef]

58. Priyadarshini, S.; Gopinath, V.; Priyadharsshini, N.M.; Mubarak, A.D.; Velusamy, P. Synthesis of anisotropic silver nanoparticles using novel strain, *Bacillus flexus* and its biomedical application. *Colloids Surf.* **2013**, *102*, 232–237. [CrossRef]
59. Lin, Y.S.E.; Vidic, R.D.; Stout, J.E.; McCartney, C.A.; Yu, V.L. Inactivation of Mycobacterium avium by copper and silver ions. *Water Res.* **1998**, *32*, 1997–2000. [CrossRef]
60. Rai, M.; Yadav, A.; Gade, A. Silver nanoparticles as a new generation of antimicrobials. *Biotechnol. Adv.* **2009**, *27*, 76–83. [CrossRef]
61. Natalello, A.; Mangione, P.P.; Giorgetti, S.; Porcari, R.; Marchese, L.; Zorzoli, I.; Relini, A.; Ami, D.; Faravelli, G.; Valli, M.; et al. Co-fibrillogenesis of Wild-type and D76N β2-Microglobulin: THE CRUCIAL ROLE OF FIBRILLAR SEEDS. *J. Biol. Chem.* **2016**, *291*, 9678–9689. [CrossRef] [PubMed]
62. Mancini, A.; Pucciarelli, S. Antibiotic activity of the antioxidant drink effective Microorganism-X (EM-X) extracts against common nosocomial pathogens: An in vitro study. *Nat. Prod. Res.* **2018**, *4*, 1–6. [CrossRef] [PubMed]

marine drugs

MDPI

Article

New Discorhabdin Alkaloids from the Antarctic Deep-Sea Sponge *Latrunculia biformis*

Fengjie Li [1], Christian Peifer [2], Dorte Janussen [3] and Deniz Tasdemir [1,4,*]

1 GEOMAR Centre for Marine Biotechnology (GEOMAR-Biotech), Research Unit Marine Natural Products Chemistry, GEOMAR Helmholtz Centre for Ocean Research Kiel, Am Kiel-Kanal 44, 24106 Kiel, Germany
2 Pharmaceutical Chemistry, Kiel University, Gutenbergstraße 76, 24118 Kiel, Germany
3 Senckenberg Research Institute and Natural History Museum, Senckenberganlage 25, D-60325 Frankfurt, Germany
4 Faculty of Mathematics and Natural Sciences, Kiel University, Christian-Albrechts-Platz 4, 24118 Kiel, Germany
* Correspondence: dtasdemir@geomar.de; Tel.: +49-431-600-4430

Received: 14 June 2019; Accepted: 22 July 2019; Published: 25 July 2019

Abstract: The sponge genus *Latrunculia* is a prolific source of discorhabdin type pyrroloiminoquinone alkaloids. In the continuation of our research interest into this genus, we studied the Antarctic deep-sea sponge *Latrunculia biformis* that showed potent in vitro anticancer activity. A targeted isolation process guided by bioactivity and molecular networking-based metabolomics yielded three known discorhabdins, (−)-discorhabdin L (**1**), (+)-discorhabdin A (**2**), (+)-discorhabdin Q (**3**), and three new discorhabdin analogs (−)-2-bromo-discorhabdin D (**4**), (−)-1-acetyl-discorhabdin L (**5**), and (+)-1-octacosatrienoyl-discorhabdin L (**6**) from the MeOH-soluble portion of the organic extract. The chemical structures of **1–6** were elucidated by extensive NMR, HR-ESIMS, FT-IR, $[\alpha]_D$, and ECD (Electronic Circular Dichroism) spectroscopy analyses. Compounds **1**, **5**, and **6** showed promising anticancer activity with IC_{50} values of 0.94, 2.71, and 34.0 μM, respectively. Compounds **1–6** and the enantiomer of **1** ((+)-discorhabdin L, **1e**) were docked to the active sites of two anticancer targets, topoisomerase I-II and indoleamine 2,3-dioxygenase (IDO1), to reveal, for the first time, the binding potential of discorhabdins to these proteins. Compounds **5** and **6** are the first discorhabdin analogs with an ester function at C-1 and **6** is the first discorhabdin bearing a long-chain fatty acid at this position. This study confirms *Latrunculia* sponges to be excellent sources of chemically diverse discorhabdin alkaloids.

Keywords: *Latrunculia*; Antarctica; deep-sea sponge; molecular networking; molecular docking; discorhabdin

1. Introduction

Latrunculia species are cold-adapted sponges commonly found in the coastlines of the southern hemisphere [1–3]. The genus *Latrunculia* has proven to be a prolific source of structurally intriguing compounds from different classes, such as norsesterterpenes [4,5], callipeltins [6,7], and various types of pyrroloiminoquinone alkaloids [8–10]. Discorhabdins represent a large and unique subclass of pyrroloiminoquinone alkaloids that have been associated with the chemical defense and greenish to brownish coloration of the sponge [11,12]. Discorhabdins exhibit strong anticancer activity against many cancer types, such as human colon cancer, adenocarcinoma, and leukemia [13–15]. However, the mechanism of their anticancer action has been poorly studied. Indeed, only the farnesyltransferase enzyme [16] and hypoxia-inducible factor 1α (HIF-1α) and transcriptional coactivator p300 interaction [17] have been shown as potential targets of discorhabdins.

As part of our research interest into deep-sea *Latrunculia* sponges from Antarctica [18], herein we investigated the in-depth chemistry of *Latrunculia biformis*, which was collected from the Antarctic Weddell Sea shelf at 291 m depth. The crude organic extract of the sponge exhibited significant in vitro anticancer activity against six cancer cell lines. A molecular networking (MN)-based metabolomics study on fractions obtained from the MeOH-soluble portion of the sponge indicated the presence of a large discorhabdin cluster with many nodes belonging to potentially new discorhabdins. Guided by anticancer activity and MN-based dereplication, six discorhabdin-type alkaloids were isolated from the MeOH subextract, including three known compounds (−)-discorhabdin L (**1**), (+)-discorhabdin A (**2**), (+)-discorhabdin Q (**3**) and three new discorhabdin derivatives, namely (−)-2-bromo-discorhabdin D (**4**), (−)-1-acetyl-discorhabdin L (**5**), and (+)-1-octacosatrienoyl-discorhabdin L (**6**). Since the amounts of the isolated compounds were very minor, only compounds **1**, **5** and **6** could be tested for their anticancer activity against the human colon cancer cell line HCT-116. We applied a structure-based docking approach on all isolated compounds and the enantiomer of **1** (**1e**) against two cancer targets reported for pyrroloiminoquinone alkaloids, i.e., topoisomerase I–II and indoleamine 2,3-dioxygenase IDO1 [19–21] to predict their anticancer potential and to suggest potential molecular mechanism(s) of action. This study reports MN and bioactivity-guided isolation of compounds **1**–**6**, their structure elucidation, and biological activities with potential target identification for their anticancer activity.

2. Results

2.1. Bioactivity and Molecular Networking-guided Purification and Structural Elucidation

The olive green-colored sponge material was freeze-dried and successively extracted with water, MeOH, and dichloromethane (DCM) subsequently. The combined organic extract was submitted to bioactivity screening against six cancer cell lines, where it showed significant activity with IC_{50} values ranging from 4.0 to 56.2 µg/mL (Table 1). The solvent partitioning of the crude organic extract between MeOH and *n*-hexane yielded the MeOH (M) and the *n*-hexane subextracts. The M subextract demonstrated strong anticancer activity (Figure 1) and was further fractionated over a C18 SPE cartridge. The anticancer activity was tracked to six SPE fractions, M2–M5, M7, and M8 (Figure 1).

Table 1. Anticancer activity of the *L. biformis* crude extract. The IC_{50} values are in µg/mL. Positive control doxorubicine.

Sample	A-375	HCT-116	A-549	MB-231	Hep G2	HT-29
Crude extract	17.4	4.8	56.2	46.8	18.2	4.0
Positive control	0.13	10.6	31.4	15.2	14.6	3.0

In order to prioritize the isolation workflow towards undescribed molecules with potential anticancer properties, we acquired tandem UPLC-QToF-MS/MS (positive-ion mode) data on these six active fractions. The generated MS/MS (MS^2) data were uploaded to the publicly available Global Natural Product Social Molecular Networking (GNPS) platform (http://gnps.ucsd.edu) and analyzed following the molecular networking (MN) online workflow [22]. Software Cytoscape (Version 3.61) was used to visualize the resulting networks. The automated dereplication on GNPS platform did not annotate any pyrroloiminoquinone alkaloids. Hence, compound annotation was based on manual dereplication by comparing the predicted molecular formulae against multiple public or commercially available databases.

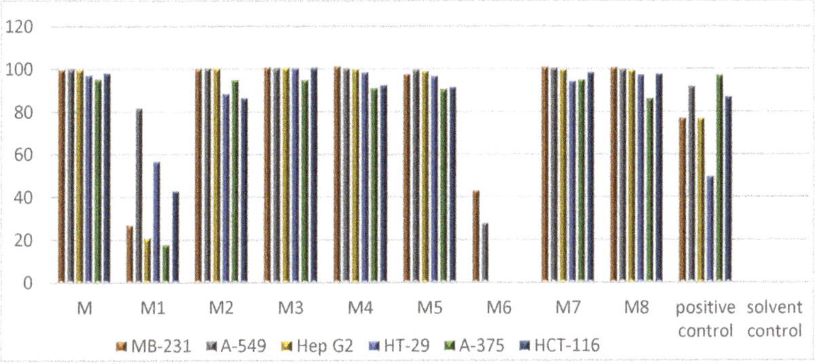

Figure 1. In vitro activity of MeOH subextract (M) and its C18 solid phase extraction (SPE) fractions (M1–M8) against six cancer cell lines. Test concentration: 100 μg/mL. Positive control: Doxorubicine. Solvent control: 0.5% DMSO.

After a comprehensive examination of the global MN of the SPE fractions, two clusters attracted our attention (Figure 2). Cluster 1 contained five nodes, four of which were annotated as known molecules discorhabdin L [13], its analog, discorhabdin D [23], and 1-methoxydiscorhabdin D [19], leaving the node at *m/z* 368.0380 to be a putatively new derivative (Figure 2). From this cluster, we were able to purify (−)-discorhabdin L (**1**), but failed to purify the potentially new discorhabdin analog (*m/z* 368.0380) due to its very minor quantity.

With 21 nodes, cluster 2 was the biggest in the generated MN, which can be further divided into three subclusters (Figure 2). Based on the elemental composition analysis, MS/MS fragmentation patterns, and biological source, two brominated alkaloids discorhabdin A [24] and discorhabdin G [25] were identified in subcluster 3. However, only discorhabdin A (**2**) was isolated in sufficient amounts for NMR and other spectroscopic analyses. Discorhabdin H2 [26] was the only annotated compound in subcluster 2. Unfortunately, neither this compound nor the remaining nodes that represent potentially new discorhabdin analogs could be purified in sufficient quantity.

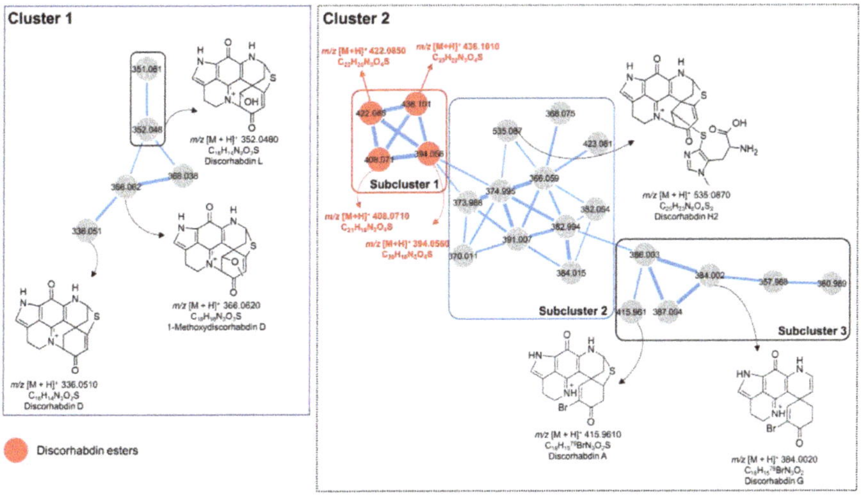

Figure 2. Molecular cluster observed in SPE fractions of *L. biformis* MeOH subextract. Numbers within the nodes indicate parent ions, and edge thickness represents the cosine similarity between nodes. Red nodes: Discorhabdin esters; Grey nodes: Other discorhabdin analogs.

The subcluster 1 (of cluster 2) contained four nonbrominated nodes at *m/z* 394.0560, 408.0710, 422.085, and 436.1010 connected with thick edges, indicating their high structural similarity. Elemental composition analysis revealed the difference of a CH_2 unit between these ions (Figure 2, in red). In-depth analysis of their MS/MS spectra revealed the presence of the same MS fragment (*m/z* 352.0766, $C_{18}H_{14}N_3O_3S$) in all four compounds, suggesting these compounds to be discorhabdin alkaloids bearing an alkyl chain with varying lengths. From subcluster 1, we isolated the compound with *m/z* 394.0560 and identified it as a new metabolite, (−)-1-acetyl-discorhabdin L (**5**), as discussed later.

In addition, we purified three compounds, namely the known compound (+)-discorhabdin Q (**3**) as well as two new compounds, namely (−)-2-bromo-discorhabdin D (**4**) and (+)-1-octacosatrienoyl-discorhabdin L (**6**), which did not appear in the MN because of the low intensity of their MS fragments. The enantiopurity of all purified compounds was further checked individually by RP-DAD-HPLC on an analytical chiral column. The sharp single peak in the UV chromatograms confirmed the enantiopurity of **1–6**.

The structure of compound **1** was elucidated as (−)-(1*R*,2*S*,6*R*,8*S*)-discorhabdin L [13], based on comparison of its 1D and 2D NMR data including NOESY spectrum (Tables 2 and 3, Supplementary Figures S1–S6). The specific rotation of compound **1** ($[\alpha]^{20}_D$ = −71, *c* 0.1, MeOH) showed the same sign as that reported for (−)-discorhabdin L ($[\alpha]^{20}_D$ = −240, *c* 0.0125, MeOH) [26]. In order to confirm the absolute configuration of compound **1**, the ECD (Electronic Circular Dichroism) spectrum was run. The experimental ECD spectrum of **1** (Supplementary Figure S8) was essentially identical to the ECD spectrum of (−)-(1*R*,2*S*,6*R*,8*S*)-discorhabdin L [26]. Hence, compound **1** was unambiguously characterized as (−)-(1*R*,2*S*,6*R*,8*S*)-discorhabdin L.

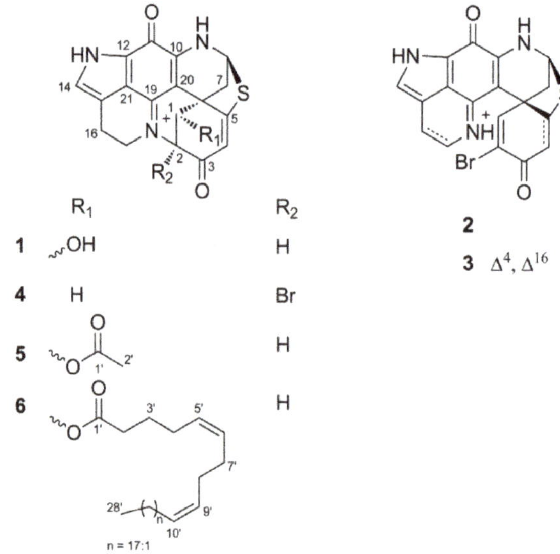

Figure 3. Chemical structures of compounds **1–6**.

Compound **2** exhibited the same ^{1}H and ^{13}C NMR resonances (Supplementary Figures S9 and S10) as (+)-discorhabdin A [24,27]. The analysis of its COSY, HSQC, and HMBC spectra (Supplementary Figures S10–S12) supported the same planar structure as discorhabdin A and NOESY spectrum confirmed the relative configuration of three stereocenters (Supplementary Figure S13). The specific rotation of compound **2** ($[\alpha]^{20}_D$ = +197, *c* 0.01, MeOH) exhibited the same sign as (+)-discorhabdin A ($[\alpha]^{20}_D$ = +400, *c* 0.05, MeOH) [24]. An early X-ray crystal analysis has confirmed the configuration of the chiral centers within (+)-discorhabdin A as 5*R*,6*S*,8*S* [27]. Thus, compound **2** was identified as (+)-(5*R*,6*S*,8*S*)-discorhabdin A (Figure 3).

Compound **3** was identified as the known compound discorhabdin Q, based on its 1D and 2D NMR data (Supplementary Figures S15–S20), which were in good agreement with those reported in the literature [26]. The examination of the ^{1}H-^{1}H NOESY spectrum of **3** (Supplementary Figure S19) allowed the assignment of the relative configuration of two stereocenters. Compound **3** exhibited a specific rotation value ($[\alpha]^{20}_{D}$ = +568, *c* 0.1, MeOH), which was similar both in the magnitude and sign to that observed for (+)-(6*S*,8*S*)-discorhabdin Q ($[\alpha]^{20}_{D}$ = +720, *c* 0.025, MeOH) [26], hence we concluded compound **3** as (+)-(6*S*,8*S*)-discorhabdin Q.

Table 2. ^{1}H NMR data of compounds **1**, **4**, **5**, and **6** in CD_3OD (trifluoroacetic acid (TFA) salts, 600 MHz, δ in ppm).

NO.	1	4	5	6
	δ_H, Mult. (*J* in Hz)	δ_H, Mult. (*J* in Hz)	δ_H, Mult. (*J* in Hz)	δ_H, Mult. (*J* in Hz)
1	4.63 d (3.6)	3.58 d (13.3) 3.23 d (13.3)	5.79 d (3.6)	5.79 d (3.6)
2	4.15 d (3.6)	-	4.36 d (3.6)	4.35 d (3.6)
4	6.14 s	6.14 s	6.23 s	6.23 s
7α	2.57 dd (1.3, 12.0)	2.66 dd (1.5, 12.1)	2.63 dd (1.4, 12.1)	2.64 d (1.2, 12.1)
7β	2.96 dd (3.6, 12.0)	2.84 dd (3.5, 12.1)	2.81 dd (3.7, 12.1)	2.76 dd (3.6, 12.1)
8	5.59 dd (1.3, 3.6)	5.68 dd (1.5, 3.5)	5.61 dd (1.4, 3.7)	5.61 dd (1.2, 3.6)
14	7.11 s	7.14 s	7.13 s	7.13 s
16	3.19 ddd (7.5, 13.0, 16.7) 3.06 ddd (3.0, 6.9, 16.7)	3.10 m	3.21 ddd (6.9, 7.5, 16.6) 3.08 ddd (2.9, 6.9, 16.6)	3.22 ddd (6.8, 7.3, 16.6) 3.08 ddd (2.7, 6.8, 16.6)
17	4.02 ddd (3.0, 7.5, 14.2) 3.91 ddd (6.9, 13.0, 14.2)	4.62 ddd (2.1, 5.6, 13.8) 3.66 td (6.3, 13.8)	4.04 ddd (2.9, 7.5, 13.8) 3.93 td (6.9, 13.8)	4.04 ddd (2.7, 7.3, 13.7) 3.93 td (6.8, 13.7)
2′	-	-	2.15 s	2.44 td (1.5, 7.5)
3′	-	-	-	1.69 m
4′	-	-	-	2.10 m
5′	-	-	-	5.34 m
6′	-	-	-	5.44 m
7′	-	-	-	2.08 m
8′	-	-	-	2.08 m
9′	-	-	-	5.37 m
10′	-	-	-	5.34 m
11′–27′	-	-	-	1.25–1.40 m; 2.00–2.06 m; 5.36 m
28′	-	-	-	0.90 t (7.0)

Compound **4** was obtained as a greenish film. The isotopic pattern of the molecule ion peaks (1:1 ratio) was indicative for the presence of one bromine atom in this molecule. The molecular formula of $C_{18}H_{13}{}^{79}BrN_3O_2S$ was established by the pseudo-molecular ion peak at *m/z* 413.9913 $[M + H]^+$ in the HR-ESIMS (Supplementary Figure S27) spectrum, requiring 14 degrees of unsaturation. The ^{1}H NMR data (Table 2, Supplementary Figure S22) together with HSQC spectrum (Supplementary Figure S23) revealed the presence of three methine resonances at δ_H 7.14 (H-14, s), δ_H 6.14 (H-4, s), and δ_H 5.68 (H-8, dd, *J* = 1.5, 3.5 Hz), four methylene groups corresponding to H_2-17 (δ_H 3.66 and 4.62), H_2-1 (δ_H 3.23 and 3.58), H_2-16 (δ_H 3.10), and H_2-7 (δ_H 2.66 and 2.84). The ^{13}C NMR spectrum (Table 3) showed 18 carbon signals including 4 methylenes (δ_C 20.0, 38.7, 42.4, and 50.2), 3 methines (δ_C 63.1, 110.9, and 126.0), and 11 quaternary carbons (δ_C 44.5, 78.1, 100.4, 119.3, 122.2, 124.0, 148.2, 150.2, 165.4, 172.8, and 176.4). By comparison with the data reported for discorhabdins [13,23], the three low-field quaternary carbon signals at δ_C 176.4, 172.8, and 165.4 were tentatively assigned to C-3, C-5, and C-11, respectively, while the high-field quaternary carbon at δ_C 44.5 was assigned to C-6. The COSY correlation between H_2-16 and H_2-17, together with the additional ^{1}H - ^{13}C HMBC correlations between H-14/C-12, C-21, C-11; H_2-16/C-14, C-21; H_2-17/C-15, C-19 confirmed the pyrroloiminoquinone motif [13,23]. Similarly, the homonuclear COSY correlation between H_2-7 and H-8, and the HMBC correlations between H_2-1/C-2, C-3, C-6, C-20; H-4/C-2, C-3, C-6; and H_2-7/C-5, C-6, C-20 suggested the position of the carbonyl group

(δ_C 176.4) at C-3, and the position of the methylene (δ_C 42.4) at C-1 (Figure 4A). A further HMBC coupling between H-8 and C-5 was indicative of a thioether bridge between C-8 and C-5, while the HMBC correlation between H_2-17 and C-2 established the bridge between N-18 and C-2 (Figure 4A). All these data, plus the lack of any further spin coupling observed for H_2-1, allowed the placement of the bromine atom on the remaining quaternary carbon, C-2. Thus the planar structure of compound **4** was elucidated as 2-bromo-discorhabdin D.

Table 3. ^{13}C NMR data of compounds **1**, **4**, **5**, and **6** in CD_3OD (150 MHz, δ in ppm).

Position	1	4	5	6
	δ_C	δ_C [a]	δ_C	δ_C
1	68.5 (CH)	42.4 (CH_2)	69.6 (CH)	69.5 (CH)
2	67.8 (CH)	78.1 (C)	64.6 (CH)	64.6 (CH)
3	184.8 (C)	176.4 (C)	183.1 (C)	183.0 (C)
4	114.1 (CH)	110.9 (CH)	114.4 (CH)	114.4 (CH)
5	171.5 (C)	172.8 (C)	171.2 (C)	171.1 (C)
6	48.6 (C)	44.5 (C)	47.0 (C)	47.1 (C)
7	37.4 (CH_2)	38.7 (CH_2)	37.4 (CH_2)	37.5 (CH_2)
8	63.7 (CH)	63.1 (CH)	63.5 (CH)	63.5 (CH)
10	148.6 (C)	148.2 (C)	149.0 (C)	149.1 (C)
11	167.5 (C)	165.4 (C)	167.1 (C)	167.1 (C)
12	125.6 (C)	124.0 (C)	125.6 (C)	125.6 (C)
14	127.2 (CH)	126.0 (CH)	127.4 (CH)	127.4 (CH)
15	119.2 (C)	119.3 (C)	119.4 (C)	119.4 (C)
16	20.6 (CH_2)	20.0 (CH_2)	20.7 (CH_2)	20.7 (CH_2)
17	52.8 (CH_2)	50.2 (CH_2)	52.9 (CH_2)	52.9 (CH_2)
19	150.3 (C)	150.2 (C)	150.4 (C)	150.4 (C)
20	101.8 (C)	100.4 (C)	100.6 (C)	100.6 (C)
21	122.7 (C)	122.2 (C)	122.7 (C)	122.7 (C)
1′	-		171.0 (C)	173.6 (C)
2′	-		20.4 (CH_3)	34.0 (CH_2)
3′	-		-	25.8 (CH_2)
4′	-		-	27.5 (CH_2)
5′	-		-	129.7 (CH)
6′	-		-	131.7 (CH)
7′	-		-	28.4 (CH_2)
8′	-		-	28.4 (CH_2)
9′	-		-	130.1 (CH)
10′	-		-	130.8 (CH)
11′–25′	-		-	28.1–30.9 (CH_2); 130.9 (CH); 131.4 (CH)
26′	-		-	32.9 (CH_2)
27′	-		-	23.7 (CH_2)
28′	-		-	14.5 (CH_3)

[a] Extracted from HSQC and HMBC spectra.

Compound **4** is a configurationally rigid molecule with seven rings and three stereocenters at C-2, C-6, and C-8. The relative configurations of these stereogenic centers were proposed by the NOE correlations as shown in Figure 4B. The specific rotation value of **4** ($[\alpha]^{20}_D$ = −246, *c* 0.05, MeOH) is opposite to that of (+)-(2*S*,6*R*,8*S*)-discorhabdin D ($[\alpha]^{20}_D$ = +80, *c* 0.025, MeOH) [26]. The experimental ECD spectrum of compound **4** (Supplementary Figure S8) showed the same cotton effects as compound **1** (−)-(1*R*,2*S*,6*R*,8*S*)-discorhabdin L. So it is reasonable to assume that compound **4** is (−)-(2*R*,6*R*,8*S*)-2-bromodiscorhabdin D.

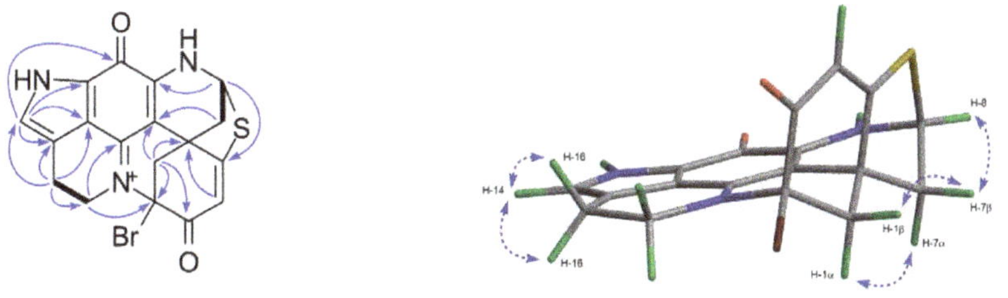

A B

Figure 4. Key 2D NMR correlations observed for compound **4**. (**A**) The COSY (in bold), key H→C HMBC (arrows); (**B**) key H→H NOESY correlations (dashed line).

Compound **5** was obtained as a green film. Its molecular formula $C_{20}H_{16}N_3O_4S$ was deduced by HR-ESIMS (*m/z* 394.0816, $[M + H]^+$) indicating 15 degrees of unsaturation. The FT-IR spectrum of compound **5** displayed the characteristic ester carbonyl absorption band at υ_{max} 1747 cm^{-1} and other similar bands as compound (**1**) at υ_{max} 1653, 1621, 1560, 1528, 1412, and 1201 cm^{-1}. The ^1H and ^{13}C NMR spectra of **5** (Tables 2 and 3) revealed high similarity with **1**, with the only difference being the presence of an extra acetyl group in **5** (δ_H 2.15; δ_C 171.0 and δ_C 20.4). The site of esterification was identified as C-1, based on strong HMBC correlations between H-1/C-1′ and a weaker HMBC coupling between H-2′/C-1 (Figure 5A). Thus, the planar structure of compound **5** was confirmed as 1-acetyl-discorhabdin L. The analysis of the full 2D NMR dataset (COSY, HSQC, and HMBC) further confirmed that the planar structure of compound **5** (Figure 5A). The relative configuration of compound **5** was elucidated by examining its NOESY spectrum (Figure 5B). The COSY correlation between H-4/H-7 (Supplementary Figure S32) indicated a planar "W" arrangement [28] of the molecule as observed in discorhabdins L [13] and D [23], thus allowing the assignment of the resonance at δ_H 2.63 to H-7α [13]. The stereochemistry at C-1 was proposed by the strong NOE correlation (Figure 5B) between H-1/H-7α. To establish the absolute configuration of (−)-**5**, its experimental ECD spectrum was compared with that of (−)-(1*R*,2*S*,6*R*,8*S*)-discorhabdin L (**1**) (Supplementary Figure S8). The same Cotton effects observed at 290, 360, and 440 nm for both compounds established the absolute configuration of **5** as 1*R*,2*S*,6*R*,8*S*. Finally, the comparison of the specific rotation values of compounds **1** ($[\alpha]^{20}_D$ = −71, *c* 0.1, MeOH) and **5** ($[\alpha]^{20}_D$ = −420, *c* 0.01, MeOH) identified the structure of **5** as (−)-(1*R*,2*S*,6*R*,8*S*)-1-acetyl-discorhabdin L.

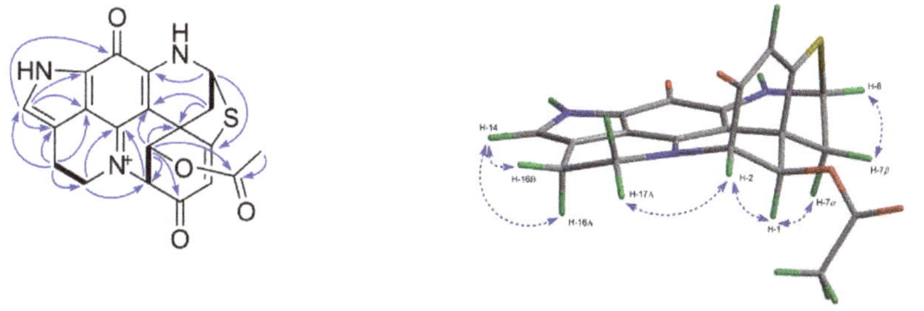

(A) **(B)**

Figure 5. Key 2D NMR correlations observed for compound **5**. (**A**) The COSY (in bold), key H→C HMBC (arrows); (**B**) key H→H NOESY correlations (dashed line).

The most nonpolar component, compound **6**, was obtained as a green film with an $[\alpha]^{20}_D$ value of + 541 (*c* 0.1, MeOH). It showed a molecular ion peak at *m/z* 752.4452 $[M + H]^+$ in the HR-ESIMS spectrum. The molecular formula of $C_{46}H_{62}N_3O_4S$ was deduced from its ^{13}C NMR and HR-ESIMS data (Table 3 and Supplementary Figure S41), indicating 18 degrees of unsaturation. The FT-IR spectrum contained absorption bands typical of an ester function (υ_{max} 1739 cm^{-1}) and an alkyl chain (υ_{max} 2927 and 2855 cm^{-1}, -CH_2 and -CH_3 stretching bands). Comparison of the 1D-NMR data of **6** with those of **1** and **5** (Tables 2 and 3) suggested **6** to be another analog of discorhabdin L esterified with a long chain fatty acid (δ_C 25–35 ppm; δ_H 1.2–1.4 ppm), which made this molecule very lipophilic. The discorhabdin L core structure that was evident from the 1D and 2D NMR data of **6** (Tables 2 and 3; Figure 6) accounted for 14 degrees of unsaturation. The additional ester carbonyl at δ_C 173.6 and six sp^2 carbons belonging to three double bonds at δ_C 129.7, 130.1, 130.8, 130.9, 131.4, and 131.7 (Supplementary Figure S36) accounted for the remaining 4 degrees of unsaturation. Hence, we concluded that the alkyl chain was an unbranched octacosa-triene-oic acid (28:3) (Tables 2 and 3). The HMBC correlation between H-1 (δ_H 5.79) and C-1′ (δ_C 173.6) supported the attachment of the fatty acid at C-1 (Figure 6A). The geometry of these three double bonds in the fatty acid portion was elucidated by analyzing the ^{13}C NMR chemical shifts of the six carbons neighboring the double bonds [29]. Carbon atoms adjacent to *cis* double bonds resonate around δ_C 26.0–28.5, whereas those adjacent to *trans* double bonds appear at higher chemical shift values, namely δ_C 29.5–38.0 [29]. The observed ^{13}C NMR shifts in (+)-**6** at δ_C 27.5, 28.1, 28.2 (× 2), 28.4 (× 2) confirmed the *cis* (*Z*) configuration of all three double bonds in the fatty acid part (Table 3). The COSY correlations from C-2′ to C-10′ and HMBC correlations between H_2-2′/C-1′, C-4′; H_2-3′/C-1′, C-4′, C-5′; H-6′/C-4′, C-7′, C-8′; H_2-7′/C-9′ (Figure 6A) allowed us to corroborate the position of two unsaturations at C-5′ and C-9′, and to assign the C-1′ to C-10′ portion of the fatty acid (Figure 3). Comparison of the 1D NMR data of (+)-**6** with the literature [30] also supports the presence of a $\Delta^{5,9}$ unsaturated fatty acid. This finding is not surprising since these *cis,cis*-5,9-dienoic lipids are common in sponges [31]. The chemical shift values of C-26′, C-27′ and C-28′ (Table 3) were also assigned by comparison with the literature data [32]. Thus, compound (+)-**6** was identified as C-1 octacosatrienoic acid (C28:3) ester of (−)-discorhabdin L (Figure 3). Due to availability of very minor amount of the compound (0.2 mg) and the failed attempts to improve the highly overlapped NMR signals through different solvents (e.g., MeOD, $CDCl_3$, and DMSO-*d6*), we were unable to confirm the position of the third double bond. However, we believe that the lipid residue in **6** is related to the well-known 5*Z*,9*Z* demospongic acids bearing another double bond at C-17, or C-19, or C-23 [31].

On the basis of a strong NOE correlation between H-1 and H-7α (Figure 6B), as well as the other NOE correlations shown in Figure 6B, the relative configuration of **6** was elucidated to be the same as compounds **1** and **5**. The absolute configuration of **6** was established by comparing its experimental ECD spectrum with those of **1** and **5** (Supplementary Figure S8). Based on the opposite sign of the specific rotation value of **6** ($[\alpha]^{20}_D$ = +541, *c* 0.1, MeOH) in comparison to compounds **1** ($[\alpha]^{20}_D$ = −71, *c* 0.1, MeOH) and **5** ($[\alpha]^{20}_D$ = −420, *c* 0.01, MeOH), **6** was identified as (+)-(1*R*,2*S*,6*R*,8*S*)-1-octacosatrienoyl-discorhabdin L (Figure 3).

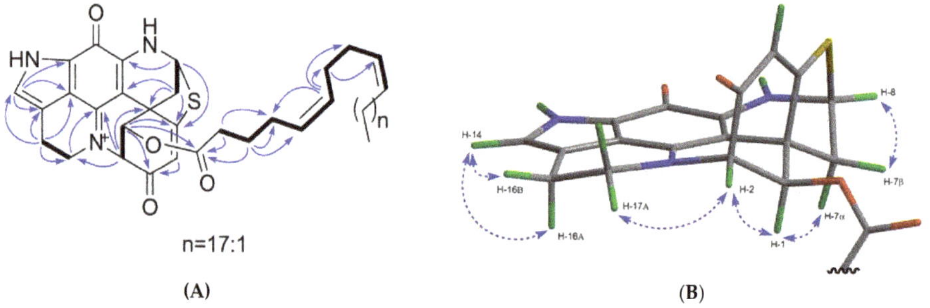

Figure 6. Key 2D NMR correlations observed for compound **6**. (**A**) The COSY (in bold), key H→C HMBC (arrows); (**B**) key H→H NOESY correlations (dashed line).

2.2. *In Vitro Bioactivity Tests and Molecular Docking on Purified Compounds*

Anticancer activity of the pyrroloiminoquinone-type alkaloids has been the main driving force for isolation of these intriguing structural types. Due to low quantities of the isolated compounds, we were only able to assess the in vitro anticancer activities of compounds **1**, **5**, and **6** against one cell line. We used HCT-116 colon cancer cells for testing, because of the observed high activity of the MeOH subextract and SPE fractions (Table 1), plus the availability of literature data for (−)-discorhabdin L (**1**) against this cell line (IC_{50} value 6.2 μM) [17]. In the current study, compound **1** showed IC_{50} value of 0.94 μM (equal to 0.33 μg/mL). The compound **5** displayed promising activity with an IC_{50} value of 2.71 μM (= 1.1 μg/mL), while compound **6** was only modestly active against the same cell line (IC_{50} value 34.0 μM, equal to 25.6 μg/mL). These results indicate that C-1 OH function is important for anti-colon cancer activity and the substitution of the C-1 OH group, especially with a long chain fatty acyl function is not favored.

Limited by the amounts of the isolated compounds, we performed a molecular modeling study (using Schrödinger software Maestro; www.schrodinger.com) on compounds **1–6** and (+)-discorhabdin L (**1e**), the (+) enantiomer of compound **1**, against two known anticancer targets (topoisomerase I/II, indoleamine 2,3-dioxygenase IDO1) to estimate their potential anticancer activity and mechanism(s) of action. Where possible, based on suitable pdb structures, docking experiments were performed. We prepared available relevant pdb protein structures, removed the original ligands, and generated receptor grids. Small molecule 3D structures of the compounds containing a quaternary nitrogen were energetically minimized and possible tautomers/protonated states were evaluated (LigPrep, counter ion not specified). Next, we docked the optimized ligand structures into respective active sites (Glide SP). Calculated 3D binding modes were illustrated, or presented as 2D ligand-interaction diagrams, for clarity.

Docking of compounds **1–5** into the active site of topoisomerase I (pdb 1T8I) yielded plausible binding modes (Figure 7), while no binding pose could be calculated for compound **6**, due to the sterically demanding side chain that did not fit into the tight binding pocket). Compared to the original ligand camptothecin, the flat, partly aromatic core of the discorhabdins **1–5** intercalated into the DNA part thereby forming aromatic π-π-stacking interactions while also addressing H-bonds towards residues of the topoisomerase I protein. Similar results were obtained by docking experiments with topoisomerase II (pdb 3QX3, original ligand etoposide) suggesting these proteins to be anticancer targets for the compounds **1–5**. Molecular docking study performed (in analogy to the procedure described above) on compound **1e**, which was reported to exhibit strong in vitro cytotoxicity [33], revealed a binding mode in the active site of topoisomerase I, too (Figure 7). Comparable to **1**, the flat core forms a DNA-intercalating complex, but the ligand is distorted by 180°. Thus, the binding modes of both compounds, **1** and **1e**, suggest those ligands to be rather non-specific DNA intercalators.

We also performed docking experiments with another reported target for pyrroloiminoquinone alkaloids, namely the indoleamine 2,3-dioxygenase (IDO1) enzyme for which structural data including ligand–protein complexes are available. As cofactor to mediate physiological substrate oxidation, IDO1 contains a heme moiety and ligands typically form interactions by complexing the iron central atom. Examples for such IDO1 inhibitors and relevant interacting moieties include NLG919 derivative (imidazole-like nitrogen in pdb 5EK2) or ligand INCB14943 (hydroxylamidine moiety in pdb 5XE1). Since the compounds lack comparable nitrogen functionalities to able to interact with heme in a similar manner, docking of the compounds into these active sites revealed no plausible binding modes. However, recent reports demonstrated that another class of potent IDO1 inhibitors such as FXB-001116 (pdb 6AZW) and BMS-978587 (pdb 6AZV) bind to the IDO1 apo structure with high affinity, thereby displacing the heme moiety. Accordingly, we performed docking experiments of compounds **1–6** and **1e** using the apo-protein. This approach suggested possible binding modes for compounds **1–4** and **1e** in the apo active site of IDO1 (Figure 8), but not for the sterically more demanding compounds **5** and **6**.

Compound **A** **B**

1

1e

2

3

4

5

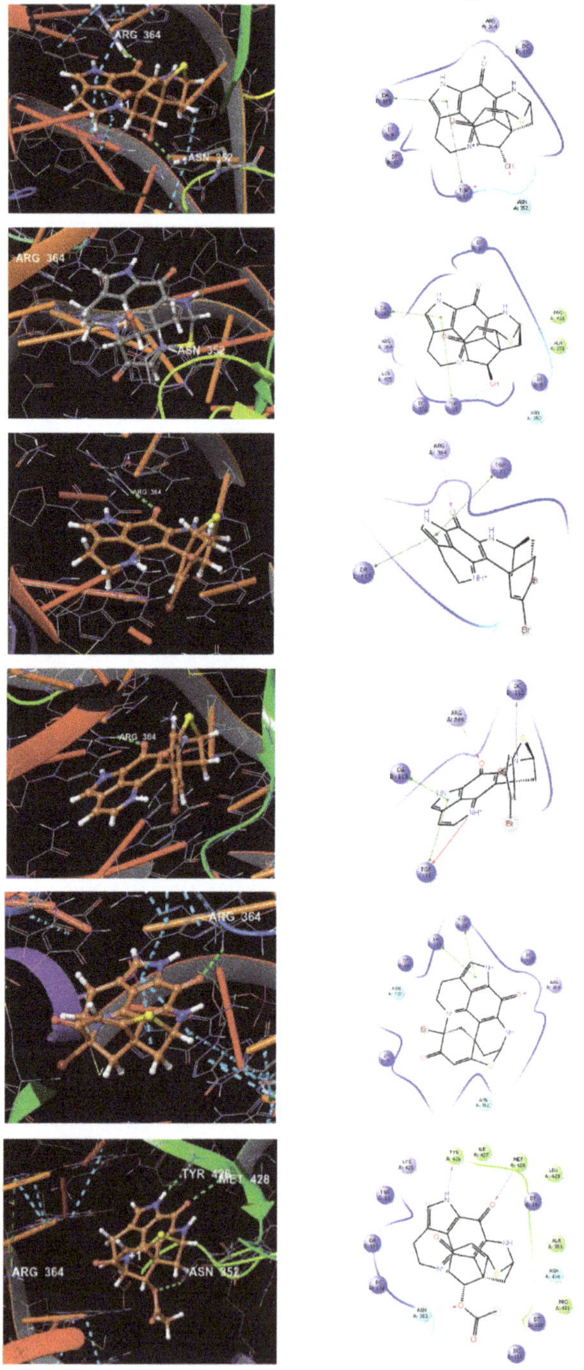

Figure 7. (**A**) Calculated 3D binding modes of compounds **1–5** and **1e** in the active site of topoisomerase I (pdb 1T8I) also containing a DNA molecule (colored in red) with a single strand break; (**B**) corresponding 2D ligand interaction diagrams showing key interactions of compounds **1–5** and **1e** towards topoisomerase I and DNA.

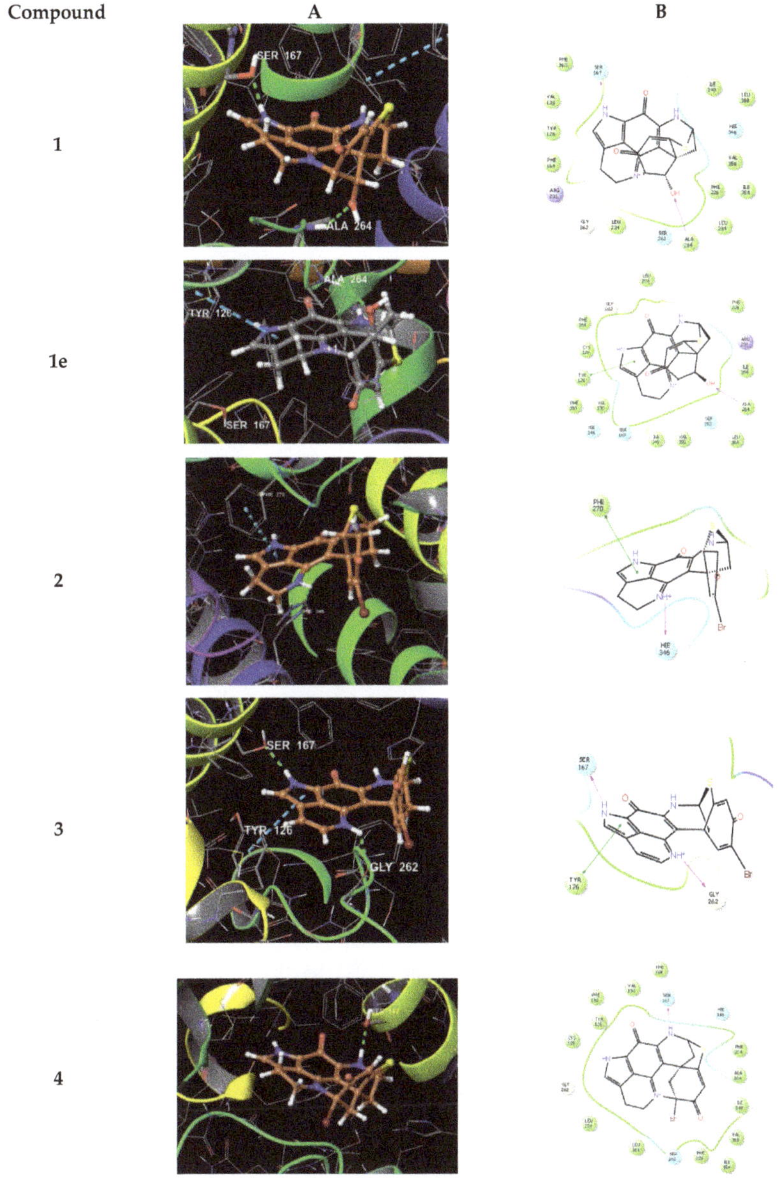

Figure 8. 3D binding poses (**A**) and ligand interaction diagrams (**B**) of compounds **1–4** and **1e** in the active site of IDO1 (pdb 6AZW). Key interactions are shown. The binding pocket is shown in a similar orientation, respectively. Ligand docking revealed plausible binding poses for compounds **1–4** and **1e**, but not for compounds **5** and **6**.

Inspecting the docking poses of **1** in the above-mentioned protein structures on a molecular level pointed towards a key role for the sterically defined OH-function in **1**, as it mediates an H-bond towards Ala264. Another key H-bond interaction occurred between aromatic NH of **1** towards Ser167 (Figure 8). Compound **1** shows a rather planar core, anchoring the ligand with a strong shape-fit into the tight binding pocket. Relative to this core, the thioether bridge sits almost rectangular on top, occupying a lipophilic area within the binding site, flanked by residues including Val350, Phe226, and Leu384. Within these small sets of compounds, docking of **1** reveals the optimal pose. We also docked (+)-discorhabdin L (**1e**), the enantiomer of **1,** into the active site of IDO1 (in analogy to the procedure described above). Interestingly, the flat core was found to again fill the rather flat pocket. In comparison to **1**, the core sits upside down in **1e**, with the key H-bond towards Ala264 being maintained. Accordingly, the NH-bond towards Ser167 was lost, but the aromatic system formed a π-interaction to Tyr126 (Figure 8). These poses suggest the flat aromatic core of this type of compounds to be the main requisite to bind into the pocket. Furthermore, stereochemistry seems to play a minor role in binding. Thus, it can be assumed the compounds are rather non-specific IDO1-ligands.

The calculated binding mode of compound **4** yielded a shifted orientation of the core, with only one H-bond towards Ser167 (Figure 8). In contrast, compounds **5** and **6** gave no plausible docking solutions, again due to the sterically demanding ester moieties, thus also preventing H-bonding by OH towards Ala264.

In summary, the molecular modeling data suggested plausible binding modes for compounds **1–5** in the target structure of topoisomerase I, and for compounds **1–4** towards IDO1, respectively. However, it is well possible that this class of compounds bind further key anticancer targets, contributing to their cytotoxic potential.

3. Discussion

Since the discovery of discorhabdin C from a New Zealand *Latrunculia* sp. in 1986 [8], more than 40 discorhabdin analogs have been reported from different marine sponge genera [34]. Some discorhabdins contain bromination at C-2, C-4, or C-14 positions (e.g., discorhabdin A, discorhabdin C, 14-bromodihydrodiscorhabdin C) [8,23,24,35], some possess a sulfur bridge between C-5 and C-8 (e.g., discorhabdin B, discorhabdin Q) [24,36]. A few discorhabdins (e.g., discorhabdin L, discorhabdin D) are heptacyclic through the formation of an extra bridge between C-2 and N-18 [13,24]. Of the six compounds obtained in the current study, two of them (**5** and **6**) are (−)-discorhabdin L esters. Compound **6** is a triunsaturated C28 fatty acid ester of discorhabdin L. To our knowledge this is the first discorhabdin alkyl ester structure being reported from a marine sponge. Notably, Zou et al. (2013) reported atkamine, a new, large pyrroloiminoquinone scaffold containing a fused epoxybenzazepin and bromophenol groups connected with a cyclic sulfide ring [37]. Between the former and the latter rings, there is a substitution with a monosaturated C20 alkyl chain. The authors suggested this alkyl group to originate from (*Z*)-15-docosenoic acid, a fatty acid commonly found in sponge species that was possibly incorporated in the very early biosynthesis stages of atkamine [37]. Compounds **5** and **6** isolated in this study instead bear an esterification at C-1 position of the pyrroloiminoquinone ring system. Compound **5** is an acetyl ester of (−)-discorhabdin L, while **6** is an ester of discorhabdin L with an unbranched octacosatrienoic acid. Marine sponges, especially demosponges, are regarded as one of the richest sources of long-chain fatty acids (LCFAs; i.e., C23–34) [38,39]. The octacosatrienoic acid (C28:3) has been reported from marine sponges and corals [40–42], but not from any *Latrunculia* species. The only study that analyzed the FAs composition of Antarctic *Latrunculia* sponges in 2015 showed that Antarctic *L. biformis* contained diverse common and LCFAs (C16, C18), however longer chain unsaturated FAs were not found [43]. This is the first report of a discorhabdin-LCFA ester from nature, and the current study adds three new and intriguing analogs to the list of discorhabdin class alkaloids.

Discorhabdins have been repeatedly studied for their in vitro anticancer activity [10,13,14]. Limited by the strong cytotoxicity and the supply issue, no molecule from this chemical family has ever proceeded to further clinical studies. A few structure–activity relationship studies (SARs) associated with discorhabdins have been conducted, revealing that the ring closure by a bridge between C2 and N18 can significantly reduce the cytotoxicity, while a substitution at C-1 (i.e., OMe, NH_2) can enhance the anticancer activity [19,26]. The discovery of C-1 esters of discorhabdin L with good to moderate inhibitory activity against HCT-116 cell line here provides further insights for the SARs of discorhabdins.

Although many discorhabdins are associated with anticancer/cytotoxic activity, little is known on their exact mechanism(s) of action. Wada et al. (2011) evaluated (+)-discorhabdin A and its synthetic oxa analog for inhibition against a set of anticancer target enzymes, such as protein kinase, histone deacetylase, farnesyltransferase, telomerase, and proteasome [16]. (+)-Discorhabdin A and its synthetic oxa analog weakly inhibited the farnesyltransferase enzyme (IC_{50} > 10μM) [16]. Geoy et al. recently tested the HIF-1α/p300 inhibition activity of several discorhabdins, including (−)-discorhabdin L (IC_{50} value 0.73 μM) concluding them to be a novel class of HIF-1α/p300 inhibitors [17]. In the current study, an *in silico* molecular modeling study revealed the plausible binding modes of discorhabdins in two additional cancer target enzymes, topoisomerase I/II and IDO1.

In summary, guided by the anticancer activity and MN-based metabolomics, the Antarctic deep-sea sponge *L. biformis* led to the isolation and characterization of three known and three new discorhabdin alkaloids. Despite the small amounts of the extract and fractions that hampered the isolation of many further new discorhabdins, MN-based metabolomics proved useful for identification of chemical inventory of the sponge in early stages. Two compounds were a new type of discorhabdin esters that yielded meaningful SARs in comparison to the parent compound discorhabdin L. Mechanistic studies based on molecular modeling showed, for the first time, the potential binding of discorhabdins to additional anticancer targets that may be involved in their anticancer activity.

4. Materials and Methods

4.1. General Procedures

Specific rotation of compounds **1–6** were measured on a Jasco P-2000 polarimeter (Jasco, Pfungstadt, Germany). FT-IR spectra were recorded using a PerkinElmer Spectrum Two FT-IR spectrometer (PerkinElmer, Boston, MA, USA). UV spectra were run on a NanoVue Plus spectrophotometer (GE Healthcare, New York, NY. USA). ECD spectra were run in MeOH on a J-810 CD spectrometer (Jasco, Pfungstadt, Germany). NMR spectra were obtained on a Bruker AV 600 spectrometer (600 and 150 MHz for ^1H and ^{13}C NMR, respectively, Bruker®, Billerica, MA, USA) equipped with 5.0 mm Shigemi tube (SHIGEMI, Co., LTD., Tokyo, Japan). The residual solvent signals were used as internal references: δ_H 3.31/δ_C 49.0 ppm (MeOD), and δ_H 2.50/δ_C 39.51 ppm (DMSO-d_6). 4-Dimethyl-4-silapentane-1-sulfonic acid (DSS) served as the internal standard. HRMS/MS data were recorded on a Waters Xevo G2-XS QTof Mass Spectrometer (Waters®, Milford, MA, USA) coupled to a Waters Acquity I-Class UPLC system (Waters®, Milford, MA, USA). HR-ESIMS was recorded on micrOTOF II-High-performance TOF-MS system (Bruker®, Billerica, MA, USA) equipped with an electrospray ionization source. Solid phase extraction (SPE) was performed on the Chromabond SPE C18 column cartridges (6 mL/2000 mg, Macherey-Nagel, Duren, Germany). HPLC separations were performed on a VWR Hitachi Chromaster system (VWR International, Allison Park, PA, USA) consisting of a 5430-diode array detector (VWR International, Allison Park, PA, USA), a 5310-column oven, a 5260 autosampler, and a 5110 pump combined in parallel with a VWR evaporative light scattering detector (ELSD 90, VWR International, Allison Park, PA, USA). The eluents used for HPLC separations were H_2O (A) and MeCN (B). Routine HPLC separations were performed on a semi-preparative C18 monolithic column (Onyx, 100 × 10 mm, Phenomenex, Torrance, CA, USA) and an analytical synergi column (250 × 4.6 mm, Phenomenex, Torrance, CA, USA). A chiral cellulose-1 column (Lux 5μ, 250 × 4.6 mm, Phenomenex, Torrance, CA, USA) was used for checking the enantiopurity of each purified compound. The organic solvents used for UPLC-QToF-MS/MS analyses were ULC/MS grade (Biosolve BV, North Brabant, Netherlands) and HPLC grade (ITW Reagents, Darmstadt, Germany) for HPLC isolation processes. The water used was MilliQ-water produced by Arium® Water Purification Systems (Sartorius, Göttingen, Germany).

4.2. Sponge Material

The sponge was collected in 2015/2016 during the Expedition PS96 of the Research Vessel POLARSTERN to the southern Weddell Sea (Antarctica). The sponge was collected by an Agassiz trawl at a depth of −291 m, and was fixated immediately after collection. Specimens were cleaned, pre-sorted, photographed, and transferred into buckets with cold seawater as soon as the catch was on deck. Subsamples were transferred into pure ethanol (96%) and the main parts were frozen at −20 °C. The sponges were transported to the Senckenberg Research Institute and Nature Museum in Frankfurt am Main, Germany. Tissue samples were taken and skeletal preparations were made for transmission light microscopy and SEM, according to standard protocols [44]. For taxonomic examination, the sponge spicules were mounted on microscope slides and studied by light microscopy and by SEM. Based on comparative morphology of skeletal characters, the sponge was identified as *Latrunculia biformis*, which is a common species in the Antarctic deeper shelf areas. For identification, the World Porifera Database [45] and relevant literature were used. A specimen (SMF 12109) is deposited in the Porifera collection of Senckenberg Research Institute and Nature Museum, electronically inventoried. The data are online available in the SESAM database.

4.3. Extraction and Isolation

The sponge material (43.615 g, frozen weight) was cut into small pieces and freeze-dried (Martin Christ, Osterode am Harz, Germany). The lyophilized biomass (5.809 g) was extracted at room temperature with water (3 × 200 mL) under agitation to yield the aqueous extract (1.892 g). The remaining sponge residue (3.572 g, dry weight) was extracted with MeOH (3 × 150 mL) and subsequently with DCM (3 × 150 mL) under the same conditions. Combined MeOH and DCM extracts were evaporated to dryness by a rotary evaporator to yield the crude organic extract (328 mg) that showed very strong anticancer activity against multiple cancer cell lines. This extract was partitioned between MeOH (100 mL) and *n*-hexane (100 mL) to yield MeOH (190 mg) and *n*-hexane (120 mg) subextracts. The MeOH-soluble portion, which exhibited strong anticancer activity was fractionated on a Chromabond SPE C18 cartridge. The elution with a step gradient MeOH:H_2O mixture (0% to 100%) afforded 8 fractions (M1–M8), of which the anticancer activity was tracked to six fractions M2–M5, M7, and M8. RP-HPLC separation of M2 (18 mg) on the analytical Synergi column gradient of H_2O:MeCN (77:22), with 0.1% TFA, flow 1.0 mL/min yielded compound **1** (1.5 mg, t_R 5.5 min). RP-HPLC analysis of M3 (10 mg) on the same column (gradient of H_2O:MeCN from 80:20 to 70:30 in 25 min, with 0.1% TFA, flow 1.0 mL/min) afforded compounds **5** (0.3 mg, t_R 15.2 min) and **3** (0.3 mg, t_R 19.0 min). M4 (16 mg) was further fractionated on a Chromabond SPE C18 cartridge to furnish 5 subfractions (M4-1 to M4-5). The subfraction M4-1 (4.4 mg) was further purified by RP-HPLC equipped with an analytical C18 column using a gradient of H_2O:MeCN (87:13 to 80:20, 0–16 min, 80:20 to 74:26, 16–27 min, with 0.1% TFA, flow 1.0 mL/min) to yield compounds **4** (0.1 mg, t_R 18.9 min) and **2** (0.1 mg, t_R 20.5 min). RP-HPLC separation of the nonpolar fraction M8 (23.9 mg) (gradient of H_2O:MeCN 25:75 to 0:100, 0–15 min, with 0.1% TFA, flow 1.0 mL/min) on an analytical C18 column yielded compound **6** (0.2 mg, t_R 14.9 min). Each purified compound was further checked, individually, for enantiopurity by RP-DAD-HPLC on a chiral analytical column using a gradient of H_2O:MeCN (99:1 to 0:100, 0–15 min, with 0.1% TFA, flow 1.5 mL/min).

(−)-(1R,2S,6R,8S)-Discorhabdin L (**1**): Greenish film; $[\alpha]^{20}{}_D = -71$ (*c* 0.1, MeOH); ^{1}H NMR (CD_3OD, 600 MHz) and ^{13}C NMR (CD_3OD, 150 MHz) Tables 2 and 3; HR-ESIMS found *m/z* $[M + H]^+$ 352.0748, $C_{18}H_{14}N_3O_3S$ requires 352.0756.

(+)-(5R,6S,8S)-Discorhabdin A (**2**): Orange film; $[\alpha]^{20}{}_D = +197$ (*c* 0.01, MeOH); HR-ESIMS found *m/z* $[M + H]^+$ 416.0065, $C_{18}H_{15}{}^{79}BrN_3O_2S$ requires 416.0068.

(+)-(6S,8S)-Discorhabdin Q (**3**): Orange film; $[\alpha]^{20}{}_D = +568$ (*c* 0.1, MeOH); HR-ESIMS found *m/z* $[M + H]^+$ 411.9733, $C_{18}H_{11}{}^{79}BrN_3O_2S$ requires 411.9759.

(−)-(2R,6R,8S)-2-Bromodiscorhabdin D (**4**): Greenish film; UV (MeOH) λ_{max} 250 (ϵ 13840), 285 (ϵ 11184), 325 (ϵ 7947), 403 (ϵ 7802) nm; $[\alpha]^{20}{}_D = -246$ (*c* 0.05, MeOH); IR (film) v_{max} 2922, 2852, 1657, 1533,

1514, 1432, 1230 cm^{-1}; ^1H NMR (CD_3OD, 600 MHz) and ^{13}C NMR (CD_3OD 150 MHz) Tables 2 and 3; HR-ESIMS found *m/z* $[M + H]^+$ 413.9913, $C_{18}H_{13}{}^{79}BrN_3O_2S$ requires 413.9912.

(−)-(1R,2S,6R,8S)-1-Acetyl-discorhabdin L (**5**): Greenish film; UV (MeOH) λ_{max} 250 (ϵ 24822), 283 (ϵ 17019), 325 (ϵ 11700), 403 (ϵ 11169) nm; $[\alpha]^{20}{}_D = -420$ (*c* 0.01, MeOH); IR (film) v_{max} 2926, 2854, 1747, 1653, 1621, 1560, 1528, 1412, 1201 cm^{-1}; ^1H NMR (CD_3OD, 600 MHz) and ^{13}C NMR (CD_3OD, 150 MHz) Tables 2 and 3; HR-ESIMS found *m/z* $[M + H]^+$ 394.0816, $C_{20}H_{16}N_3O_4S$ requires 394.0861.

(+)-(1R,2S,6R,8S)-1-Octacosatrienoyl-discorhabdin L (**6**): Greenish film; UV (MeOH) λ_{max} 203 (ϵ 19890), 249 (ϵ 19439), 285 (ϵ 15904), 325 (ϵ 13122), 403 (ϵ 11543) nm; $[\alpha]^{20}{}_D = +541$ (*c* 0.1, MeOH); IR (film) v_{max} 3007, 2927, 2855, 1739, 1678, 1621, 1566, 1527, 1441, 1206, 1185, 1135 cm^{-1}; ^1H NMR (CD_3OD, 600 MHz) and ^{13}C NMR (CD_3OD, 150 MHz) Tables 2 and 3; HR-ESIMS found *m/z* $[M + H]^+$ 752.4452, $C_{46}H_{62}N_3O_4S$ requires 752.4461.

4.4. UPLC-QToF-MS/MS Analysis

The six active C18 SPE fractions of the MeOH soluble portion were analyzed on an ACQUITY UPLC I-Class System coupled to the Xevo G2-XS QToF Mass Spectrometer (Waters®, Milford, Massachusetts, USA) equipped with an electrospray ionization (ESI) source operating with a positive polarity at a mass range of *m/z* 50–1600 Da. The 0.1 mg/mL MeOH solution of the fractions were filtered through a 0.2 µm PTFE syringe filter (Carl Roth, Karlsruhe, Germany) and then injected (injection volume: 1.0 µL) into the system equipped with Acquity UPLC HSS T3 column (high-strength silica C18, 1.8 µm, 100 × 2.1 mm I.D., Waters®) operating at 40 °C. Separation was achieved with a binary LC solvent system controlled by MassLynx® (version 4.1) using mobile phase A 99.9% water/0.1% formic acid (ULC/MS grade) and B 99.9% ACN/0.1% formic acid (ULC/MS grade), pumped at a rate of 0.6 mL/min with the following gradient: Initial, 1% B; 0.0–12.0 min to 100% B; 12.0–13.0 min 100% B, and a column reconditioning phase until 15 min.

ESI conditions were set with the capillary voltage at 0.8 kV, sample cone voltage at 40.0 V, source temperature at 150 °C, desolvation temperature at 550 °C, cone gas flow in 50 L/h, and desolvation gas flow in 1200 L/h. MS/MS setting was linear collision energy (CE) at 30 eV. As a control, solvent (methanol) was injected. MassLynx® (Waters®, V4.1) was used to analyze the achieved MS and MS^2 data.

4.5. Molecular Networking

The network was created using the UPLC-HRMS/MS data generated from the six active MeOH subfractions of *L. biformis*. All raw MS/MS data were converted from files (.raw) to mzXML file format using MSConvert (Version 3.6.10051, Vanderbilt University, Nashville, TN, USA). The converted data files were uploaded to the Global Natural Products Social molecular networking (http://gnps.ucsd.edu) platform using FileZilla (https://filezilla-project.org/) and a molecular network was created using the online workflow at GNPS [22]. The data were filtered by removing all MS/MS peaks within +/− 17 Da of the precursor *m/z*. MS/MS spectra were window filtered by choosing only the top 6 peaks in the +/− 50Da window throughout the spectrum. The data were then clustered with MS-Cluster with a parent mass tolerance of 0.1 Da and an MS/MS fragment ion tolerance of 0.05 Da to create consensus spectra. Further, concensus spectra that contained less than 2 spectra were discarded. A network was then created where edges were filtered to have a cosine score above 0.6 and more than 3 matched peaks. Further edges between two nodes were kept in the network if and only if each of the nodes appeared in each other's respective top 10 most similar nodes. The spectra in the network were then searched against GNPS' spectral libraries. The library spectra were filtered in the same manner as the input data. All matches kept between network spectra and library spectra were required to have a score above 0.7 and at least 6 matched peaks. The output molecular networking data were analyzed and visualized using Cytoscape (ver. 3.61) [46].

4.6. Cytotoxicity Assay

Crude extract of *L. biformis* and downstream fractions were tested in vitro at a final concentration of 100 μg/mL against 6 human cancer cell lines, Hep G2 (liver cancer cell line, DSMZ, Braunschweig, Germany), HT29 (colorectal adenocarcinoma cell line, DSMZ, Braunschweig, Germany), A375 (malignant melanoma cell line, CLS, Eppelheim, Germany), HCT116 (colon cancer cell line, DSMZ, Braunschweig, Germany), A549 (lung carcinoma cell line, CLS, Eppelheim, Germany), and MDA-MB231 (human breast cancer line, CLS, Eppelheim, Germany). Cells were supplemented at 37 °C and 5% CO_2 in RPMI 1640 medium (Life Technologies, Darmstadt, Germany) with 10% fetal bovine serum, 100 U/mL penicillin and 100 mg/mL streptomycin. A stock solution of 20 mg/mL in DMSO was prepared for each test sample. After 24 h incubation in 96-well plates, the medium in the cells was replaced by 100 μL fresh medium containing the test samples and cells were incubated for another 24 h at 37 °C. Doxorubicin was used as positive control, while 0.5% DMSO and growth media served as negative controls. All samples were prepared in duplicates. The assay was performed according to the manufacturer's instructions (Promega, Madison, WI, USA). Cells were incubated for 2 h at 37 °C and fluorescence at an excitation wavelength of 560 nm and emission at 590 nm was measured. For the determination of IC_{50} values, a dilution series of the extracts were tested following the same procedure as described before. IC_{50} values were calculated by using Excel to determine the concentration that shows 50% inhibition of the viability.

4.7. Molecular Modeling and Docking

Molecular modeling was performed on a DELL Precision T3610 four core workstation using Schrödinger Maestro (version 11.3, 2017, Schrödinger, LLC, New York, NY, USA). The following RCSB protein data bank (pdb) crystal structures were used for modeling studies: 1T8I, 3QX3, 5EK2, 5XE1, 6AZV, 6AZW. Each protein structure was initially prepared by standard settings of the Protein Preparation Wizard 2015-4 (Epik version 2.4, Schrödinger, LLC, 2015; Impact version 5.9, Schrödinger, LLC, 2015; Prime version 3.2, Schrödinger LLC, 2015). For energy minimizations of the small-molecule ligands, MacroModel (version 11.0, Schrödinger, LLC, 2015) was used. Ionization states and tautomers were generated with LigPrep (version 3.6, Schrödinger, LLC, 2015). Ligand docking and receptor grid generation was performed with Glide (version 6.9, Schrödinger, LLC, 2015). Figures and ligand interaction diagrams (LID) were generated by Maestro.

Supplementary Materials: The following are available online at http://www.mdpi.com/1660-3397/17/8/439/s1, HR-ESIMS and NMR spectra of compounds **1–6**. ECD spectra of compounds **1**,**4**,**5**, and **6**.

Author Contributions: Design of the work, D.T. and F.L.; sample provision, D.J.; extraction, purifications of compounds, F.L.; data analysis, F.L. and D.T.; molecular docking experiment, C.P.; writing original manuscript, F.L. and D.T.; editing, D.T.; supervision, D.T.

Funding: This research received no external funding.

Acknowledgments: Fengjie Li thanks the China Scholarship Council for a Ph.D. fellowship. The Deutsche Forschungsgemeinschaft (DFG) is acknowledged by Dorte Janussen for financial support to her Antarctic sponge research (JA 1063/17-1). We thank Daniel Kersken for his dedicated effort in collection and fixation of these sponges during the PS96 expedition, thanks are due also to the captain and crew of RV POLARSTERN. We are grateful to Arlette Wenzel-Storjohann and Jana Heumann for performing anticancer assays. Joachim Grötzinger is acknowledged for offering the J-810 CD spectrometer for ECD spectrum measurement. We acknowledge financial support by Land Schleswig-Holstein within the funding program Open Access Publikationsfonds.

Conflicts of Interest: The authors declare no conflict of interest.

References

1. Alvarez, B.; Bergquist, P.R.; Battershill, C.N. Taxonomic revision of the genus *Latrunculia* du Bocage (Porifera: Demospongiae: Latrunculiidae) in New Zealand. *N. Z. J. Mar. Freshw. Res.* **2002**, *36*, 151–184. [CrossRef]

2. Samaai, T.; Gibbons, M.J.; Kelly, M.; Davies-Coleman, M. South African Latrunculiidae (Porifera: Demospongiae: Poecilosclerida): Descriptions of new species of *Latrunculia* du Bocage, *Strongylodesma* Lévi, and *Tsitsikamma* Samaai & Kelly. *Zootaxa* **2003**, *371*, 1.
3. Kelly, M.; Sim-Smith, C.; Stone, R.; Samaai, T.; Reiswig, H.; Austin, W. New taxa and arrangements within the family Latrunculiidae (Demospongiae, Poecilosclerida). *Zootaxa* **2016**, *4121*, 1. [CrossRef] [PubMed]
4. Capon, R.; MacLeod, J.K.; Willis, A.C. Trunculins A and B, norsesterterpene cyclic peroxides from a marine sponge, *Latrunculia brevis*. *J. Org. Chem.* **1987**, *52*, 339–342. [CrossRef]
5. Butler, M.; Capon, R.; Capon, R. Trunculin-F and Contrunculin-A and -B: Novel oxygenated norterpenes From a Southern Australian marine sponge, *Latrunculia conulosa*. *Aust. J. Chem.* **1993**, *46*, 1363. [CrossRef]
6. Zampella, A.; Randazzo, A.; Borbone, N.; Luciani, S.; Trevisi, L.; Debitus, C.; D'Auria, M.V. Isolation of callipeltins A–C and of two new open-chain derivatives of callipeltin A from the marine sponge *Latrunculia* sp. A revision of the stereostructure of callipeltins. *Tetrahedron Lett.* **2002**, *43*, 6163–6166. [CrossRef]
7. Sepe, V.; D'Orsi, R.; Borbone, N.; D'Auria, M.V.; Bifulco, G.; Monti, M.C.; Catania, A.; Zampella, A. Callipeltins F–I: New antifungal peptides from the marine sponge *Latrunculia* sp. *Tetrahedron* **2006**, *62*, 833–840. [CrossRef]
8. Perry, N.B.; Blunt, J.W.; McCombs, J.D.; Munro, M.H.G. Discorhabdin C, a highly cytotoxic pigment from a sponge of the genus *Latrunculia*. *J. Org. Chem.* **1986**, *51*, 5476–5478. [CrossRef]
9. Ford, J.; Capon, R.J. Discorhabdin R: A new antibacterial pyrroloiminoquinone from two latrunculiid marine sponges, *Latrunculia* sp. and Negombata sp. *J. Nat. Prod.* **2000**, *63*, 1527–1528. [CrossRef]
10. Hu, J.-F.; Fan, H.; Xiong, J.; Wu, S.-B. Discorhabdins and pyrroloiminoquinone-related alkaloids. *Chem. Rev.* **2011**, *111*, 5465–5491. [CrossRef] [PubMed]
11. Miller, K.; Alvarez, B.; Battershill, C.; Northcote, P.; Parthasarathy, H. Genetic, morphological, and chemical divergence in the sponge genus *Latrunculia* (Porifera: Demospongiae) from New Zealand. *Mar. Biol.* **2001**, *139*, 235–250. [CrossRef]
12. Furrow, F.B.; Amsler, C.D.; McClintock, J.B.; Baker, B.J. Surface sequestration of chemical feeding deterrents in the Antarctic sponge *Latrunculia apicalis* as an optimal defense against sea star spongivory. *Mar. Boil.* **2003**, *143*, 443–449. [CrossRef]
13. Reyes, F.; Martín, R.; Rueda, A.; Fernandez, R.; Montalvo, D.; Gomez, C.; Sánchez-Puelles, J.M. Discorhabdins I and L, cytotoxic alkaloids from the sponge *Latrunculia brevis*. *J. Nat. Prod.* **2004**, *67*, 463–465. [CrossRef] [PubMed]
14. Gunasekera, S.P.; Zuleta, I.A.; Longley, R.E.; Wright, A.E.; Pomponi, S.A. Discorhabdins S, T, and U, new cytotoxic pyrroloiminoquinones from a deep-water Caribbean sponge of the genus *Batzella*. *J. Nat. Prod.* **2003**, *66*, 1615–1617. [CrossRef] [PubMed]
15. Jeon, J.-E.; Na, Z.; Jung, M.; Lee, H.-S.; Sim, C.J.; Nahm, K.; Oh, K.-B.; Shin, J. Discorhabdins from the Korean Marine Sponge *Sceptrella* sp. *J. Nat. Prod.* **2010**, *73*, 258–262. [CrossRef] [PubMed]
16. Wada, Y.; Harayama, Y.; Kamimura, D.; Yoshida, M.; Shibata, T.; Fujiwara, K.; Morimoto, K.; Fujioka, H.; Kita, Y. The synthetic and biological studies of discorhabdins and related compounds. *Org. Biomol. Chem.* **2011**, *9*, 4959–4976. [CrossRef] [PubMed]
17. Goey, A.K.L.; Chau, C.H.; Sissung, T.M.; Cook, K.M.; Venzon, D.J.; Castro, A.; Ransom, T.R.; Henrich, C.J.; McKee, T.C.; McMahon, J.B.; et al. Screening and biological effects of marine pyrroloiminoquinone alkaloids: Potential inhibitors of the HIF-1α/p300 interaction. *J. Nat. Prod.* **2016**, *79*, 1267–1275. [CrossRef]
18. Li, F.; Janussen, D.; Peifer, C.; Pérez-Victoria, I.; Tasdemir, D. Targeted isolation of tsitsikammamines from the antarctic deep-sea sponge *Latrunculia biformis* by molecular networking and anticancer activity. *Mar. Drugs* **2018**, *16*, 268. [CrossRef]
19. Antunes, E.M.; Beukes, D.R.; Kelly, M.; Samaai, T.; Barrows, L.R.; Marshall, K.M.; Sincich, C.; Davies-Coleman, M.T. Cytotoxic Pyrroloiminoquinones from four new species of South African Latrunculid Sponges. *J. Nat. Prod.* **2004**, *67*, 1268–1276. [CrossRef]
20. Delfourne, E. Analogues of marine pyrroloiminoquinone alkaloids: Synthesis and antitumor properties. *Anti-Cancer Agents Med. Chem.* **2008**, *8*, 910–916. [CrossRef]
21. Dolušić, E.; Larrieu, P.; Meinguet, C.; Colette, D.; Rives, A.; Blanc, S.; Ferain, T.; Pilotte, L.; Stroobant, V.; Wouters, J.; et al. Indoleamine 2,3-dioxygenase inhibitory activity of derivatives of marine alkaloid tsitsikammamine A. *Bioorg. Med. Chem. Lett.* **2013**, *23*, 47–54. [CrossRef]

22. Wang, M.; Carver, J.J.; Phelan, V.V.; Sanchez, L.M.; Garg, N.; Peng, Y.; Nguyen, D.D.; Watrous, J.; A Kapono, C.; Luzzatto-Knaan, T.; et al. Sharing and community curation of mass spectrometry data with Global Natural Products Social Molecular Networking. *Nat. Biotechnol.* **2016**, *34*, 828–837. [CrossRef]
23. Perry, N.B.; Blunt, J.W.; Munro, M.H.G.; Higa, T.; Sakai, R. Discorhabdin D, an antitumor alkaloid from the sponges *Latrunculia brevis* and Prianos sp. *J. Org. Chem.* **1988**, *53*, 4127–4128. [CrossRef]
24. Perry, N.B.; Blunt, J.W.; Munro, M.H.G. Cytotoxic pigments from New Zealand sponges of the genus *Latrunculia*: Discorhabdin A, discorhabdin B and discorhabdin C. *Tetrahedron* **1988**, *44*, 1727–1734. [CrossRef]
25. Yang, A.; Baker, B.J.; Grimwade, J.; Leonard, A.; McClintock, J.B. Discorhabdin Alkaloids from the Antarctic Sponge *Latrunculia apicalis*. *J. Nat. Prod.* **1995**, *58*, 1596–1599. [CrossRef]
26. Grkovic, T.; Pearce, A.N.; Munro, M.H.G.; Blunt, J.W.; Davies-Coleman, M.T.; Copp, B.R. Isolation and characterization of diastereomers of discorhabdins H and K and assignment of absolute configuration to discorhabdins D, N, Q, S, T, and U. *J. Nat. Prod.* **2010**, *73*, 1686–1693. [CrossRef]
27. Kobayashi, J.; Cheng, J.-F.; Ishibashi, M.; Nakamura, H.; Ohizumi, Y.; Hirata, Y.; Sasaki, T.; Lu, H.; Clardy, J. Prianosin A, a novel antileukemic alkaloid from the okinawan marine sponge Prianos melanos. *Tetrahedron Lett.* **1987**, *28*, 4939–4942. [CrossRef]
28. Sternhell, S. Correlation of interproton spin?spin coupling constants with structure. *Q. Rev. Chem. Soc.* **1969**, *23*, 236. [CrossRef]
29. Choudhury, S.R.; Traquair, J.A.; Jarvis, W.R. New extracellular fatty acids in culture filtrates of Sporothrix flocculosa and S. rugulosa. *Can. J. Chem.* **1995**, *73*, 84–87. [CrossRef]
30. Makarieva, T.N.; Santalova, E.A.; Gorshkova, I.A.; Dmitrenok, A.S.; Guzii, A.G.; Gorbach, V.I.; Svetashev, V.I.; Stonik, V.A. A new cytotoxic fatty acid (5Z,9Z)-22-methyl-5,9-tetracosadienoic acid and the sterols from the far Eastern sponge Geodinella robusta. *Lipids* **2002**, *37*, 75–80. [CrossRef]
31. Kornprobst, J.-M.; Barnathan, G. Demospongic acids revisited. *Mar. Drugs* **2010**, *8*, 2569–2577. [CrossRef]
32. Gunstone, F.; Pollard, M.; Scrimgeour, C.; Vedanayagam, H. Fatty acids. Part 50. 13C nuclear magnetic resonance studies of olefinic fatty acids and esters. *Chem. Phys. Lipids* **1977**, *18*, 115–129. [CrossRef]
33. Grkovic, T.; Ding, Y.; Li, X.-C.; Webb, V.L.; Ferreira, D.; Copp, B.R. Enantiomeric discorhabdin alkaloids and establishment of their absolute configurations using theoretical calculations of electronic circular dichroism spectra. *J. Org. Chem.* **2008**, *73*, 9133–9136. [CrossRef]
34. Botić, T.; Defant, A.; Zanini, P.; Žužek, M.C.; Frangež, R.; Janussen, D.; Kersken, D.; Knez, Ž.; Mancini, I.; Sepčić, K. Discorhabdin alkaloids from Antarctic *Latrunculia* spp. sponges as a new class of cholinesterase inhibitors. *Eur. J. Med. Chem.* **2017**, *136*, 294–304.
35. Hooper, G.J.; Davies-Coleman, M.T.; Kelly-Borges, M.; Coetzee, P.S. New alkaloids from a South African latrunculid sponge. *Tetrahedron Lett.* **1996**, *37*, 7135–7138. [CrossRef]
36. Dijoux, M.-G.; Gamble, W.R.; Hallock, Y.F.; Cardellina, J.H.; Van Soest, R.; Boyd, M.R. A new discorhabdin from two sponge genera. *J. Nat. Prod.* **1999**, *62*, 636–637. [CrossRef]
37. Zou, Y.; Hamann, M.T. Atkamine: A New Pyrroloiminoquinone scaffold from the cold water Aleutian Islands *Latrunculia* sponge. *Org. Lett.* **2013**, *15*, 1516–1519. [CrossRef]
38. Litchfield, C.; Greenberg, A.J.; Noto, G.; Morales, R.W. Unusually high levels of C24–C30 fatty acids in sponges of the class demospongiae. *Lipids* **1976**, *11*, 567–570. [CrossRef]
39. Řezanka, T.; Sigler, K. Odd-numbered very-long-chain fatty acids from the microbial, animal and plant kingdoms. *Prog. Lipid Res.* **2009**, *48*, 206–238. [CrossRef]
40. Litchfield, C.; Marcantonio, E.E. Occurrence of 5,9,19-octacosatrienoic, 5,9-hexacosadienoic and 17-hexacosenoic acids in the marine spongeXestospongia halichondroides. *Lipids* **1978**, *13*, 199–202. [CrossRef]
41. Imbs, A.B.; Demidkova, D.A.; Dautova, T.N.; Latyshev, N.A. Fatty acid biomarkers of symbionts and unusual inhibition of tetracosapolyenoic acid biosynthesis in corals (Octocorallia). *Lipids* **2009**, *44*, 325–335. [CrossRef]
42. Thiel, V.; Blumenberg, M.; Hefter, J.; Pape, T.; Pomponi, S.; Reed, J.; Reitner, J.; Wörheide, G.; Michaelis, W. A chemical view of the most ancient metazoa—Biomarker chemotaxonomy of hexactinellid sponges. *Naturwissenschaften* **2002**, *89*, 60–66. [CrossRef]
43. Botic, T.; Cör, D.; Anesi, A.; Guella, G.; Sepčić, K.; Janussen, D.; Kersken, D.; Knez, Ž. Fatty acid composition and antioxidant activity of Antarctic marine sponges of the genus *Latrunculia*. *Polar Boil.* **2015**, *38*, 1605–1612. [CrossRef]
44. Boury-Esnault, N.; Rützler, K.; Ruetzler, K. Thesaurus of sponge morphology. *Smithson. Contrib. Zool.* **1997**, *596*, 1–55. [CrossRef]

45. Samaai, T.; Gibbons, M.J.; Kelly, M. Revision of the genus *Latrunculia* du Bocage, 1869 (Porifera: Demospongiae: Latrunculiidae) with descriptions of new species from New Caledonia and the Northeastern Pacific. *Zootaxa* **2006**, *1127*, 1–71. [CrossRef]
46. Shannon, P.; Markiel, A.; Ozier, O.; Baliga, N.S.; Wang, J.T.; Ramage, D.; Amin, N.; Schwikowski, B.; Ideker, T. Cytoscape: A software environment for integrated models of biomolecular interaction networks. *Genome Res.* **2003**, *13*, 2498–2504. [CrossRef]

marine drugs

Article

The First Genome Survey of the Antarctic Krill (*Euphausia superba*) Provides a Valuable Genetic Resource for Polar Biomedical Research

Yuting Huang [1,2,3,†], Chao Bian [2,3,†], Zhaoqun Liu [1,†], Lingling Wang [1,†], Changhu Xue [4], Hongliang Huang [5], Yunhai Yi [2,3], Xinxin You [2,3], Wei Song [5], Xiangzhao Mao [4], Linsheng Song [1,*] and Qiong Shi [1,2,3,*]

1. Liaoning Key Laboratory of Marine Animal Immunology, Dalian Ocean University, Dalian 116023, China; huangyuting@genomics.cn (Y.H.); liuzhaoqun@dlou.edu.cn (Z.L.); wanglingling@dlou.edu.cn (L.W.)
2. Shenzhen Key Lab of Marine Genomics, Guangdong Provincial Key Lab of Molecular Breeding in Marine Economic Animals, BGI Academy of Marine Sciences, BGI Marine, BGI, Shenzhen 518083, China; bianchao@genomics.cn (C.B.); yiyunhai@genomics.cn (Y.Y.); youxinxin@genomics.cn (X.Y.)
3. BGI Education Center, University of Chinese Academy of Sciences, Shenzhen 518083, China
4. Ocean University of China, Qingdao 266100, China; xuech@ouc.edu.cn (C.X.); xzhmao@ouc.edu.cn (X.M.)
5. East China Sea Fisheries Research Institute, Chinese Academy of Fishery Sciences, Shanghai 200090, China; ecshhl@163.com (H.H.); songw@ecsf.ac.cn (W.S.)

* Correspondence: lshsong@dlou.edu.cn (L.S.); shiqiong@genomics.cn (Q.S.); Tel.: +86-155-4269-9991 (L.S.); +86-185-6627-9826 (Q.S.); Fax: +86-755-3630-7273 (Q.S.)

† These authors contributed equally to this work.

Received: 29 February 2020; Accepted: 25 March 2020; Published: 31 March 2020

Abstract: The world-famous Antarctic krill (*Euphausia superba*) plays a fundamental role in the Antarctic food chain. It resides in cold environments with the most abundant biomass to support the Antarctic ecology and fisheries. Here, we performed the first genome survey of the Antarctic krill, with genomic evidence for its estimated genome size of 42.1 gigabases (Gb). Such a large genome, however, is beyond our present capability to obtain a good assembly, although our sequencing data are a valuable genetic resource for subsequent polar biomedical research. We extracted 13 typical protein-coding gene sequences of the mitochondrial genome and analyzed simple sequence repeats (SSRs), which are useful for species identification and origin determination. Meanwhile, we conducted a high-throughput comparative identification of putative antimicrobial peptides (AMPs) and antihypertensive peptides (AHTPs) from whole-body transcriptomes of the Antarctic krill and its well-known counterpart, the whiteleg shrimp (*Penaeus vannamei*; resident in warm waters). Related data revealed that AMPs/AMP precursors and AHTPs were generally conserved, with interesting variations between the two crustacean species. In summary, as the first report of estimated genome size of the Antarctic krill, our present genome survey data provide a foundation for further biological research into this polar species. Our preliminary investigations on bioactive peptides will bring a new perspective for the in-depth development of novel marine drugs.

Keywords: Antarctic krill *(Euphausia superba)*; genome survey; mitochondrial genome; whiteleg shrimp (*Penaeus vannamei*); antimicrobial peptide (AMP); antihypertensive peptide (AHTP)

1. Introduction

The Antarctic krill (*Euphausia superba*), widely distributed in the Southern Ocean, provides the most abundant biomass for Antarctic ecology and fisheries [1]. It establishes a critical link between primary producers (phytoplankton) and apex predators (such as fishes, squids, penguins, and seals) in the Antarctic food chains [2,3], with an estimated biomass of 100~500 million tons [3]. With such a large number of Antarctic krill, the Southern Ocean supports an unprecedented abundance of upper trophic-level predators. Field observations have reported that population trends of some krill predators are in part influenced by the abundance changes in Antarctic krill [4]. Human beings are also benefited by many extracted products from the Antarctic krill, such as pharmaceuticals, nutraceutical health foods, and aquaculture feeds [5]. Thus, getting insight into the genetic resources of the Antarctic krill is necessary for species protection, as well as for the development of related fisheries and industry. Studies on the genetic resources of the Antarctic krill primarily focus on transcriptomes [1,3], simple sequence repeats (SSRs) [1], and the mitochondrial genome [6,7]. These data provide valuable foundation for in-depth genetic research on this polar species. However, no complete genome assembly is available for this important crustacean.

Recently, a high-quality genome assembly of its famous counterpart, the whiteleg shrimp (*Penaeus vannamei*), was published [8]. As we know, this shrimp species predominantly inhabits tropical and subtropical areas, and has been extensively cultivated in Asian countries. Resident in such remarkably different environments, the Antarctic krill and the whiteleg shrimp may have undergone differential genetic variances. Since the genome size of the Antarctic krill is huge (over 40 Gb; see more details in our Results), we had to stop our genome project temporarily with only a genome survey available. However, these genomic data are still useful for uncovering short sequences, such as bioactive peptides encoded by entire or partial genes.

For example, antimicrobial peptides (AMPs) are short with broad-spectrum antimicrobial activities; most of them can be classified into either own gene type or proteolysis type (derived from immune related genes) [9]. They are usually less than 10 kDa while acting as the major components of the innate immune defense system in marine invertebrates [10,11], and habitat-related variances in AMPs/AMP precursors are likely to exist in various crustaceans [11]. Although AMPs in the Antarctic krill have received some attention [12], researchers still know little of the overall AMPs in such an important crustacean species and other marine animals from diverse habitats. Looking into the connection between AMPs/AMP precursors and creatures from various environments may help us to identify novel peptides and even apply them for species protection and human health.

Angiotensin converting enzyme (ACE) inhibitors are preferred antihypertensive drugs, and antihypertensive peptides (AHTPs), another important representative with short sequences, are the most effective and popularly studied ACE inhibitory peptides [13]. A lot of AHTPs are usually digested from natural products, and they most frequently contain 2~10 amino acids. Endogenous AHTPs can be hydrolyzed and degraded with assistance of digestive enzymes from in vivo proteins; by binding to ACEs or related receptors, they may adjust the renin angiotensin system for antihypertensive effects [14]. In recent years, several AHTPs have been isolated from Antarctic krill, and some of them have been used for mechanism studies [15,16]. However, general knowledge of *E. superba* AHTPs from the genomic or transcriptomic perspective is still limited. Comparative investigations on AHTPs between the Antarctic krill and the whiteleg shrimp may make contribution to our better understanding of AHTPs in various animals and identification of candidates for practical utilization as pharmaceuticals.

In the present study, we performed the first genome survey of the Antarctic krill. Such a large genome, however, is difficult for us to obtain a good assembly, although our sequencing data are a valuable genetic resource for subsequent polar biomedical research. Partial mitochondrial genome and many SSRs were able to be extracted for species identification and origin determination. Moreover, a comparative study on AMPs and AHTPs, based on available transcriptome and genome sequences from both the Antarctic krill and the whiteleg shrimp, was conducted. Here, our main aim is to establish a basic genomic and genetic foundation for future polar biomedical studies on the Antarctic krill, especially to initiate a preliminary exploration of bioactive peptides in a polar animal for the development of novel marine drugs.

2. Results

2.1. A Genome Survey of the Antarctic Krill

In total, we obtained 911.0 Gb of raw reads sequenced by a BGISeq500 platform (BGI-Shenzhen, Shenzhen, China) from all the constructed libraries (400 bp in length). A detailed K-mer analysis [14] was performed to estimate the genome size, and a survey peak was visible with high heterozygosity in Antarctic krill (see Figure 1). We calculated the genome size (G) of the Antarctic krill according to the following formula: G = K_num/K_depth [17]. In our present study, the total number of K-mers (K_num) was 758,531,899,196 and the K_depth was 18 (Table 1 and Figure 1). Therefore, we estimated that the genome size of *E. superba* was 42.1 Gb; the sequencing depth (X) of the clean data is therefore ~21 of the estimated genome size (Table 1).

Table 1. Statistics of 17–mers for the genome size estimation.

K-mer	K_num	K_depth	Genome Size	Clean Base (bp)	Depth (X)
17	758,531,899,196	18	42,140,661,066	902,660,212,000	21

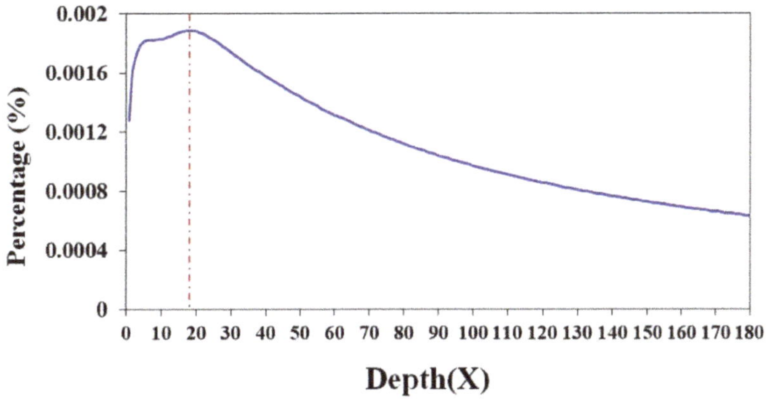

Figure 1. A 17-mer distribution curve of the Antarctic krill (*E. superba*). The *x*-axis is the sequencing depth (X) of each unique 17-mer, and the *y*-axis is the percentage of these unique 17–mers.

2.2. Assembly of Extracted Partial Mitochondrial Genome

A roughly complete mitochondrial genome of the Antarctic krill was assembled to be 12,272 bp in length, while the entire length was 15,498 bp in a previous report [6]. Based on these sequences, we extracted all the 13 typical mitochondrial protein-coding genes from our genomic raw sequences, although certain gene sequences are still partial (see File S1). These genes include cytochrome c oxidase subunit I (*coxI*), cytochrome c oxidase subunit II (*coxII*), cytochrome c oxidase subunit III (*coxIII*), ATPase subunit 8 (*atp8*), ATPase subunit 6 (*atp6*), NADH dehydrogenase subunit 3 (*nad3*), NADH dehydrogenase subunit 5 (*nad5*), NADH dehydrogenase subunit 4 (*nad4*), NADH dehydrogenase subunit 4L (*nad4L*), NADH dehydrogenase subunit 6 (*nad6*), cytochrome b (*Cytb*), NADH dehydrogenase subunit 1 (*nad1*), and NADH dehydrogenase subunit 2 (*nad2*). More details about the gene map can be seen in Figure S1, in which the order of these genes was arranged manually, in accordance with the previous report [6].

2.2.1. Annotation and Analysis of Our Extracted Mitochondrial Genes

These mitochondrial genes were assigned into six Kyoto Encyclopedia of Genes and Genomes (KEGG) pathways (see Tables S1 and S2) by using the BLASTp [18] to map against the public KEGG database [19]. Energy metabolism pathway, as the representative one, consists of 11 genes (Table S2), such as *nad5*, *nad4*, *nad1*, *coxI*, and *coxII* (Figure S2A). The functions of these extracted mitochondrial genes were predicted with classifications by searching the public Gene Ontology (GO) databases [20]. Based on the GO annotation, we assigned them into 13 subcategories under three main categories, including biological process (3), cellular component (7), and molecular function (3). The "catalytic activity" terms (8; 53.3%) were obviously dominant in the "molecular function" (Figure S2B).

2.2.2. Multiple Sequence Alignment and Phylogenetic Analysis of the Representative Mitochondrial Gene *nad4L*

The representative mitochondrial gene *nad4L* from both Antarctic krill and whiteleg shrimp (a good counterpart from warm waters) were chosen to perform multiple sequence alignment (Figure 2). We observed 6 and 30 different residues between the Antarctic krill in this study and the sample collected from Prydz Bay (*E. superba* PB) [6], and between our Antarctic krill and the whiteleg shrimp, respectively. Obviously, both Antarctic krill samples were more conserved; however, their sequence variances may represent various origins.

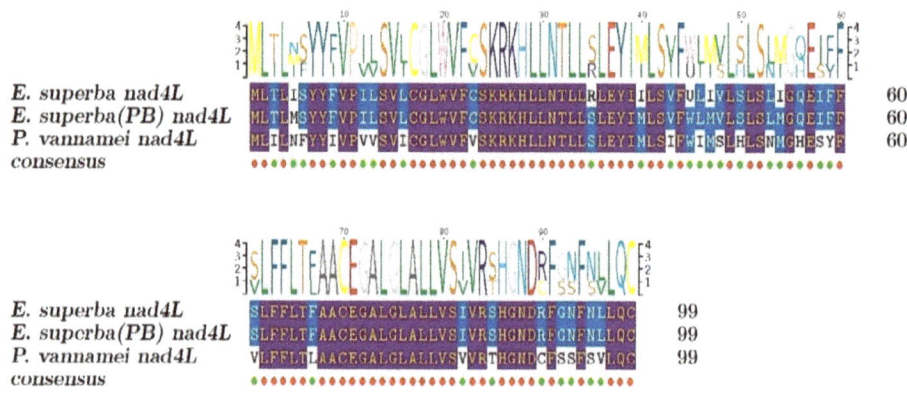

Figure 2. Multiple sequence alignment of the putative *nad4L* genes. Red circles at the bottom stand for the same residues. Blue and purple colors on the sequences represent the alignment with identity >50% and >80%, respectively.

To confirm the Antarctic krill in the present study is the same species as reported *E. superba* (PB) [6] and to provide more evidence for the phylogenetic relationship between Penaeidae and Euphausiacea, we used the *nad4L* sequence of Australian freshwater crayfish (*Cherax destructor*; NCBI Gene ID: 2827710) as an out-group and constructed a phylogenetic tree of *nad4L* among the Antarctic krill, the whiteleg shrimp, and several other representative shrimps. The established phylogenetic topology was divided into two main groups of Penaeidae and Euphausiacea (Figure 3). The *nad4L* identified for the Antarctic krill in the present study was not surprised to be much closer to the reported *E. superba* (PB)'s [6]. That is to say, the *nad4L* is practicable for the Antarctic krill in species identification and has potential for origin determination.

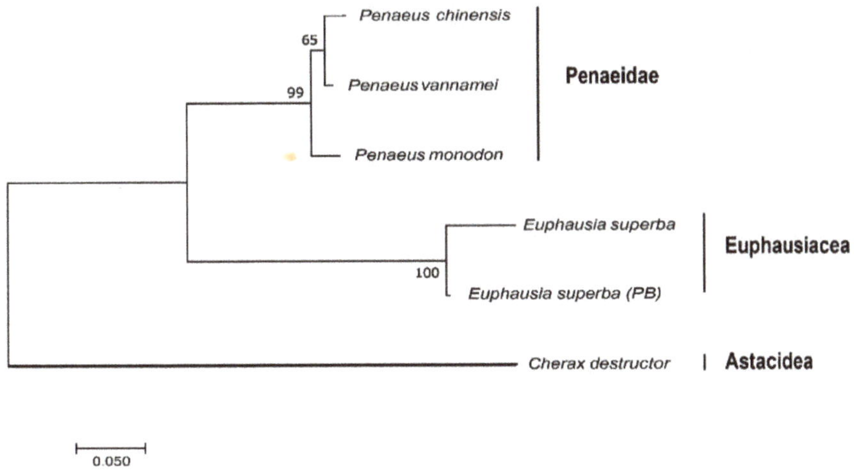

Figure 3. Phylogenetic topology of *nad4L* derived from the Neighbor–Joining method [21]. The bootstrap test employed 1,000 replicates, and the numbers next to branches were replicate percentage of taxa clustering [22]. Corresponding amino acid sequences were analyzed in MEGA7 [23].

2.3. *Assemblies of Reported Transcriptomes of the Antarctic Krill and the Whiteleg Shrimp*

Raw data of the Antarctic krill transcriptomes were downloaded from the National Center for Biotechnology Information (NCBI; accession number PRJNA307639). Total RNA was isolated from six whole specimens that were collected from the Southern Ocean. High-throughput transcriptome sequencing (pair-ended at 2 × 150 bp) on an Illumina HiSeq 3000 platform generated ~77.9 million of raw reads, equal to 11.8 Gb [1]. Here, we assembled these available public transcriptome sequences. After removal of low-quality reads and trimming adapter sequences, we collected 10.6 million of clean reads corresponding to 1.5 Gb, and generated 16,797 unigenes with a GC rate of 37.6% for the Antarctic krill. As summarized in Table 2 for the transcriptome assembly, the average length was 637 bp and the N50 was 923 bp.

Table 2. Summary of our de novo assembly of the previously reported *E. superba* transcriptomes [1].

Parameter	Value
Total Number (unigene)	16,797
Total Length (bp)	10,715,598
Mean Length (bp)	637
N50 (bp)	923
GC (%)	37.63

The raw data of the whiteleg shrimp transcriptomes were downloaded from NCBI under the accession number PRJNA288849. In the corresponding report [24], whole-body adult shrimps at three molting stages (including inter-molt, pre-molt and post-molt) were collected from a laboratory culture, and an Illumina HiSeq 2500 platform was used for the sequencing of cDNA libraries. Here, we assembled the publicly available transcriptome sequences. Finally, a total of 90.9 million clean reads (equal to 3.1 Gb) were obtained after data filtering. In the transcriptome assembly, 3,768 unigenes were annotated; the average length was 574 bp and the N50 value was 759 bp, with an average GC content of 51.0% (Table 3).

Table 3. Summary of our de novo assembly of the reported *P. vannamei* transcriptomes [24].

Parameter	Value
Total Number (unigene)	3,768
Total Length (bp)	2,165,058
Mean Length (bp)	574
N50 (bp)	759
GC (%)	50.95

These assemblies of reported transcriptomes were set for high-throughput SSR identification in the Antarctic krill (Section 2.4) and further comparisons of AMPs and AHTPs between the Antarctic krill and the whiteleg shrimp (Sections 2.5 and 2.6).

2.4. High-throughput SSR Identification in the Antarctic Krill

In order to investigate whether genomic data of the Antarctic krill can be used for the development of genetic markers for species identification and origin determination, we picked SSR as a trial example. Interestingly, a total of 1,026 and 74,661 SSRs were identified from our transcriptome (Section 2.3) and partial genome raw data (Section 2.1) of the Antarctic krill, respectively (Table S3). These SSRs ranged from 2 to 6 bp.

In the transcriptome assembly, the most abundant type of SSRs was the trinucleotide repeats. As shown in Figure 4A, the total number of SSRs with trinucleotide repeats was 577, and their percentage reached 75.62%; the second highest number of SSRs, 160, was with dinucleotide repeats. However, in our partial genome raw data, the situation seemed to be different. The most abundant SSRs were with dinucleotide repeats (33,737), accounting for 52.9%; SSRs with trinucleotide repeats were dropped down to the second highest number, 25,120 (see more details in Figure 4B).

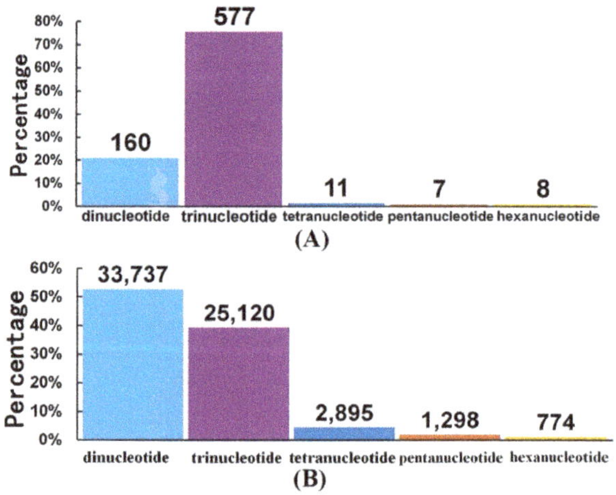

Figure 4. SSR classification in the Antarctic krill. Data were analyzed in our transcriptome assembly (**A**; Section 2.3) and our partial genome raw data (**B**; Section 2.1). The *x*-axis is the nucleotide type of each SSR, and the *y*-axis is the percentages of these SSRs. The number on the top of each bar is the total amount of corresponding SSRs.

2.5. Comparisons of AMPs between the Antarctic Krill and the Whiteleg Shrimp

Employing our previously collected list of active AMPs (Table S4) and analysis pipeline [9], we employed BLAST to search the Antarctic krill and the whiteleg shrimp transcripts (Section 2.3) and identified 85 and 78 putative AMPs (Table S5), respectively. These AMPs/AMP precursors were classified into 16 groups (Figure 5). Interestingly, in the present study, CcAMP1_insect was only identified in the Antarctic krill transcripts, but not in the transcriptome and genome sequences of the whiteleg shrimp (the third group in Figure 5). We also noted that histone 2 (one of the six histones; with the mapped AMP of Buforin I) and ubiquitin/ribosomal S27 fusion protein (with the mapped AMP of cgUbiquitin) were the top two AMP precursors with the highest transcription values in the Antarctic krill (Table S6; not detectable in the whiteleg shrimp). PvHCt, corresponding to the C-terminal fragment in hemocyanin of *P. vannamei* [25], presented high transcription values in our assembled whiteleg shrimp whole-body transcriptomes (see Table S6).

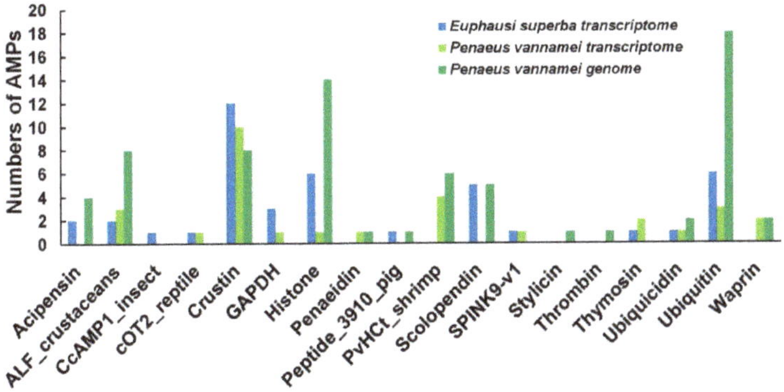

Figure 5. Summary of the identified anti-microbial peptides (AMPs)/AMP precursors from the Antarctic krill transcriptome and the whiteleg shrimp transcriptome and genome assemblies. Blue bars represent those identified in the former (*E. superba*), and green bars represent those retrieved from the latter (*P. vannamei*).

Meanwhile, we observed that the homologous sequence of the CcAMP1_insect extracted from the Antarctic krill transcriptomes in the present study had one different residue (K) from that of insect *Coridius chinensis*'s (V) (Figure 6). The predicted 3D structure of *E. superba* CcAMP1_insect (Figure 6B) was different from the *C. chinensis*'s (Figure 6A), although both contained strands and coils.

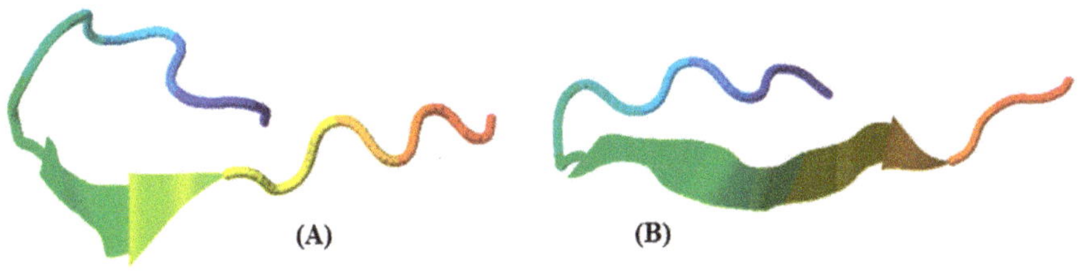

Figure 6. Predicted 3D structures of CcAMP1_insect in insect *C. chinensis* (**A**) and the Antarctic krill (**B**). They were predicted by I-TASSER with high confidence (see more details in Section 3.2).

An important AMP category, crustin, abundantly existed in both crustaceans (Figure 5). Some of them, named CrusEs, belong to a group of cysteine-rich antibacterial peptides with whey acidic protein (WAP) domains, including two four-disulfide core domains and each domain with 8 conserved cysteine residues. The WAP domains also contain a KXGXCP motif [26,27]. Multiple sequence alignments of crustin (CrusEs; Figure 7A) demonstrated that both the Antarctic krill and the whiteleg shrimp possessed conserved cysteines. Another CXXP motif of the WAP domain could also be identified in the Antarctic krill, while it was incomplete in the whiteleg shrimp (see the detailed *P. vannamei* CrusEs (genome) sequence in Figure 7A). A phylogenetic analysis of the representative CrusEs between the two crustaceans was performed for more comparison (Figure S3; data from Figure 7A).

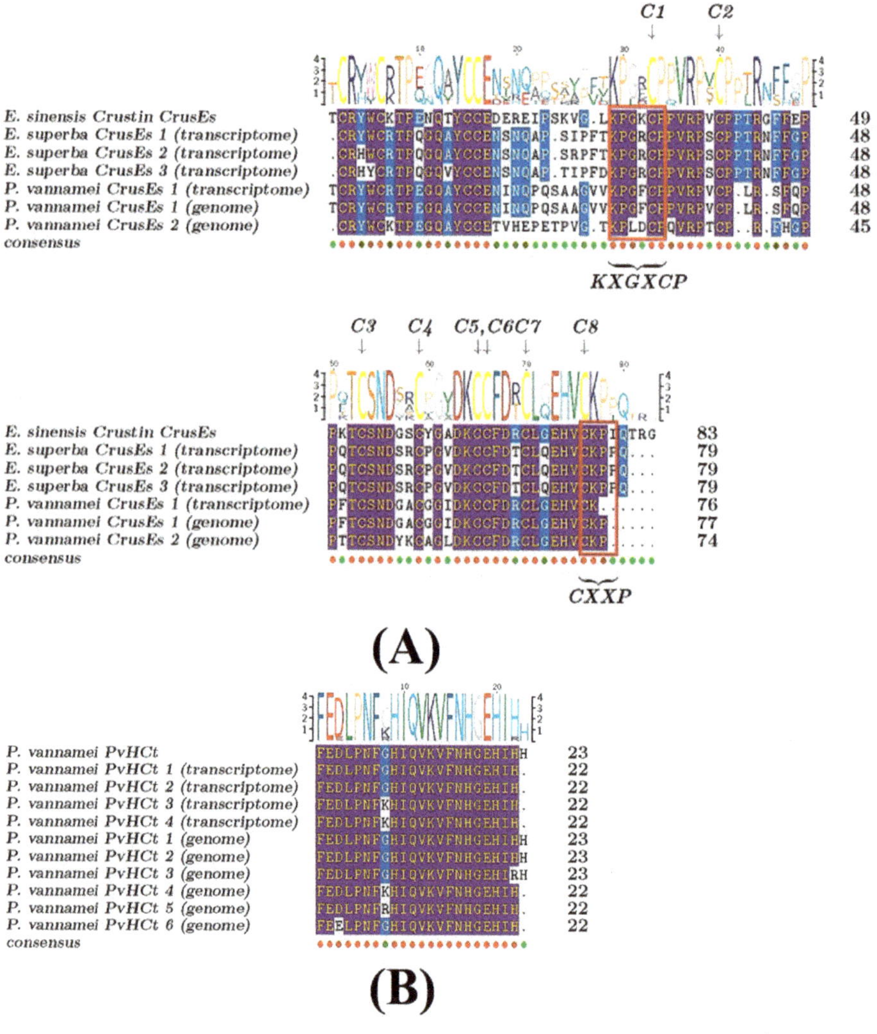

Figure 7. Multiple sequence alignment of representative AMPs/AMP precursors. (**A**) Crustins from different species. The eight cysteine residues, conserved in all crustaceans with the consensus sequences of whey-acidic proteins [26], were also present in the CrusE sequences, as indicated by arrows and C1~C8. (**B**) PvHCt from the whiteleg shrimp (*P. vannamei*). Red circles at the bottom stand for the same residues. Blue marks represent the alignment with identity >50%.

The transcription levels of crustin (such as CrusEs and MrCrs) were usually very high in the Antarctic krill, whereas they were not detectable in the whiteleg shrimp (see more details in Table S6). Interestingly, we observed three CrusEs in the former but only one in the latter. Similarly, another crustin category (MrCrs) was highly transcribed in the Antarctic krill but not detectable in the whiteleg shrimp; there were nine MrCrs in the former but only two in the latter (Table S6). There were also some *P. vannamei* unique crustins including Crustin*Pm*1, Crustin*Pm*7 as well as other AMPs including CqCrs,

SWDPm2, PvHCt, penaeidin, and waprin were obtained from the whiteleg shrimp transcriptome and genome, although their transcriptions were not detectable either (see Table S6). We noted that sylicin and thrombin were not identified in the transcriptome but only in the genome of the whiteleg shrimp in this study (Figure 5, Table S6). As expected, penaeidins of the whiteleg shrimp were the same as those of the reported penaeid shrimp [28]. The sequence of PvHCt identified in the present study was also highly conserved in comparison to that in previous studies [25] with minor variances (Figure 7B).

2.6. Prediction and Analysis of AHTPs in both Crustacean Species

To identify potential AHTPs in the translated proteomes (from the genome or transcriptome data) of the Antarctic krill and the whiteleg shrimp, we built a local AHTP-searching database [13]. Most of the known AHTPs searched in this database have been verified in reported studies, and they are usually tripeptides with less than 10 amino acids; the top 50 AHTPs with the highest activity were chosen to identify AHTPs in the two crustacean species, as reported in our previous study [14]. Finally, in the Antarctic krill, 23 AHTP sequences were identified from the transcriptomes; in the whiteleg shrimp, AHTP numbers were 20 and 29 from the reported transcriptomes [1] and genome assembly [8] (Table S9). The detailed location(s) of each matched AHTP sequence in its corresponding protein was listed in Table S7. It seems that AHTPs are almost overlapped between the two crustaceans (Figure 8, Table S9).

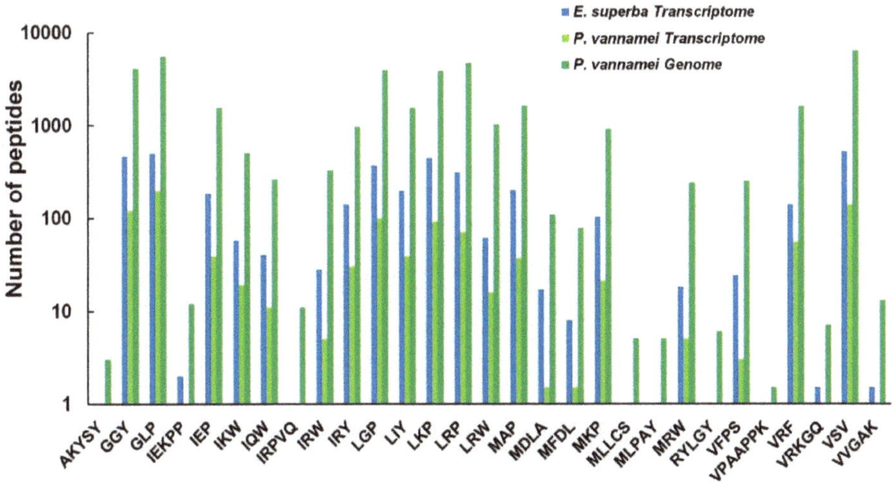

Figure 8. A comparative overview of the identified antihypertensive peptides (AHTPs) in both crustaceans. Blue bars denote the AHTPs identified from *E. superba* transcriptome [1]; green bars represent the *P. vannamei* AMPs retrieved from both transcriptome [24] and genome [8] data.

In the Antarctic krill, we observed that involucrin had the most abundant AHTP hit numbers (14; Table S8). In the whiteleg shrimp, however, it is the collagen alpha-1 chain-like protein that possessed the most AHTP hits (27; see Table S8). As shown in Figure 8, the richest AHTP categories were VSV, GLP, LRP, GGY, LGP, LKP in both crustacean species. Some AHTPs were identified only in the genome of whiteleg shrimp but were not detectable in the transcripts of Antarctic krill and whiteleg shrimp, such as AKYSY, IRPVQ, MLLCS, MLPAY, RYLGY, as well as VPAAPPK (Figure 8, Table S9).

3. Discussion

3.1. Importance to Characterize the Genome Size, Mitochondrial Genome and SSRs in the Antarctic Krill

Our genome survey in the present study first calculated the estimated genome size of the Antarctic Krill as 42.1 Gb (Figure 1). This result is consistent with a previous report of 47.5 Gb from both flow cytometry and Feulgen image analysis densitometry [29]. However, such a large genome is beyond our present capacity to obtain a good assembly. We had to stop our genome project temporally, without wasting more time and money, until we figure out practicable assemble strategies.

Mitochondrial genes have been widely used for species identification. In the present study, sequence alignment and phylogenetic analysis of the representative *nad4L* between two sources of Antarctic krill and the whiteleg shrimp (Figures 2 and 3) revealed the phylogenetic relationship between Penaeidae and Euphausiacea (Figure 3). We also mapped the 13 typical protein-coding genes (Figure S1), which were similar to a previous report in *E. superba* (PB) [1]. It seems that the extraction of mitochondrial genes from the genome survey data can be used for origin determination, which will be informative for in-depth studies on various sources of Antarctic krill. Meanwhile, the mitochondrial roles for cold adaptation have been studied in cod. The overall COX activities in liver were reported to be higher in the cold-adapted population, although they were not affected by cold acclimation [30]. Similarly, the mitochondrial genes in the Antarctic krill may also benefit from the examination of cold adaptive mechanisms to polar environments.

SSRs, also called microsatellite markers, are a class of repetitive DNA sequences. They usually consist of tandem repeating units of mon-, di-, tri-, and tetra-nucleotide types. They have become well-known markers for identifying and classifying species from various resources [31]. In diverse shrimps, SSRs have been developed for potential applications in genetic studies, kinship analysis, origin determination, etc. [32]. Dinucleotide repeats were the most abundant type in reported Antarctic krill transcriptomes [1] and our partial genome raw data (Figure 4B). With the availability of more genome-wide SSRs from other resources of Antarctic krill, we may determine the origin of any commercial frozen products in the future.

3.2. Similarities and Differences of AMPs between the Two Examined Crustacean Species

Our present study also provided a valuable genetic resource for AMP comparisons between Antarctic krill and whiteleg shrimp. It seems that AMPs and AMP precursors were generally conserved, while being differentially various between the two crustacean species, possibly due to their residency in significantly different waters.

The Antarctic krill unique CcAMP1 was originally extracted from *C. chinensis* [33]. However, there is no document revealing the correlation of CcAMP1 and environmental adaptation. According to previous reports, there were five hydrophobic amino acids (VAWVL) on its surface, which might construct an α-helix to destroy the cell member integrity of bacteria [25] for stronger antimicrobial effects. However, since the predicted 3D structures of CcAMP1 of *E. superba* and *C. chinensis* in the present study were different (without the critical helix structures; Figure 6), thereby leading to uncertainty of the putative antimicrobial activity. As highly transcribed in the Antarctic krill, a specific protease was reported to be responsible for the generation of AMP buforin I from the histone 2 [34]. Buforin I was originally identified from Asian toad and showed strong antimicrobial activities against a broad spectrum of bacteria [35]. The AMP cgUbiquitin, mapped in the ubiquitin/ribosomal S27 fusion protein, was originally isolated from the gill of the Pacific oyster, and its precursor mRNA was reported to be significantly upregulated after *Vibrio* stimulation [36]. We therefore propose that these Antarctic krill's unique and highly transcribed AMPs were possibly important for the survival of aquatic animals in a cold environment.

For the crustin (CrusEs) from both Antarctic krill and whiteleg shrimp, the CXXP motif was identified completely from the former, while incomplete in the latter. This may cause non-functionality or neo-functionality in the whiteleg shrimp. Furthermore, the cDNA sequences of CrusEs, previously identified from Chinese mitten crab with the validation of purified proteins to inhibit the growth of Gram-positive bacteria [26], and the cDNA encoding MrCrs, with a first report in a freshwater prawn *Macrobrachium rosenbergii*, could be inductively expressed when the host was affected by bacteria [37]. Their high transcription levels and the greater number present in Antarctic krill compared to whiteleg shrimp suggest their more important roles in Antarctic krill.

The whiteleg shrimp's unique AMPs, identified in the present study, were from a preliminary exploration. It will be necessary to perform a double check when the genome assembly of the Antarctic krill is available. Crustin*Pm*1, crustin*Pm*7, CqCrs, and stylicin were previously identified from black tiger shrimp (*Penaeus monodon*), red claw crayfish (*Cherax quadricarinatus*) and Pacific blue shrimp (*Litopenaeus stylirostris*), and exhibited antimicrobial activities against bacterial and fungal invasions [37–39]. SWD*Pm*2, originally identified from hemocytes of the black tiger shrimp, is another group of WAP domains containing protein similar to crustin; it was up-regulated after an injection of white spot syndrome virus (WSSV) [40]. PvHCt, a histidine-rich antimicrobial peptide with antimicrobial activity to fungal cells, was originally found in whiteleg shrimp. It has potentially been derived in large quantities by the proteolytic cleavage of the hemocyanin protein [25]. Unlike gene-encoded cationic defense peptides such as crustins and penaeidins, PvHCt can be obtained massively by hemocyanin proteolytic cleavage without any recombinant production or purification system and is the most abundant plasma protein in crustaceans [25]. The whiteleg shrimp's unique AMPs identified in our present study were potentially more important for this species. Furthermore, those genes with high transcription levels, such as AMP precursor histone 2, ubiquitin/ribosomal S27 fusion protein, and the WAP-domain-containing proteins including crustin and waprin, as well as hemocyanins-derived PvHCt, may be promising antimicrobial candidates and potentially good sources for the development of AMP-based drugs. Regarding the stylicin [39] and thrombin [41], which were only identified in the *P. vannamei* genome in our present study, we guess that they may not be well transcribed.

Meanwhile, the environmental specificity of the AMPs in both Antarctic krill and whiteleg shrimp were also investigated. Interestingly, we found that some AMPs that are unique to the Antarctic krill or in both crustaceans may not show environmental specificity, because the habitats of their derived species and the bacteria inhibited by them were not coincident with Antarctic krill's distribution areas [35,36,38,42,43]. However, some AMPs only identified in whiteleg shrimp in the present study (such as crustin*Pm*1) may play important roles in special responses to warm environments due to the fact that their originally sourced species were geographically consistent with whiteleg shrimp [44].

3.3. Conservations of AHTPs between the Two Crustacean Species

AHTPs were investigated in the present study for the potential development of antihypertensive drugs from the Antarctic krill. Although from different environments, unlike AMPs, the most abundant AHTPs (such as VSV) were the same, and most of the AHTPs can be found both in the datasets of the Antarctic krill as well as the whiteleg shrimp. These data indicate that the AHTPs may be highly conserved in both crustaceans, which is consistent with our previous report of marine mammals [14]. However, those AHTPs identified only in the genome of the whiteleg shrimp also need to be retrieved from the genome of the Antarctic krill once its good assembly is made available in future.

Interestingly, the AHTP mapping ratio in involucrin was higher than other proteins in the Antarctic krill, with AHTP hits to 14. The Involucrin with the most abundant AHTPs is a keratinocyte protein [45], and keratinocytes is the major constituent of the epidermis tissue [46] of the skin's outer layer [47]. As for the whiteleg shrimp, however, both collagen alpha-1(V) chain-like protein and collagen alpha-1(XI) chain-like protein were the most abundant AHTP-containing proteins, which were revealed previously by us in fishes [13]. In fact, ACE-inhibitory peptides had been obtained from the collagen hydrolysates of many animals [48–53]. Based on our present work, we propose to apply the epidermis tissues of the Antarctic krill and collagen alpha chain proteins of shrimps as a promising resource to obtain AHTP production. Of course, similarly to the AMPs, the ACE inhibitory activity can be evaluated after the comprehensive prediction results are available, once the genome of the Antarctic krill is assembled with high quality.

4. Materials and Methods

4.1. Genomic DNA Extraction and Genome Sequencing for the Antarctic Krill

Our experimental procedures complied with the current laws on animal welfare and research in China. Alive Antarctic krill specimens were collected from the Argentine Sea area (45°92′S,61°82′W). Genomic DNAs were extracted from the whole bodies of pooled specimens with a Qiagen GenomicTip100 kit (Qiagen, Germanton, MD, USA) according to the manufacturer's protocol. With the traditional whole-genome shotgun sequencing strategy [14], we used 1 μg of normalized DNA to prepare a paired-end short-insert library (400 bp). Quantification and size estimations of the library were performed on a Zebra Flowcell 3.1 chip. Finally, the library was normalized to 15 ng/μL for paired-end sequencing (100 bp in length) on a BGISeq500 platform (BGI, Shenzhen, China). Raw genome sequencing reads have been deposited in the NCBI and China National GeneBank (CNGB) under the project IDs PRJNA598052 and CNP0000808, respectively.

4.2. Assembly of the Antarctic Krill Mitochondrial Genome and Transcriptomes

At first, we estimated the genome size of the Antarctic krill using a routine K–mer analysis method [14] with the following formula: G = K_num/K_depth, where K_num is the total number of K–mers, and K_depth indicates the frequency of reads occurring more frequently than others [17].

BGI paired-end reads were filtered with SOAPnuke1.5.6 [54] and the common adapter sequences were trimmed. A roughly complete mitochondrial genome of the Antarctic krill was assembled. Firstly, the mitochondrial genome of a congeneric *E. superba* (downloaded from the NCBI with an accession number EU583500.1) was employed [6]. Those sequencing reads with a high similarity to the reference mitochondrial genome were identified by SOAP2 (version 2.21) [55]. Subsequently, SPAdes (version 3.10.0) was employed [56] to assemble all these highly similar reads. Finally, Blast (version 2.6.1) [57] was applied to compare the archived assembly with the reference mitochondrial genome. The scaffolds containing a low length (<200 bp) were removed and the filtered scaffolds were combined into one sequence as a mitochondrial genome sequence. The redundancy sequences were also manually deleted. Then, the mitochondrial genome sequence was annotated with AGORA [58] to get the 13 protein-coding genes nucleotide sequences.

The *E. superba* and *P. vannamei* transcriptome sequences were downloaded from the NCBI with accession numbers PRJNA307639 (SRR3089571) [1] and PRJNA288849 [24], respectively. SOAPnuke 1.5.6 [54] was employed to filter the paired-end short reads of transcriptomes with the removal of contaminants, adapters and those low-quality reads (with over 5% non-sequenced bases or more than 20% of bases with quality score ≤ 10). We then employed Trinity v2.5.1 [59] to assemble the remaining clean reads, which were clustered by using TGICL v2.1 [60] based on sequence similarity and assembled to consensus unigenes. Clean reads were aligned to the de novo assemblies with a Bowtie 2 read aligner [61] to calculate gene transcription values in the assembled transcriptomes. Finally, we used RNA–Seq by Expectation Maximization (RSEM) v1.2.31 [62] to estimate transcript abundance in term of FPKM (fragments per kilobase of transcript per million mapped reads) values. The candidate coding regions from the assembled transcripts were identified with TransDecoder (http://transdecoder.sourceforge.net/), and then were translated into amino acid sequences using the standard codon table.

4.3. Functional Annotation of the Extracted Mitochondrial Genome and the Reported Transcriptomes

The amino acid sequences of Antarctic krill mitochondrial protein-coding genes from AGORA [58] annotation results were mapped to KEGG [19] pathway annotations using Diamond [18] with an *E*-value threshold of 1.0×10^{-5}. Blast2GO v4.1 [63] was employed to perform GO [20] annotation of NCBI

Nr blast results. Unigene sequences from the Antarctic krill and the whiteleg shrimp transcriptomes were searched using Diamond [18] and blastn [57] against the NCBI Nr and UniProtKB/Swiss-Prot [64] databases (E–value $\leq 1.0 \times 10^{-5}$) to retrieve protein functional annotations based on sequence similarity.

4.4. Phylogenetic Analysis and Multiple Sequence Alignment

Along with the *nad4L* sequence extracted from the Antarctic krill mitochondrial genome, we also extracted several other malacostracan *nad4L* sequences from the NCBI for a subsequent phylogenetic analysis. Examined species include *Penaeus chinensis, P. vannamei, P. monodon, E. superba* (from the present study), *E. superba* (PB), and *Cherax destructor* (as the out group). The translated protein sequences from these species were aligned using mafft v7.158b [65] with default parameters. The phylogenetic tree was constructed with the Neighbor Joining (NJ) of pairwise distances using MEGA 7.0 [23]. Multiple sequence alignment was performed using MEGA 7.0 [23], and the archived results were further analyzed and visualized by TEXshade (version 2.12.14) [66].

4.5. SSR Analysis

We employed our own script SSR.sh to search known SSRs from the reported transcriptome and our randomly selected partial genome raw data of the Antarctic krill. Our own script filter_ssr.pl was used to calculate SSR ratio, and the SSR distribution map was plotted with our own script draw_ssr.pl and Excel.

4.6. AMP Analysis

A total of 3073 AMP sequences were used as a local AMPs searching list as previously reported [9,67]. Standard homology searches were performed against the *E. superba* [1] and *P. vannamei* transcriptomes [24] as well as *P. vannamei* genome [8] to predict putative AMP sequences. In brief, index transcriptome and genome databases were built by running a makeblastdb command in ncbi-blast-2.6.0 [57]. Subsequently, the tBLASTn (E-value of 1.0×10^{-5}) in ncbi-blast-2.6.0 [57] was employed to search our reference AMP list from the index transcriptome and genome databases with filtering of those with a query align ratio less than 0.5.

4.7. AHTP Analysis

The AHTPs with the top 50 inhibitory activities were compiled as a local searching reference as described in our previous study [13]. Employing a local custom Perl script pipeline, we identified matched AHTPs sequences and locations from target proteins in the transcriptomes of *E. superba* [1] and *P. vannamei* [24], as well as the genome of *P. vannamei* [8]. AHTPs hit numbers in the mapped proteins were summarized for comparison between the two crustacean species.

4.8. Tertiary Structure Prediction

To predict the 3D structures of AMPs, I–TASSER [68] was employed and the high confidence model is supported by high C-score. The top ten starting threading templates for the predicted 3D structures of CcAMP1_insect in *C. chinensis* were 3hiaB, 5lqwX, 1jy4A, 3mlqE, 6et5A, 1jy4A, 3hiaB, 1e0nA, 1jy4A and 3hiaB, and the first starting template was 3HIA, a crystal structure of the choline-binding domain of Spr1274 in *Streptococcus pneumoniae*. The top ten starting threading templates for the CcAMP1_insect in the Antarctic krill were 5af7A, 5lqwX, 1jy4A, 3mlqE, 1udyA, 1jy4A, 3hiaB, 6pz9D, 5jscA and 3hiaB, and the first starting template was 5AF7 for the 3-Sulfinopropionyl-coenzyme A (3SP-CoA) desulfinase from *Advenella mimigardefordensis* DPN7T: crystal structure and function of a desulfinase with an acyl-CoA dehydrogenase fold. In our present work, the C-scores with a range between –5 and 2 were collected as confidence indexes for model estimation.

5. Conclusions

At first, we reported a genome survey of Antarctic krill, the most fundamental animal in the Antarctic food chain. Partial mitochondrial genome and abundant SSRs were extracted from our archived partial genome raw data and reported transcriptomes, which may be useful for the species identification and origin determination of this important polar crustacean species. A high-throughput identification and comparison of AMPs/AMP precursors and AHTPs between Antarctic krill and its famous counterpart, the whiteleg shrimp from warm waters, revealed general conservation with interesting variations between the two species. In summary, as the first report of the estimated genome size of Antarctic krill, our present genome survey data provide a foundation for further biological research of this economically and ecologically important invertebrate species. Our primary investigations on bioactive peptides (including AMPs and AHTPs) on a large-scale from such a polar species will bring new a perspective for in-depth predictions and the development of novel marine drugs in the future.

Supplementary Materials: The following are available online at http://www.mdpi.com/1660-3397/18/4/185/s1. Figure S1. A sketch map for the 13 mitochondrial protein-coding genes of the Antarctic krill. The orders of these genes are in a clockwise direction, except for *nad1*, *nad4*, *nad4L*, and *nad5*. Figure S2. Functional classification of the *E. superba* mitochondrial genome. Figure S3. A phylogenetic analysis of the representative AMP precursors, CrusEs, from both crustaceans. File S1. Representative sequences of the 13 mitochondrial protein-coding genes of the Antarctic krill, using the reported entire mitochondrial genome sequence as the reference. Table S1. KEGG analysis of the Antarctic krill extracted mitochondrial genes. Table S2. KEGG2Gene of the *E. superba* extracted mitochondrial genes. Table S3. SSRs extracted from *E. superb* reported transcriptome sequences and part of our genome raw reads. Table S4. Collection of reported AMPs. Table S5. Putative AMPs identified from the *E. superba* and *P. vannamei* transcriptomes. Table S6. Summary of the identified AMPs/AMP precursors in both crustacean species with transcription levels (FPKM values). Table S7. Specific alignments of all mapped proteins and their corresponding matched AHTPs in both crustacean species. Table S8. Identified proteins with hit numbers of matched AHTPs in the Antarctic krill and whiteleg shrimp. Table S9. Number of mapped AHTPs in both crustacean species from transcriptome or genome data.

Author Contributions: L.S., C.X., H.H., and Q.S. conceived and designed the project. Y.H., C.B., and L.W. analyzed the data; Z.L., Y.Y., and X.Y. participated in data analysis and manuscript preparation. C.X., H.H., W.S., and X.M. collected samples. Y.H. and Q.S. wrote the manuscript. Q.S., L.W., C.X., and L.S. revised the manuscript. All authors have read and agreed to the published version of the manuscript.

Acknowledgments: The work was supported by China National Key R & D Program (No. 2018YFC0310802), Shenzhen Dapang Special Program for Industrial Development (Nos. KY20180205 and PT201901-08), and Shenzhen Special Project for High-Level Talents (No. SZYSGZZ-2018001).

Conflicts of Interest: The authors declare no conflict of interest.

References

1. Ma, C.; Ma, H.; Xu, G.; Feng, C.; Ma, L.; Wang, L. De novo sequencing of the Antarctic krill *(Euphausia superba)* transcriptome to identify functional genes and molecular markers. *J. Genet.* **2018**, *97*, 995–999. [CrossRef]
2. Ikeda, T.; Dixon, P. The influence of feeding on the metabolic activity of Antarctic krill (*Euphausia superba* Dana). *Polar Biol.* **1984**, *3*, 1–9. [CrossRef]
3. Sales, G.; Deagle, B.E.; Calura, E.; Martini, P.; Biscontin, A.; De Pitta, C.; Kawaguchi, S.; Romualdi, C.; Meyer, B.; Costa, R. KrillDB: A *de novo* transcriptome database for the Antarctic krill (*Euphausia superba*). *PLoS ONE* **2017**, *12*, e0171908. [CrossRef]
4. Friedlaender, A.S.; Johnston, D.W.; Fraser, W.R.; Burns, J.; Costa, D.P. Ecological niche modeling of sympatric krill predators around Marguerite Bay, Western Antarctic Peninsula. *Deep Sea Res. Part II Top. Stud. Oceanogr.* **2011**, *58*, 1729–1740. [CrossRef]
5. Nicol, S.; Foster, J.; Kawaguchi, S. The fishery for Antarctic krill–recent developments. *Fish Fish.* **2012**, *13*, 30–40. [CrossRef]
6. Shen, X.; Wang, H.; Ren, J.; Tian, M.; Wang, M. The mitochondrial genome of *Euphausia superba* (Prydz Bay) (Crustacea: Malacostraca: Euphausiacea) reveals a novel gene arrangement and potential molecular markers. *Mol. Biol. Rep.* **2010**, *37*, 771. [CrossRef]

7. Machida, R.J.; Miya, M.U.; Yamauchi, M.M.; Nishida, M.; Nishida, S. Organization of the mitochondrial genome of Antarctic krill *Euphausia superba* (Crustacea: Malacostraca). *Mar. Biotechnol.* **2004**, *6*, 238–250. [CrossRef]
8. Zhang, X.; Yuan, J.; Sun, Y.; Li, S.; Gao, Y.; Yu, Y.; Liu, C.; Wang, Q.; Lv, X.; Zhang, X. Penaeid shrimp genome provides insights into benthic adaptation and frequent molting. *Nat. Commun.* **2019**, *10*, 356. [CrossRef]
9. Yi, Y.; You, X.; Bian, C.; Chen, S.; Lv, Z.; Qiu, L.; Shi, Q. High-throughput identification of antimicrobial peptides from amphibious mudskippers. *Mar. Drugs* **2017**, *15*, 364. [CrossRef]
10. Tincu, J.A.; Taylor, S.W. Antimicrobial peptides from marine invertebrates. *Antimicrob. Agents Chemother.* **2004**, *48*, 3645–3654. [CrossRef]
11. Sperstad, S.V.; Haug, T.; Blencke, H.-M.; Styrvold, O.B.; Li, C.; Stensvag, K. Antimicrobial peptides from marine invertebrates: Challenges and perspectives in marine antimicrobial peptide discovery. *Biotechnol. Adv.* **2011**, *29*, 519–530. [CrossRef]
12. Zhao, L.; Yin, B.; Liu, Q.; Cao, R. Purification of antimicrobial peptide from Antarctic Krill (*Euphausia superba*) and its function mechanism. *J. Ocean. Univ. China* **2013**, *12*, 484–490. [CrossRef]
13. Yi, Y.; Lv, Y.; Zhang, L.; Yang, J.; Shi, Q. High throughput identification of antihypertensive peptides from fish proteome datasets. *Mar. Drugs* **2018**, *16*, 365. [CrossRef]
14. Jia, K.; Bian, C.; Yi, Y.; Li, Y.; Jia, P.; Gui, D.; Zhang, X.; Lin, W.; Sun, X.; Lv, Y.; et al. Whole genome sequencing of Chinese white dolphin (*Sousa chinensis*) for high-throughput screening of antihypertensive peptides. *Mar. Drugs* **2019**, *17*, 504. [CrossRef]
15. Park, S.Y.; Je, J.-Y.; Kang, N.; Han, E.J.; Um, J.H.; Jeon, Y.-J.; Ahn, G.; Ahn, C.-B. Antihypertensive effects of Ile–Pro–Ile–Lys from krill (*Euphausia superba*) protein hydrolysates: Purification, identification and in vivo evaluation in spontaneously hypertensive rats. *Eur. Food Res. Technol.* **2017**, *243*, 719–725. [CrossRef]
16. Zhao, Y.-Q.; Zhang, L.; Tao, J.; Chi, C.-F.; Wang, B. Eight antihypertensive peptides from the protein hydrolysate of Antarctic krill (*Euphausia superba*): Isolation, identification, and activity evaluation on human umbilical vein endothelial cells (HUVECs). *Food Res. Int.* **2019**, *121*, 197–204. [CrossRef]
17. Yu, Y.; Zhang, X.; Yuan, J.; Li, F.; Chen, X.; Zhao, Y.; Huang, L.; Zheng, H.; Xiang, J. Genome survey and high-density genetic map construction provide genomic and genetic resources for the Pacific White Shrimp *Litopenaeus vannamei*. *Sci. Rep.* **2015**, *5*, 15612. [CrossRef]
18. Buchfink, B.; Xie, C.; Huson, D.H. Fast and sensitive protein alignment using DIAMOND. *Nat. Methods* **2015**, *12*, 59–60. [CrossRef]
19. Kanehisa, M.; Goto, S. KEGG: Kyoto encyclopedia of genes and genomes. *Nucleic Acids Res.* **2000**, *28*, 27–30. [CrossRef]
20. Consortium, G.O. The Gene Ontology (GO) database and informatics resource. *Nucleic Acids Res.* **2004**, *32*, D258–D261. [CrossRef]
21. Saitou, N.; Nei, M. The neighbor-joining method: A new method for reconstructing phylogenetic trees. *Mol. Biol. Evol.* **1987**, *4*, 406–425.
22. Felsenstein, J. Confidence limits on phylogenies: An approach using the bootstrap. *Evolution* **1985**, *39*, 783–791. [CrossRef]
23. Kumar, S.; Stecher, G.; Tamura, K. MEGA7: Molecular evolutionary genetics analysis version 7.0 for bigger datasets. *Mol. Biol. Evol.* **2016**, *33*, 1870–1874. [CrossRef]
24. Gao, Y.; Zhang, X.; Wei, J.; Sun, X.; Yuan, J.; Li, F.; Xiang, J. Whole transcriptome analysis provides insights into molecular mechanisms for molting in *Litopenaeus vannamei*. *PLoS ONE* **2015**, *10*, e0144350. [CrossRef]
25. Petit, V.W.; Rolland, J.-L.; Blond, A.; Cazevieille, C.; Djediat, C.; Peduzzi, J.; Goulard, C.; Bachère, E.; Dupont, J.; Destoumieux-Garzón, D. A hemocyanin-derived antimicrobial peptide from the penaeid shrimp adopts an alpha-helical structure that specifically permeabilizes fungal membranes. *Biochim. Biophys. Acta* **2016**, *1860*, 557–568. [CrossRef]
26. Mu, C.; Zheng, P.; Zhao, J.; Wang, L.; Zhang, H.; Qiu, L.; Gai, Y.; Song, L. Molecular characterization and expression of a crustin-like gene from Chinese mitten crab, *Eriocheir sinensis*. *Dev. Comp. Immunol.* **2010**, *34*, 734–740. [CrossRef]
27. Ranganathan, S.; Simpson, K.J.; Shaw, D.C.; Nicholas, K.R. The whey acidic protein family: A new signature motif and three-dimensional structure by comparative modeling. *J. Mol. Graph. Model.* **1999**, *17*, 106–113. [CrossRef]

28. Destoumieux, D.; Munoz, M.; Bulet, P.; Bachere, E. Penaeidins, a family of antimicrobial peptides from penaeid shrimp (Crustacea, Decapoda). *Cell. Mol. Life Sci.* **2000**, *57*, 1260–1271. [CrossRef]
29. Jeffery, N.W. The first genome size estimates for six species of krill (Malacostraca, Euphausiidae): Large genomes at the north and south poles. *Polar Biol.* **2012**, *35*, 959–962. [CrossRef]
30. Lucassen, M.; Koschnick, N.; Eckerle, L.; Pörtner, H.-O. Mitochondrial mechanisms of cold adaptation in cod (*Gadus morhua* L.) populations from different climatic zones. *J. Exp. Biol.* **2006**, *209*, 2462–2471. [CrossRef]
31. Sundaray, J.K.; Rasal, K.D.; Chakrapani, V.; Swain, P.; Kumar, D.; Ninawe, A.S.; Nandi, S.; Jayasankar, P. Simple sequence repeats (SSRs) markers in fish genomic research and their acceleration via next-generation sequencing and computational approaches. *Aquacult. Int.* **2016**, *24*, 1089–1102. [CrossRef]
32. Perez, F.; Ortiz, J.; Zhinaula, M.; Gonzabay, C.; Calderon, J.; Volckaert, F.A. Development of EST-SSR markers by data mining in three species of shrimp: *Litopenaeus vannamei*, *Litopenaeus stylirostris*, and *Trachypenaeus birdy*. *Mar. Biotechnol.* **2005**, *7*, 554–569. [CrossRef]
33. Li, S.; Zhao, B. Isolation, purification, and detection of the antimicrobial activity of the antimicrobial peptide CcAMP1 from *Coridius chinensis* (Hemiptera: Dinidoridae). *Acta Entomol. Sin.* **2015**, *58*, 610–616.
34. Kim, H.S.; Park, C.B.; Kim, M.S.; Kim, S.C. cDNA cloning and characterization of buforin I, an antimicrobial peptide: A cleavage product of histone H2A. *Biochem. Biophys. Res. Commun.* **1996**, *229*, 381–387. [CrossRef]
35. Park, C.B.; Kim, M.S.; Kim, S.C. A novel antimicrobial peptide from *Bufo bufo* gargarizans. *Biochem. Biophys. Res. Commun.* **1996**, *218*, 408–413. [CrossRef]
36. Seo, J.-K.; Lee, M.J.; Go, H.-J.; Do Kim, G.; Do Jeong, H.; Nam, B.-H.; Park, N.G. Purification and antimicrobial function of ubiquitin isolated from the gill of Pacific oyster, *Crassostrea gigas*. *Mol. Immunol.* **2013**, *53*, 88–98. [CrossRef]
37. Krusong, K.; Poolpipat, P.; Supungul, P.; Tassanakajon, A. A comparative study of antimicrobial properties of crustin*Pm*1 and crustin*Pm*7 from the black tiger shrimp *Penaeus monodon*. *Dev. Comp. Immunol.* **2012**, *36*, 208–215. [CrossRef]
38. Yu, A.-Q.; Shi, Y.-H.; Wang, Q. Characterisation of a novel type i crustin involved in antibacterial and antifungal responses in the red claw crayfish, *Cherax quadricarinatus*. *Fish. Shellfish Immunol.* **2016**, *48*, 30–38. [CrossRef]
39. Rolland, J.A.M.; Dupont, J.; Lefevre, F.; Bachère, E.; Romestand, B. Stylicins, a new family of antimicrobial peptides from the Pacific blue shrimp *Litopenaeus stylirostris*. *Mol. Immunol.* **2010**, *47*, 1269–1277. [CrossRef]
40. Amparyup, P.; Donpudsa, S.; Tassanakajon, A. Shrimp single WAP domain (SWD)-containing protein exhibits proteinase inhibitory and antimicrobial activities. *Dev. Comp. Immunol.* **2008**, *32*, 1497–1509. [CrossRef]
41. Papareddy, P.; Rydengård, V.; Pasupuleti, M.; Walse, B.; Mörgelin, M.; Chalupka, A.; Malmsten, M.; Schmidtchen, A. Proteolysis of human thrombin generates novel host defense peptides. *PLoS Pathog.* **2010**, *6*, e1000857. [CrossRef]
42. Low, B.W.; Ng, N.K.; Yeo, D.C. First record of the invasive Chinese mitten crab, *Eriocheir sinensis* H. Milne Edwards, 1853 (Crustacea: Brachyura: Varunidae) from Singapore. *BioInvas. Rec* **2013**, *2*, 73–78. [CrossRef]
43. Thanh, N.M.; Ponzoni, R.W.; Nguyen, N.H.; Vu, N.T.; Barnes, A.; Mather, P.B. Evaluation of growth performance in a diallel cross of three strains of giant freshwater prawn (*Macrobrachium rosenbergii*) in Vietnam. *Aquaculture* **2009**, *287*, 75–83. [CrossRef]
44. Benzie, J.; Ballment, E.; Forbes, A.; Demetriades, N.; Sugama, K.; Moria, S. Mitochondrial DNA variation in Indo-Pacific populations of the giant tiger prawn, *Penaeus monodon*. *Mol. Ecol.* **2002**, *11*, 2553–2569. [CrossRef]
45. Eckert, R.L.; Green, H. Structure and evolution of the human involucrin gene. *Cell* **1986**, *46*, 583–589. [CrossRef]
46. McGrath, J.; Eady, R.; Pope, F. Anatomy and organization of human skin. *Rook's Textb. Dermatol.* **2004**, *10*, 9781444317633.
47. Sotiropoulou, P.A.; Blanpain, C. Development and homeostasis of the skin epidermis. *Cold Spring Harb. Perspect. Biol.* **2012**, *4*, a008383. [CrossRef]
48. Saiga, A.; Iwai, K.; Hayakawa, T.; Takahata, Y.; Kitamura, S.; Nishimura, T.; Morimatsu, F. Angiotensin I-converting enzyme-inhibitory peptides obtained from chicken collagen hydrolysate. *J. Agric. Food Chem.* **2008**, *56*, 9586–9591. [CrossRef]
49. Kim, S.-K.; Byun, H.-G.; Park, P.-J.; Shahidi, F. Angiotensin I converting enzyme inhibitory peptides purified from bovine skin gelatin hydrolysate. *J. Agric. Food Chem.* **2001**, *49*, 2992–2997. [CrossRef]

50. Fu, Y.; Young, J.F.; Rasmussen, M.K.; Dalsgaard, T.K.; Lametsch, R.; Aluko, R.E.; Therkildsen, M. Angiotensin I–converting enzyme–inhibitory peptides from bovine collagen: Insights into inhibitory mechanism and transepithelial transport. *Food Res. Int.* **2016**, *89*, 373–381. [CrossRef]
51. Zhuang, Y.; Sun, L.; Li, B. Production of the angiotensin-I-converting enzyme (ACE)-inhibitory peptide from hydrolysates of jellyfish (*Rhopilema esculentum*) collagen. *Food. Bioproc. Tech.* **2012**, *5*, 1622–1629. [CrossRef]
52. Fahmi, A.; Morimura, S.; Guo, H.-C.; Shigematsu, T.; Kida, K.; Uemura, Y. Production of angiotensin I converting enzyme inhibitory peptides from sea bream scales. *Process. Biochem.* **2004**, *39*, 1195–1200. [CrossRef]
53. Liu, Z.-Y.; Chen, D.; Su, Y.-C.; Zeng, M.-Y. Optimization of hydrolysis conditions for the production of the angiotensin-I converting enzyme inhibitory peptides from sea cucumber collagen hydrolysates. *J. Aquat. Food Prod. Technol.* **2011**, *20*, 222–232. [CrossRef]
54. Chen, Y.; Chen, Y.; Shi, C.; Huang, Z.; Zhang, Y.; Li, S.; Li, Y.; Ye, J.; Yu, C.; Li, Z. SOAPnuke: A MapReduce acceleration-supported software for integrated quality control and preprocessing of high-throughput sequencing data. *Gigascience* **2017**, *7*, gix120. [CrossRef]
55. Li, R.; Yu, C.; Li, Y.; Lam, T.-W.; Yiu, S.-M.; Kristiansen, K.; Wang, J. SOAP2: An improved ultrafast tool for short read alignment. *Bioinformatics* **2009**, *25*, 1966–1967. [CrossRef]
56. Bankevich, A.; Nurk, S.; Antipov, D.; Gurevich, A.A.; Dvorkin, M.; Kulikov, A.S.; Lesin, V.M.; Nikolenko, S.I.; Pham, S.; Prjibelski, A.D. SPAdes: A new genome assembly algorithm and its applications to single-cell sequencing. *J. Comput. Biol.* **2012**, *19*, 455–477. [CrossRef]
57. Mount, D.W. Using the basic local alignment search tool (BLAST). *Cold Spring Harb. Protoc.* **2007**, *2007*, pdb.top17. [CrossRef]
58. Jung, J.; Kim, J.I.; Jeong, Y.-S.; Yi, G. AGORA: Organellar genome annotation from the amino acid and nucleotide references. *Bioinformatics* **2018**, *34*, 2661–2663. [CrossRef]
59. Haas, B.J.; Papanicolaou, A.; Yassour, M.; Grabherr, M.; Blood, P.D.; Bowden, J.; Couger, M.B.; Eccles, D.; Li, B.; Lieber, M. De novo transcript sequence reconstruction from RNA-seq using the Trinity platform for reference generation and analysis. *Nat. Protoc.* **2013**, *8*, 1494–1512. [CrossRef]
60. Pertea, G.; Huang, X.; Liang, F.; Antonescu, V.; Sultana, R.; Karamycheva, S.; Lee, Y.; White, J.; Cheung, F.; Parvizi, B. TIGR Gene Indices clustering tools (TGICL): A software system for fast clustering of large EST datasets. *Bioinformatics* **2003**, *19*, 651–652. [CrossRef]
61. Langmead, B.; Salzberg, S.L. Fast gapped-read alignment with Bowtie 2. *Nat. Methods* **2012**, *9*, 357–359. [CrossRef] [PubMed]
62. Li, B.; Dewey, C.N. RSEM: Accurate transcript quantification from RNA-Seq data with or without a reference genome. *BMC Bioinform.* **2011**, *12*, 323. [CrossRef] [PubMed]
63. Conesa, A.; Götz, S.; García-Gómez, J.M.; Terol, J.; Talón, M.; Robles, M. Blast2GO: A universal tool for annotation, visualization and analysis in functional genomics research. *Bioinformatics* **2005**, *21*, 3674–3676. [CrossRef] [PubMed]
64. Boeckmann, B.; Bairoch, A.; Apweiler, R.; Blatter, M.-C.; Estreicher, A.; Gasteiger, E.; Martin, M.J.; Michoud, K.; O'Donovan, C.; Phan, I. The SWISS-PROT protein knowledgebase and its supplement TrEMBL in 2003. *Nucleic Acids Res.* **2003**, *31*, 365–370. [CrossRef]
65. Katoh, K.; Standley, D.M. MAFFT multiple sequence alignment software version 7: Improvements in performance and usability. *Mol. Biol. Evol.* **2013**, *30*, 772–780. [CrossRef]
66. Beitz, E. TEXshade: Shading and labeling of multiple sequence alignments using LATEX2 epsilon. *Bioinformatics* **2000**, *16*, 135–139. [CrossRef]
67. Wang, G.; Li, X.; Wang, Z. APD3: The antimicrobial peptide database as a tool for research and education. *Nucleic Acids Res.* **2015**, *44*, D1087–D1093. [CrossRef]
68. Yang, J.; Yan, R.; Roy, A.; Xu, D.; Poisson, J.; Zhang, Y. The I-TASSER Suite: Protein structure and function prediction. *Nat. Methods* **2015**, *12*, 7–8. [CrossRef]

MDPI
St. Alban-Anlage 66
4052 Basel
Switzerland
Tel. +41 61 683 77 34
Fax +41 61 302 89 18
www.mdpi.com

Marine Drugs Editorial Office
E-mail: marinedrugs@mdpi.com
www.mdpi.com/journal/marinedrugs

www.ingramcontent.com/pod-product-compliance
Lightning Source LLC
LaVergne TN
LVHW070432100526
838202LV00014B/1583

* 9 7 8 3 0 3 6 5 0 5 6 4 0 *